Endoscopic Imaging Techniques and Tools

Vani J.A. Konda • Irving Waxman
Editors

Endoscopic Imaging Techniques and Tools

Springer

Editors
Vani J.A. Konda
Department of Medicine
University of Chicago Medicine
Chicago, IL, USA

Irving Waxman
Biological Sciences
University of Chicago Medicine
Chicago, IL, USA

Videos to this book can be accessed at http://link.springer.com/book/978-3-319-30053-5

ISBN 978-3-319-30051-1 ISBN 978-3-319-30053-5 (eBook)
DOI 10.1007/978-3-319-30053-5

Library of Congress Control Number: 2016941327

Printed on acid-free paper

This Springer imprint is published by Springer Nature
The registered company is Springer International Publishing AG Switzerland

Preface

The field of endoscopy burgeoned from a simple tube with lenses and a light source that could visualize the gross lining of the stomach to a myriad of different platforms and technologies. The endoscopes themselves have evolved over the generations where now high-resolution endoscopy provides on the order of eight hundred thousand to one million pixels to discriminate finer details. Chromoendoscopy dyes and virtual chromoendoscopy have provided details in the mucosal surface and the superficial vasculature. This quest for detail has delved beyond the gross architecture, to be able to provide an optical biopsy with micro-architectural detail with confocal laser endomicroscopy, optical coherence tomography-based technologies, and endocytoscopy. Other strategies have widened our endoscopic field of view and provide surface area visible to us that may otherwise be hidden in a retroflexed position or behind folds in the colon. Or, new developments may allow access to places where standard scopes may not reach such as in the pancreas or in the bile ducts.

These tools may be used for lesion *detection* in the case of screening. They also may be used for lesion *classification* during screening, surveillance, diagnosis, or therapy. The diagnostic performance characteristics will guide how we can best complement histology when we utilize these imaging modalities including options such as decreasing number of negative biopsies, targeting tissue acquisition, or predicting depth of lesions prior to therapy. In these areas where tissue acquisition yield may be limited or inadequate such as in the bile ducts or pancreatic cysts, the novel imaging modality itself may potentially serve as a surrogate marker for histology in diagnosis.

Novel technologies integrate into clinical practice typically in certain stages. Many new devices first go through assessments of feasibility and safety. The technical aspect of obtaining images often has a relatively quick learning curve. The associated cognitive aspect of interpretation of the images is often a longer and more variable learning curve. The accuracy of image interpretation may also be impacted by the quality of the images and confidence of the interpretation.

It is important to appreciate the goals and limitations of image interpretation compared to standard histology. For example, often the image interpretation often may start with normal versus abnormal and then demonstrate benign versus classically malignant features. However, there may be limitations in determining grades of dysplasia or depth of invasion in superficial neoplasia in a specific imaging modality. Furthermore, similar to histology, inflammation can play a confounding role in the determination of dysplasia.

Most importantly, one must understand there if there is clinical impact. This often entails not only being able to provide accuracy in image interpretation but providing information which is beyond that what at this time high-resolution endoscopy may provide that can be clinically relevant. As the generations of endoscopes themselves provide a higher resolution, the bar for imaging modalities raises substantially. Finally, cost-effectiveness plays an important role in decision making prior to widespread adoptability. These technologies must be rigorously interrogated with all of the aspects before they can transform from a new technology to a clinically useful tool in endoscopic practice.

The concept of the optical biopsy has reached our endoscopy suites. The world of endoscopic imaging is an evolving bridge between endoscopy and histology. This book outlines the advanced endoscopic imaging modalities currently available and on the horizon. We thank all of contributors who have shared their expertise with us in the preparation of this book.

Chicago, IL, USA Vani J.A. Konda
Chicago, IL, USA Irving Waxman

Acknowledgments

We would like to thank all of our endoscopy unit staff for their dedication and hard work.

Contents

Contributors

Editors

Vani J.A. Konda, M.D. Department of Medicine, Center for Endoscopic Research and Therapeutics, University of Chicago Medicine, Chicago, IL, USA

Irving Waxman, M.D., F.A.S.G.E. Biological Sciences, The University of Chicago Medicine, Chicago, IL, USA

Authors

Sharmila Anandasabapathy, M.D. Medicine and Gastroenterology, Baylor College of Medicine, Houston, TX, USA

Christopher D. Atkinson, M.D. Section of Gastroenterology & Hepatology, Department of Medicine VA Boston Healthcare System, Boston, MA, USA

Valerio Balassone, M.D. Digestive Disease Center, Showa University Koto Toyosu Hospital,Tokyo, Japan

Daniel K. Chan, M.D. Division of Gastroenterology and Hepatology, Mayo Clinic, Rochester, MN, USA

Monica Gaidhane, M.D. Division of Gastroenterology and Hepatology, Weill Cornell Medical College, New York, NY, USA

Tian Gao, M.D. Boston University Medical Center, Boston Medical Center, Boston, MA, USA

Marc Giovannini, M.D. Department of Gastroenterology and Endoscopy, Paoli-Calmettes Institute, Marseille, France

Nina R. Gupta, M.D. Department of Medicine, Center for Endoscopic Research and Therapeutics, University of Chicago Medicine, Chicago, IL, USA

Haruhiro Inoue, M.D., Ph.D., F.A.S.G.E. Digestive Diseases Center, Showa University Koto Toyosu Hospital, Tokyo, Japan

Michel Kahaleh, M.D., A.G.A.F., F.A.C.G., F.A.S.G.E. Division of Gastroenterology and Hepatology, Weill Cornell Medical Center, New York, NY, USA

Tonya Kaltenbach, M.D., M.S. Veteran Affairs Palo Alto Health Care System and Stanford University School of Medicine, Palo Alto, CA, USA

Kunal Karia, M.D. Division of Gastroenterology and Hepatology, Weill Cornell Medical College, New York, NY, USA

Masayuki Kitano, M.D., Ph.D. Department of Gastroenterology and Hepatology, Kinki University Faculty of Medicine, Osaka-sayama, Osaka, Japan

Ammar O. Kheir, M.B.B.S., M.R.C.P., F.R.A.C.P. Department of Gastroenterology, Queen Elizabeth II Jubilee Hospital, Brisbane, QLD, Australia

School of Medicine and Public Health, University of Newcastle, Newcastle, NSW, Australia

Masatoshi Kudo, M.D., Ph.D. Department of Gastroenterology and Hepatology, Kinki University Faculty of Medicine, Osaka, Japan

Cadman L. Leggett, M.D. Division of Gastroenterology and Hepatology, Mayo Clinic, Rochester, MN, USA

Dileep Mangira, M.B.B.S (F.R.A.C.P.) The Lyell McEwin Hospital and The University of Adelaide, Adelaide, SA, Australia

Kosuke Minaga, M.D. Department of Gastroenterology and Hepatology, Kinki University Faculty of Medicine, Osaka, Japan

Ioannis S. Papanikolaou, M.D., Ph.D., F.E.B.G.H. Hepatogastroenterology Unit, Second Department of Internal Medicine and Research Unit, "Attikon" University General Hospital, University of Athens, Athens, Greece

Daniel P. Perl, M.D. Internal Medicine, University of Michigan Health System, Ann Arbor, MI, USA

Massimiliano di Pietro, M.D. MRC Cancer Unit, University of Cambridge, Cambridge Biomedical Campus, Cambridge, UK

Krish Ragunath, M.D., F.R.C.P., F.A.S.G.E. NIHR Biomedical Research Unit in Gastrointestinal and Liver Diseases, Nottingham University Hospitals NHS Trust and the University of Nottingham, Nottingham, UK

Hemant K. Roy, M.D. Boston University Medical Center, Boston, MA, USA

Angela Saul, M.D. Division of Gastroenterology and Hepatology, Weill Cornell Medical College, New York, NY, USA

Prateek Sharma, M.D. The Lyell McEwin Hospital and The University of Adelaide, SA, Australia

Peter D. Siersema, M.D., Ph.D., F.A.S.G.E. Department of Gastroenterology and Hepatology, University Medical Center Utrecht, Utrecht, The Netherlands

Department of Gastroenterology and Hepatology, Radboud University Medical Center, Nijmegen, GA, The Netherlands

Rajvinder Singh, F.R.A.C.P., A.M., F.R.C.P. The Lyell McEwin Hospital and The University of Adelaide, SA, Australia

Satish K. Singh, M.D., A.G.A.F. Section of Gastroenterology and Hepatology, Department of Medicine, VA Boston Healthcare System, Boston, MA, USA

Section of Gastroenterology, Department of Medicine, Boston University School of Medicine and Department of Biomedical Engineering, Boston University College of Engineering, Boston, MA, USA

Roy Soetikno, M.D., M.S. Department of Gastroenterology and Hepatology, Singapore General Hospital, Singapore, Singapore

National Cancer Center Singapore, Singapore, Singapore

Duke–National University Singapore Graduate Medical School, Singapore, Singapore

Amy Tyberg, M.D. Division of Gastroenterology and Hepatology, Weill Cornell Medical College, New York, NY, USA

Kenneth K. Wang, M.D. Barrett's Esophagus Unit, Division of Gastroenterology and Hepatology, Mayo Clinic, Rochester, MN, USA

Stephanie Wong, M.B.B.S. The Lyell McEwin Hospital and The University of Adelaide, SA, Australia

Chapter 1
High-Resolution Endoscopy and Magnification Endoscopy

Nina R. Gupta and Vani J.A. Konda

Technology Overview

Endoscopic imaging is the cornerstone of modern gastroenterology. The tools used in endoscopy had humble beginnings with the earliest gastroscope design accredited to Adolf Kussmaul in 1868 [1]. He employed a simple metal tube fed over a wire and illuminated a dark lumen by shining a turpentine lamp against a lens and reflector. This simple system morphed through an era of rapid technological advancement into the first flexible fiber endoscope in 1958 [1] and ultimately the high definition, high magnification video endoscopes that have widespread use today.

The quality of the image produced by the modern endoscope is governed by two fundamental variables; resolution and magnification. Image resolution is the level of detail an image possesses. When defined technically, image resolution quantifies two-point discrimination—a measure of how close two points in the image can be while still being perceived as separate by the naked eye observer. For digital images, resolution is correlated with pixels (picture elements), which are the smallest controllable units of a digital image. Smaller pixel size and higher pixel density (number of pixels width × number of pixels length) produce a higher resolution image.

Magnification refers to the factor by which the image is enlarged from the actual size of the object creating it. During optical magnification, a moveable lens at the end of the endoscope slides nearer to the area of interest (controlled by a lever on the endoscope handle), thus altering the ratio of internal lenses and changing focal length in order to produce a magnified image. This allows for an observer to appreciate a

N.R. Gupta, M.D. • V.J.A. Konda, M.D. (✉)
Department of Medicine, Center for Endoscopic Research and Therapeutics, University of Chicago Medicine, 5871 S. Maryland Ave, MC 4076, Chicago, IL 60615, USA
e-mail: vkonda@bsd.uchicago.edu

V.J.A. Konda, I. Waxman (eds.), *Endoscopic Imaging Techniques and Tools*,
DOI 10.1007/978-3-319-30053-5_1

finer level of detail at, for example, a mucosal surface. Standard endoscopes can enlarge an image ×30, while high magnification or "zoom" endoscopes can magnify ×100 or greater [2]. However, if magnification is used, the surface area visualized at a given time decreases. This is in contrast to digital magnification where the image is enlarged electronically. In this process, the image is essentially sequentially cropped and pixels are interpolated as the image is magnified. The digital magnification feature of most endoscopes can magnify ×1.5–2 [3], but comes at a cost of decreased pixel density and thus poorer image resolution.

Standard definition (SD) systems generate images with 300,000–400,000 total pixels (640–700 horizontal pixels × 480–525 vertical pixels) based on the CCD (charge coupled device) chip. The CCD essentially senses light intensity from an optical image and converts it to electrical signals via an integrated circuit. A major advance in endoscope design has been the development of increasingly smaller CCD chips with greater numbers of pixels. SD images generally have a 4:3 aspect ratio as this allows for the highest pixel density and resolution given the round shape of the endoscope [3].

High-definition (HD) video is characterized by three main variables; "lines" of resolution, image scanning method, and frame speed. The number of lines of resolution equates to the number of vertical pixels that make up the image. HD images typically have a resolution with 720 or 1080 lines and boast a total pixel count between 850,000 and 1,000,000. HD images constantly refresh on a line-by-line scan using either a progressive (p) or intercalated (i) scanning system. Broadcast HD TV, for example, is available in 720p, 1080i, and 1080p. The number of frames per second can also differ among HD formats and can range from 24 to 60 frames/s (Hz). Commonly, 50 Hz is used in Europe and 60 Hz used in the USA. While HD TV formats produce images in a 19:9 aspect ratio, HD endoscopes produce images with a 4:3 or 5:4 aspect ratio [4].

Techniques

Equipment

Currently, three different HD videoendoscope systems are available in the United States. Olympus America endoscopes were designed for output onto HDTVs and include both 1080i and 1080p options. Images are displayed in a 1280 × 1024 pixel frame. Some Olympus HD endoscopes feature dual-focus imaging in which the endoscopist can switch from normal focus to near focus with the push of a button [5]. Most high-resolution Olympus endoscopes also support narrow-band imaging (NBI), a contrast enhancement feature. Absorption of light in specific wavelengths allows for visual characterization of various mucosal elements [5]. Pentax endoscopes are designed for output onto computer displays. Images are displayed in a 1920 × 1080 pixel frame. High-resolution Pentax endoscopes feature i-Scan™, a digital post-processing image enhancement technology with three modes that highlight different mucosal features [6]. Fujinon endoscopes are also designed for output onto computer displays, but display images in a 1280 × 960 pixel frame. These endoscopes provide a built-in feature for contrast enhancement called Fujinon Intelligent Contrast Enhancement (FICE). FICE utilizes spectral post-image processing for enhanced visual delineation during mucosal inspection [7]. All three of these companies produce high magnification endoscopes.

Basic Set-Up

Imaging systems consist of endoscopes, processors, light sources, and monitors. The standard light source used in HD systems is a 300 W Xenon lamp. In order to utilize HD imaging, most of these components including the endoscope, processor, and monitor must be HD compatible. The transmission cables must also have specific compatibility. For HDTV displays, HD serial digital interface cables are required, while for computer monitor displays digital video interface cables are required. Highest resolution images will be produced when the pixel density and aspect ratio of the video source match the display. If an SD endoscope is used as the video source, HD processors and monitors can up-convert the images; however, image quality will be reduced.

Operation

HD endoscopes are operated in the same manner as their SD counterparts. When HD and magnification endoscopy is utilized, supplemental techniques for tissue examination may be employed including device-specific contrast enhancement features and chromoendoscopy. Chromoendoscopy refers to the use of dyes (such as indigo carmine or methylene blue) to stain tissue and aid in the identification of normal and abnormal mucosa.

Key Clinical Indications

Esophagus

High-resolution and high magnification endoscopy has an established role in facilitating the identification of Barrett's esophagus epithelial metaplasia and squamous cell neoplasia. Additionally, the increased visualization of mucosal features (such as glandular and vascular structure) allows the operator to more accurately predict areas of dysplasia and malignancy for tissue acquisition.

Stomach

HD and magnification endoscopy has several potential indications for use in the stomach, including the identification of H. Pylori gastritis, gastric atrophy, and intestinal metaplasia. With the ability to analyze capillary morphology and subtle surface changes, normal mucosa may be able to be differentiated from metaplasia and early or advanced gastric adenocarcinoma.

Small Intestine

Superior visualization of duodenal villi form by high resolution and magnification endoscopy allows for in vivo characterization of several malabsorbtive states. This is especially relevant for targeting biopsies in patients who have patchy disease. Like in other areas of the gastrointestinal tract, high-resolution endoscopy can help to identify fine endoscopic changes associated with early malignancy; particularly duodenal ampullary and non-ampullary carcinoma.

Colon

High-definition imaging facilitates the detection of colonic lesions and polyps. Additionally, high magnification features allow validated classification schemes such as Kudo pit pattern analysis to be utilized in order to delineate potential neoplasia and colonic adenocarcinoma. This has particular significance in the screening of high-risk patients, such as those with inflammatory bowel disease.

Assessment

Esophagus

High-resolution and high magnification endoscopy is often used in conjunction with chromoendoscopy or other contrast enhancement techniques; however, even the use of these endoscopic systems alone has shown a benefit over standard definition endoscopy. Diagnosing Barrett's esophagus with standard endoscopy can be difficult since the associated specialized intestinal metaplasia (SIM) may be patchy, particularly in short-segment Barrett's esophagus. The yield of detecting intestinal metaplasia on biopsy can range from 25 to 50 % [8] with conventional endoscopy. In a study of 49 patients, high magnification endoscopy was shown to improve the accuracy in visual diagnosis of Barrett's esophagus (in vivo diagnosis confirmed with SIM on histology) by facilitating the classification of mucosal surface patterns into four different types [9]. The four patterns represent a progression of mucosal architecture from regular round pits to a villous convoluted shape. The last two patterns—villous (III) and ridged (IV)—were associated with Barrett's esophagus. They respectively had an 87 and 100 % yield of SIM when biopsied [9]. Mucosal classification can allow for targeted biopsies in the setting of patchy metaplasia, thus reducing sampling error. The basic system described continues to be used by other groups, though it has undergone some revisions. In the same study when acetic acid instillation was used along with high magnification endoscopy, the ability to detect an endoscopic pattern increased further from 38 to 100 % [9]. Similarly, a prospective randomized trial found a 1.4-fold increase in diagnostic accuracy of biopsies guided by magnification endoscopy and acetic acid. This could lead to a theoretical 55 % decrease in number of biopsies needed to diagnose Barrett's esophagus with the same accuracy as standard endoscopy and random four-quadrant biopsies [10]. In a retrospective cohort study utilizing HD endoscopy and acetic acid, a dramatic 14.7-fold increase in neoplasia detection was found compared to standard random biopsy protocol [11]. Agents such as methylene blue and indigo carmine have also been used in conjunction with HD magnification endoscopy to detect and characterize Barrett's esophagus. For example, the absorption of methylene blue has been linked to certain mucosal patters (pit patterns) appreciated on magnification endoscopy. These pit patterns have in turn been shown to correlate with intestinal metaplasia [12]. Studies utilizing indigo carmine have used analogous architectural classification schemes to aid in the identification of Barrett's esophagus and subsequent dysplasia [13, 14].

HD magnification endoscopy also allows for the use of narrow-band imaging (NBI). Compared with SD endoscopy, magnification endoscopy with NBI offers superior visualization of fine mucosal patterns and capillary morphology. This aids the endoscopist in visually distinguishing normal mucosa, specialized intestinal metaplasia, high-grade dysplasia, and adenocarcinoma [15–17]. When using NBI, one of three validated classifications systems (Amsterdam, Kansas, Nottingham) is generally used [18]. In a prospective validation study of the three systems, the Amsterdam classification system was found to have the highest global accuracy and intraobserver agreement (51 %, $k=0.47$) as compared to the Nottingham (46 %, $k=0.34$) and Kansas (47 %, $k=0.44$) systems. However, accuracy for dysplastic tissue did not vary between the systems. High-magnification endoscopy with NBI and targeted biopsy was compared to standard resolution white light endoscopy with random biopsy in a prospective, blinded, tandem endoscopy trial [19]. The former method detected dysplasia in 57 % of patients as opposed to 43 % with SD endoscopy. The high-magnification NBI exam also found a higher stage of dysplasia in 18 % of patients [19]. Notably, fewer biopsies were taken with magnification with NBI than with the standard endoscopy method. Dual focus imaging, a feature of the Olympus Exera III endoscopic system, has been analyzed in conjunction with NBI. In one study, abnormal areas of mucosa were identified by regular NBI technique and then NBI coupled with dual focus imaging was used for second-pass characterization with biopsy of suspicious areas. Study results indicated that with this two-step procedure all areas of high-grade dysplasia and early cancer were identified and 86 % of superfluous biopsies could have been avoided [20].

In addition to identifying metaplastic and dysplastic changes, high-magnification endoscopy can highlight esophageal squamous cell dysplasia and carcinoma. Endoscopes with ×80 or greater magnification power have the ability to show intrapapillary capillary loops (IPCL) [21]. Changes to the normal IPCL architecture such as increased tortuosity and dilation were classified in a five-type system based on number of changes and were found to signify the presence of malignancy; specifically superficial esophageal squamous cell cancers. When IPCLs become deformed, interconnecting, or destroyed, the affected length has been shown to correlate with depth of invasion [21]. Additionally, a study which examined magnification endoscopy with NBI found that the addition of NBI improved the accuracy of IPCL subclassification by experienced endoscopists from 81.5 % to 85.2 %. The difference was even greater for novice endoscopist, whose accuracy rose from 61 % to 77.8 % [22]. IPCL classification and assessment of superficial squamous cell carcinoma depth have particular importance in identifying endoscopic mucosal resection (EMR) candidates.

Stomach

There are several common etiologies of inflammation in the stomach. A few studies have evaluated the ability of high-resolution magnification endoscopy to aid in identifying changes specifically associated with H. Pylori-induced gastritis. With conventional endoscopy, histopathology is required for the diagnosis of H. Pylori infection. However, new high-resolution and high-magnification endoscopes allow the diagnosis to be made in vivo with a high degree of accuracy. The classification system used for identifying *H. pylori* gastritis is based on the morphology of gastric pits, collecting venules, and capillaries. It has been found to correlate with histopathology, culture, and urease testing for *H. pylori* infection in several studies [23–25]. Moreover, the classification system used for identifying *H. pylori* gastritis as well as normal mucosa and gastric atrophy was found to have high inter- and intraobserver reliability (kappa values of 0.86 and 0.91, respectively) [26]. A study utilizing this system during high-resolution endoscopic exams in 129 patients found that mucosal patterns identifying *H. pylori* gastritis could be assessed with 93.9 % sensitivity and 90.3 % specificity [23]. These values increased to 100 % and 97.6 %, respectively, with the addition of indigo carmine [23]. In addition to diagnosing inflammation, magnification endoscopy has been shown to have a role in other types of gastric examinations. For example, in patients with bleeding peptic ulcers, it was found that magnification endoscopy could allow non-bleeding visible vessels to be more readily identified and intervened upon; thus decreasing the risk of rebleeding [27].

Magnification endoscopy also has an important role in diagnosing gastric neoplasia and adenocarcinoma. In a large Japanese study of 318 patients, magnification endoscopy allowed for a diagnostic accuracy of 100 % for elevated lesions and 95 %

for depressed lesions as opposed to 80 % and 84 %, respectively, with conventional endoscopy [28]. Sensitivity and specificity were also high (96 %, 95.5 %) when examinations were performed with high-magnification endoscopes [28]. Some studies have specifically examined the ability of magnification endoscopy to identify early malignant gastric lesions, as gastric cancer often initially presents as a sublet flat lesion undiagnosed until a late stage with high morbidity and mortality. The ability to magnify ×80 and greater has been shown to allow for visualization of microvessels, which take on a specific tortuous form in malignant transformation [29]. A study of 136 patients utilizing magnification endoscopy in conjunction with chromoendoscopy (methylene blue) found that the technique and associated classification system could diagnose both gastric metaplasia and dysplasia with accuracy of 82–85 % as well as high intra- and interobserver agreement ($k=0.86$, $k=0.74$) [30]. The technique and classification system were externally validated by a similar study, which found it to have a diagnostic validity of 80 % for diagnosis of intestinal metaplasia and 99 % for intraepithelial neoplasia [31]. When high-magnification chromoendoscopy and high-magnification endoscopy with NBI were testing against conventional endoscopy, both types of high-magnification exams were found to detect early gastric cancer with higher accuracy (91–94 %) and specificity (93–94 %) than the conventional method (69 % accuracy, 63 % specificity) [32]. High-resolution magnification endoscopy used with contract enhancement techniques can aid the endoscopist in correctly stratifying patients between endoscopic and surgical therapy. Additionally, the completeness of resection can be more accurately assessed as compared to conventional endoscopy [33].

Small Intestine

Most data regarding the use of high-resolution and high-magnification endoscopy in the small bowel is limited to duodenal examination. One study with 191 patients aimed to determine the general efficacy of high-resolution magnification endoscopy in the duodenum and specifically analyzed duodenal villi. It was found that HD magnification endoscopy could not only accurately determine the presence or absence of duodenal villi, but could also distinguish villous abnormalities such as flattening and irregular shape or arrangement. Interobserver agreement was excellent ($k=0.93$), while sensitivity (95 %), specificity (99 %), positive predictive value (95 %), and negative predictive value (99 %) were all high as well [34]. Detection of these abnormalities is especially important in patients with malabsorption as it can guide biopsy for diagnosis and lead to selection of appropriate therapy. When a cohort of patients with suspected celiac disease or sprue were evaluated with combined magnification endoscopy and chromoendoscopy, 88 % of patients were correctly identified as having villous atrophy whereas only 35 % were correctly identified when standard endoscopy was performed [35]. Additionally, magnification endoscopy was found to provide superior discriminatory detail for villous architecture [35]. In studies specifically of celiac disease patients, magnification endoscopy has been used to assess villous destruction and has been found to have a sensitivity of 90–100 % and specificity of 63–91 % [36, 37]. One cohort study of 27 patients even found that magnification endoscopy identified patchy villous atrophy in 16 patients when standard endoscopy was normal [38]. High-resolution magnification endoscopy has also been implicated as a tool for identifying other small intestinal malabsorbtive processes such as primary intestinal lymphangiectasia [39].

Though duodenal cancers are rare and many are found incidentally on routine endoscopy, patients with familial adenomatous polyposis carry an increased risk for these malignancies. There has been interest in using high-resolution endoscopy to help identify these lesions at an early stage. High-resolution endoscopy has been found to be a reliable method for utilizing the Spigelman classification—a scoring system based on polyp number, polyp size, histology, and dysplasia—which stages duodenal adenomatosis in FAP patients. One study compared high-resolution endoscopy to NBI in a FAP cohort and found that NBI "second look" exams detected additional duodenal polyps in 35.6 % of patients with upstage in Spigelman score in 4.4 % [40].

Colon

A major potential benefit of high-resolution endoscopy is the decrease in false negative rate of screening colonoscopies. This has strong implications considering colonoscopy is a widespread screening tool with a false negative rate reported as high as 24 % [41]. In two large studies, including one with 630 patients [42, 43], high-resolution colonoscopy was shown to yield significantly higher polyp detection rates [42, 43] and more accurate real-time histology prediction [43] compared to SD colonoscopy. A meta-analysis with five studies and 4422 patients found that HD colonoscopy resulted in a 3.5 % higher adenoma detection rate than SD colonoscopy [44]. The difference was greatest for detection of small colonic polyps [42] and flat lesions [43]. A study which directly compared two high-resolution endoscopic systems found that megapixel density affected outcomes. The system higher megapixel system detected 66 % of polyps, whereas the lower megapixel system only detected 44 % [42].

The high magnification feature of many high-resolution endoscopes also increases the utility and accuracy of colonoscopy. High magnification allows for mucosal pit patterns to be discerned by the endoscopist, and similarly to mucosal patterns in the esophagus, these patterns have been shown to correlate with histologic changes such as dysplasia and eventual neoplasia. With sufficient magnification, the endoscope becomes akin to a low-power microscope. This is particularly important for small, flat, or depressed lesions, which may be more inconspicuous than polyps and more easily missed as a source of potential malignancy. Kudo et al. examined 2050 colorectal lesions and proposed that magnification of at least ×100 could allow several distinct mucosal pit patterns to be discerned [45]. The patterns identified by magnification endoscopy were fundamentally similar to those seen

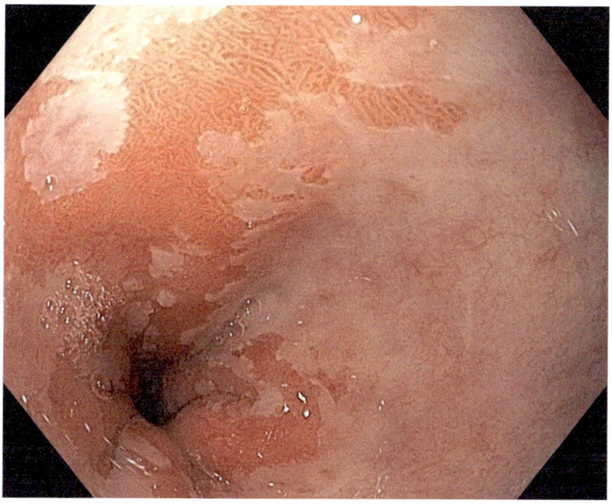

Fig. 1.1 High-resolution endoscopy can demonstrate mucosal pit patterns in Barrett's esophagus. Note the regular villiform or ceribriform pattern noted in this area of non-dysplastic Barrett's esophagus

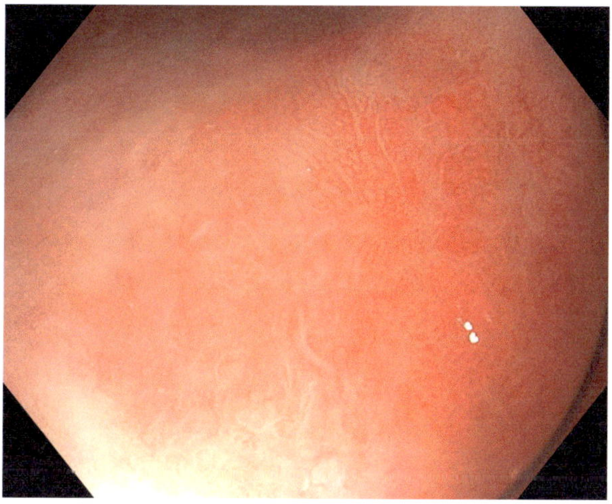

Fig. 1.2 Note the irregular mucosal pit pattern in this segment of Barrett's esophagus on high-resolution endoscopy that was subsequently diagnosed as high-grade dysplasia

with stereomicroscopy and they correlated strongly with histology—81 % of lesions had agreement in diagnosis [45]. These patterns are outlined in Figs. 1.1, 1.2, 1.3, and 1.4. Studies utilizing the Kudos pit pattern scheme have found that magnification colonoscopy more accurately identified colorectal lesions as compared to non-magnifying colonoscopy [45, 46], with a difference in accuracy as high as 24 % [46]. In a study of 660 patients, high magnification exams had a sensitivity of 97 % and specificity of 100 % as compared to 90 % and 61 %, respectively, for non-magnifying exams [46]. The comparative data was particularly strong for small (<5 mm) and flat lesions [45], but a significant difference was still observed when only polyps were examined [47]. Additionally, magnification colonoscopy has been

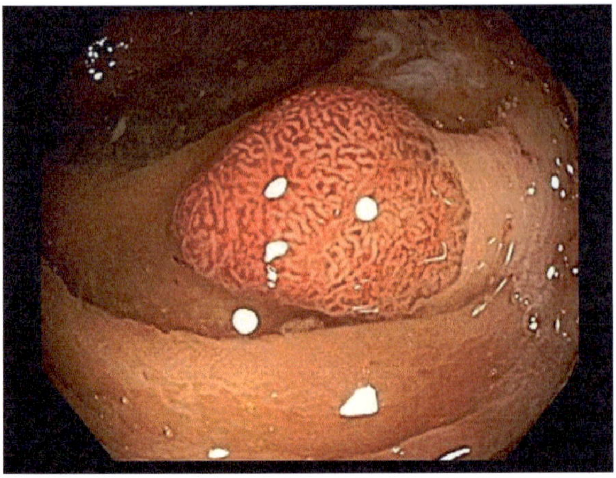

Fig. 1.3 High-resolution endoscopy can demonstrate mucosal pit patterns in colon polyps. Note regular villiform pattern seen in this colon tubular adenoma

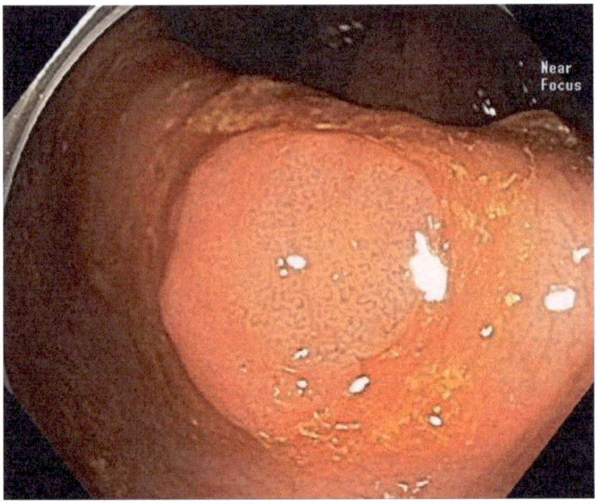

Fig. 1.4 High-resolution endoscopy with magnification can demonstrate more subtle mucosal pit patterns in colon polyps. Note regular villiform pattern seen in this colon tubular adenoma with near focus

shown to aid in the detection of earlier, more superficial cancers [48]; which is useful for guiding patients toward either endoscopic or surgical resection [49].

When magnification colonoscopy was studied in conjunction chromoendoscopy, similar results were obtained. Studies comparing high-magnification chromoendoscopy (indigo carmine-based) with non-magnification chromoendoscopy or conventional endoscopy alone showed that the high-magnification examinations had 6–11 % better accuracy for detecting neoplastic lesions [50, 51]. By using magnification not only can early cancers be detected at a higher frequency, but the morbidity associated with unnecessary polypectomy could potentially be avoided.

Magnification endoscopy has also been studied in conjunction with NBI in the colon. When magnification endoscopy with NBI was compared to standard white-light endoscopy, superior visualization of vascular networks improved the diagnostic value of pattern classification by increasing accuracy from 66 to 92 % [52]. The level of magnification power appears to be important. High-magnification colonoscopy utilizing NBI or chromoendoscopy (indigo carmine) was found to have 5–13 % superior accuracy compared to the same examinations done with low magnification [53]. However, both low and high magnifications were superior to conventional colonoscopy done without magnification. When magnification colonoscopy is being performed, the concurrent use of different contrast enhancement techniques appears to be similar in efficacy. Magnification endoscopy with NBI was found to yield similar diagnostic results as magnification endoscopy with indigo carmine dye [54]. A meta-analysis focused on optical biopsy of diminutive polyps (<5 mm) specifically analyzed 20 NBI studies and found that this contrast enhancement technique had a pooled negative predictive value of 91 % for predicting adenomatous histology [55]. This implies that NBI could serve as reliable method for optical biopsy.

A few studies have examined HD and magnification colonoscopy specifically in the setting of inflammatory bowel disease. In this high-risk population, subtle mucosal changes may represent pre-cancerous or cancerous lesions. Surveillance colonoscopy with biopsy is a mainstay of clinical management. In a retrospective cohort study, high-definition colonoscopy was found to detect significantly more dysplastic lesions in patients with IBD when compared to standard definition colonoscopy during multiple regression analysis (prevalence ratio = 2.30) [56]. This was especially true for the right side of the colon, which often houses flat lesions [56]. Studies evaluating the role of high-magnification colonoscopy in IBD patients have found that these examinations can allow for improved prediction of histopathological inflammation [57] and disease relapse [58]. Magnification endoscopy has also been tested with indigo carmine chromoendoscopy in ulcerative colitis patients and this method was found to detect 59 % more intraepithelial neoplasias as compared to conventional colonoscopy [59].

Safety and Cost Considerations

None of the studies reviewed reported any adverse events associated with utilizing high-resolution or high-magnification endoscopic systems.

The financial considerations associated with utilizing high-resolution or high-magnification endoscopy include the cost of upgrading to specialized endoscopes as well as compatible monitors and processors. To date, there had been no cost-effectiveness analyses on the use of HD endoscopic systems. However, software-based algorithmic image analysis has been proposed in conjunction with high-resolution imaging to overcome issues of training and expertise in resource-poor settings [60].

Conclusions

The use of high-resolution and high-magnification endoscopes is quickly becoming the standard of care in most clinical settings. Almost all new endoscopic systems offer these features and standard definition endoscopes are likely to become obsolete in the near future. High-resolution and high-magnification systems have been objectively shown to provide superior image quality which allows the observer to delineate fine mucosal features; from crypt and pit patterns to capillary and villous architecture. In all parts of the gastrointestinal tract, studies have validated the correlation between observable changes in surface morphology and histopathologic diagnoses. Additionally, high-resolution and high-magnification endoscopic systems increase the efficacy of contrast enhancement techniques such as chromoendoscopy. Other techniques such as narrow-band imaging depend entirely on a high-resolution, high-magnification system and cannot be utilized without it. The benefits of high-resolution and high-magnification endoscopy with or without adjuvant contrast enhancement have profound implications in terms of screening, diagnostic, and therapeutic endoscopy. While random biopsy is still a part of many gastrointestinal screening protocols, high-resolution and high-magnification endoscopy had been shown to allow for targeted biopsies and to decrease the overall number of biopsies that are needed for establishing a diagnosis. Tissue oversampling is not without associated morbidity, and patients may be spared unnecessary harm if only 'red flag' areas identified by advanced endoscopy are sampled. High-resolution and high-magnification endoscopy has also been shown to increase the accuracy and yield of many diagnostic exams, especially in high-risk populations. Throughout the literature, high-resolution and high-magnification endoscopy has been proven superior to conventional endoscopy in identifying pre-malignant lesion and early cancers. Because of this, routine use of these endoscopic methods may improve prognosis as well as afford patients with a wider range of therapeutic options. Additionally, patients may be better stratified to endoscopic therapy versus more invasive treatment, thus saving some patients with early-stage disease from surgical morbidity.

Future Directions

There is no doubt that the technology behind high-resolution and high-magnification endoscopes will continue to evolve at a fast pace. CCD chips will continue to advance, so image resolution and clarity will follow suit. This, along with advances in magnification optics, will bring endoscopy closer and closer to real-time microscopy or "optical biopsy". As high-resolution and magnification endoscopy becomes more widespread, the use of standardized classification systems will become routine. It will be increasingly important to confirm high intra- and interobserver reliability in these classification schemes with large-scale studies. Also, many studies on high-resolution and high-magnification endoscopy utilize classification systems that were developed within regionally limited populations. As such, further investigation needs to be done to determine if these classifications systems can be reliably applied to settings outside of those initially studied.

References

1. Sivak MV. Gastrointestinal endoscopy: past and future. Gut. 2006;55(8):1061–4.
2. Tanaka S, Kaltenbach T, Chayama K, Soetikno R. High magnification colonoscopy (with videos). Gastrointest Endosc. 2006;64:604–13.
3. Udagawa TAM, Okada F. Development of magnifying video endoscopes with high resolution. Dig Endosc. 2001;13:163–9.
4. ASGE Technology Committee. High definition and high magnification endoscopes. Gastrointest Endosc. 2014;80(6):919–27.
5. Olympus America Gastroenterology. [Internet]. 2015. http://medical.olympusamerica.com
6. Pentax I-Scan Mini Atlas for Gastroenterology. [Internet]. Pentax Medical. http://www.pentaxmedical.com
7. Fuji Intelligent Color Enhancement Atlas. [Internet]. Fujinon. http://www.fujinon.at
8. Chalasani N, Wo JM, Hunter JG, Waring JP. Significance of intestinal metaplasia in different areas of the esophagus including esophagogastric junction. Dig Dis Sci. 1997;42:603–7.
9. Guelrud M, Herrera I, Essenfeld H, Castro J. Enhanced magnification endoscopy: a new technique to identify specialized intestinal metaplasia in Barrett's esophagus. Gastrointest Endosc. 2001;53:559.
10. Hoffman A, Kiesslick R, Bender A, Neurath MF, Nafe B, Hermann G, et al. Acetic acid guided biopsies after magnifying endoscopy compares with random biopsies in the detection of Barrett's esophagus: a prospective randomized trial with crossover design. Gastrointest Endosc. 2006;64(1):1–8.
11. Tholoor S, Bhattacharyya R, Tsagkournis O, Longcroft-Wheaton G, Bhandari P. Acetic acid chromoendoscopy in Barrett's esophagus surveillance is superior to the standardized random biopsy protocol: results from a large cohort study (with video). Gastrointest Endosc. 2014;80:417.
12. Endo T, Awakawa T, Takahashi H, Arimura Y, Itoh F, Yamashita K, et al. Classification of Barrett's epithelium by magnifying endoscopy. Gastrointest Endosc. 2002;55:641–7.
13. Sharma P, Weston AP, Topalovski M, Cherian R, Bhattacharyya A, Sampliner RE. Magnification chromoendoscopy for the detection of intestinal metaplasia and dysplasia in Barrett's oesophagus. Gut. 2003;52:24–7.
14. Stevens PD, Lightdale CJ, Green PH, Siegel LM, Garcia-Carrasquillo RJ, Rotterdam H. Combined magnification endoscopy with chromoendoscopy for evaluation of Barrett's esophagus. Gastorintest Endosc. 2002;55:641–7.
15. Kara MA, Ennahachi M, Fockens P, ten Kate FJ, Bergman JJ. Detection and classification of the mucosal and vascular patterns (mucosal morphology) in Barrett's esophagus by using narrow band imaging. Gastrintest Endosc. 2006;64:155–66
16. Goda K, Tajiri H, Ikegami M, Urashima M, Nakayoshi T, Kaise M. Usefulness of magnification endoscopy with narrow band imaging for the detection of specialized intestinal metaplasia in columnar-lined esophagus and Barrett's adenocarcinoma. Gastrointest Endosc. 2007;65:36–46.
17. Anagnostopoulos GK, Yao K, Kaye P, Hawkey CJ, Ragunath K. Novel endoscopic observation in Barrett's esophagus using high resolution magnification endoscopy and narrow band imaging. Aliment Pharmacol Ther. 2007;26:501–7.
18. Silva FB, Dinis-Ribeiro M, Vieth M, Rabenstein T, Goda K, Kiesslich R, et al. Endoscopic assessment and grading of Barrett's esophagus using magnification endoscopy and narrow-band

imaging: accuracy and interobserver agreement of different classification systems (with videos). Gastrointest Endosc. 2011;73:7–14.
19. Wolfsen HC, Crook JE, Krishna M, Achem SR, Devault KR, Bouras EP, et al. Prospective, controlled tandem endoscopy study of narrow band imaging for dysplasia detection in Barrett's esophagus. Gastroenterology. 2008;135:24–31.
20. Singh R, Shahzad MA, Tam W, Goda K, Yu LH, Fujishiro M, et al. Preliminary feasibility study using a novel narrow-band imaging system with dual focus magnification capability in Barrett's esophagus: is the time ripe to abandon random biopsies? Dig Endosc. 2013;25 Suppl 2:151–6.
21. Inoue H, Kumagai Y, Yoshida T, Kawano T, Endo M, Iwai T. High magnification endoscopic diagnosis of the superficial esophageal cancer. Dig Endosc. 2000;12:32–5.
22. Yoshida T, Inoue H, Usui S, Satodate H, Fukami N, Kudo SE. Narrow-band imaging system with magnifying endoscopy for superficial esophageal lesions. Gastrointest Endosc. 2004; 59:288–95.
23. Gonen C, Simsek I, Sarioglu S, Akpinar H. Comparison of high resolution magnifying endoscopy and standard video endoscopy for the diagnosis of Helicobacter pylori gastritis in routine clinical practice: a prospective study. Helicobacter. 2009;14:12–21.
24. Yagi K, Nakamura A, Sekine A. Comparison between magnifying endoscopy and histological, culture, and urease test findings from the gastric mucosa of the corpus. Endoscopy. 2002; 34:76–81.
25. Yagi K, Nakamura A, Sekine A. Characteristic endoscopic and magnified endoscopic findings in the normal stomach without H. Pylori infection. J Gastroenterol Hepatol. 2002;17:39–45.
26. Anagnostropoulos GK, Yao K, Kayne P, Fogden E, Fortun P, Shonde A, et al. High resolution magnification endoscopy can reliably identify normal gastric mucosa, H. Pylori associated gastritis, and gastric atrophy. Endoscopy. 2007;39:202–7.
27. Cipolletta L, Bianco MA, Salerno R, Prisco A, Marmo R, Cipolleta F, et al. Improved characterization of visible vessels in bleeding ulcers by using magnification endoscopy: results of a pilot study. Gastrointest Endosc. 2010;72:413–8.
28. Tajiri H, Doi T, Endo H, Nishina T, Terao T, Hyodo I, et al. Routine endoscopy using a magnifying endoscope for gastric cancer diagnosis. Endoscopy. 2002;34:772–7.
29. Yao K, Oishi T, Matsui T, Yao T, Iwashita A. Novel magnified endoscopic findings of microvascular architecture in intramucosal gastric cancer. Gastrointest Endosc. 2002;56:279–84.
30. Dinis-Riberio M, da Costa-Pereira A, Lopes C, Lara-Santos L, Guilherme M, Moreira-Dias L, et al. Magnification chromoendoscopy for the diagnosis of gastric intestinal metaplasia and dysplasia. Gastrointest Endosc. 2003;57:498–504.
31. Areia M, Amaro P, Dinis-Ribeiro M, Cipriano MA, Marinho C, Costa-Pereira A, et al. External validation of a classification for methylene blue magnification chromoendoscopy in premalignant gastric lesions. Gastrointest Endosc. 2008;67:1011–8.
32. Zhang J, Guo SB, Duan ZJ. Application of magnifying narrow-band imaging endoscopy for diagnosis of early gastric cancer and precancerous lesion. BMC Gastroenterology. 2011;11:135.
33. Sumiyama K, Kaise M, Nakayoshi T, Kato M, Mashiko T, Uchiyama Y, et al. Combined use of a magnifying endoscope with narrow-band imaging and a multibending endoscope for en bloc EMR of early stage gastric cancer. Gastrointest Endosc. 2004;60:79–84.
34. Cammarota G, Martino A, Pirozzi GA, Cianci R, Cremonini F, Zuccalà G, et al. Direct visualization of intestinal villi by high-resolution magnifying upper endoscopy: a validation study. Gastrointest Endosc. 2004;60:732–8.
35. Cammarota G, Fedeli P, Gasbarrini A. Emerging technologies in upper gastrointestinal endoscopy and celiac disease. Nat Clin Pract Gastroenterol Hepatol. 2009;6:47–56.
36. Badreldin R, Barrett P, Wooff DA, Mansfield J, Yiannakou Y. How good is zoom endoscopy for assessment of villous atrophy in celiac disease? Endoscopy. 2005;37:994–8.
37. Banerjee R, Shekharan A, Ramji C, Puli SR, Kalapala R, Ramachandani M, et al. Role of magnification endoscopy in the diagnosis and evaluation of suspected celiac disease: Correlation with histology. Indian J Gastroenterol. 2007;26:67–9.

38. Lo A, Guelrud M, Essenfeld H, Bonis P. Classification of villous atrophy with enhanced magnification endoscopy in patients with celiac disease and tropical sprue. Gastrointest Endosc. 2007;66:377–82.
39. Cammarota G, Cianci R, Gasbarrini G. High-resolution magnifying video endoscopy in primary intestinal lymphangiectasia: a new role for endoscopy? Endoscopy. 2005;37:607.
40. Lopez-Ceron M, van den Broek FJ, Mathus-Vliegen EM, Boparai KS, van Eeden S, Fockens P, et al. The role of high-resolution endoscopy and narrow-band imaging in the evaluation of upper GI neoplasia in familial adenomatous polyposis. Gastrointest Endosc. 2013; 77(4):542–50.
41. Rex DK, Cutler CS, Lemmel GT, Rahmani EY, Clark DW, Helper DJ, et al. Colonoscopic miss rates of adenomas determined by back-to-back colonoscopies. Gastroenterology. 1997; 112:24–8.
42. Banks MR, Haidry R, Butt MA, Whitley L, Stein J, Langmead L, et al. High resolution colonoscopy in a bowel cancer screening program improves polyp detection. World J Gastroenterol. 2011;17:4308–13.
43. Rastogi A, Early DS, Gupta N, Bansal A, Singh V, Ansstas M, et al. Randomized, controlled trial of standard-definition white-light, high-definition white-light, and narrow-band imaging colonoscopy for the detection of colon polyps and prediction of polyp histology. Gastrointest Endosc. 2011;74:593–602.
44. Subramanian V, Mannath J, Hawkley CJ, Ragunath K. High definition colonoscopy vs. standard video endoscopy for the detection of colonic polyps: a meta-analysis. Gastrointest Endosc. 2011;43(6):1021–8.
45. Kudo S, Tamura S, Nakajima T, Yamano H, Kusaka H, Watanabe H. Diagnosis of colorectal tumorous lesions by magnifying endoscopy. Gastointest Endosc. 1996;44(1):8–14.
46. Konishi K, Kaneko K, Kurahashi T, Yamamoto T, Kushima M, Kanda A, et al. A comparison of magnifying and nonmagnifying colonoscopy for diagnosis of colorectal polyps: a prospective study. Gastrointest Endosc. 2003;57:48–53.
47. Togashi K, Konishi F, Ishizuka T, Sato T, Senba S, Kanazawa K. Efficacy of magnifying endoscopy in the differential diagnosis of neoplastic and non-neoplastic polyps of the large bowel. Dis Colon Rectum. 1999;42:1602–8.
48. Tanaka S, Haruma K, Ito M, Nagata S, Oh-e H, Hirota Y, et al. Detailed colonoscopy for detecting early superficial carcinoma: recent developments. J Gastroenterol. 2000;35 Suppl 12:121–5.
49. Bianco MA, Rotondano G, Marmo R, Garofano ML, Piscopo R, de Gregorio A. Predictive value of magnification chromoendoscopy for diagnosing invasive neoplasia in nonpolypoid colorectal lesions and stratifying patients for endoscopic resection or surgery. Endoscopy. 2006;38:470–6.
50. Emura F, Saito Y, Taniguchi M, Fujii T, Tagawa K, Yamakado M. Further validation of magnifying chromocolonoscopy for differentiating colorectal neoplastic polyps in a health screening center. J Gastroenterol Hepatol. 2007;22:1722–7.
51. Fu K, Sano Y, Kato S, Fujii T, Nagashima F, Yoshino T, et al. Chromoendoscopy using indigo carmine dye spraying with magnifying observation is the most reliable method for differential diagnosis between non-neoplastic and neoplastic colorectal lesions: a prospective study. Endoscopy. 2004;36:1089–93.
52. Tischendorf JJ, Wasmuth HE, Koch A, Hecker H, Trautwein C, Winograd R, et al. Value of magnifying chromoendoscopy and narrow band imaging (NBI) in classifying colorectal polyps: a prospective controlled study. Endoscopy. 2007;39:1092–6.
53. Chiu HM, Chang CY, Chen CC, Lee YC, Wu MS, Lin JT, et al. A prospective comparative study of narrow-band imaging, chromoendoscopy, and conventional colonoscopy in the diagnosis of colorectal neoplasia. Gut. 2007;56:373–9.
54. Okamoto Y, Watanabe H, Tominaga K, Oki R, Yamagata M, Yokotuska F, et al. Evaluation of microvessels in colorectal tumors by narrow band imaging magnification: including comparison with magnifying chromoendoscopy. Dig Dis Sci. 2011;56:532–8.

55. ASGE Technology Committee, Abu Dayyeh BK, Thosani N, Konda V, Wallace MB, Rex DK, et al. ASGE Technology Committee systematic review and meta-analysis assessing the ASGE PIVI thresholds for adopting real-time endoscopic assessment of the histology of diminutive colorectal polyps. Gastrointest Endosc. 2015;81(3):502–16.
56. Subramanian V, Ramappa V, Telakis E, Mannath J, Jawhari AU, Hawkey CJ, et al. Comparison of high definition with standard white light endoscopy for detection of dysplastic lesions during surveillance colonoscopy in patients with colonic inflammatory bowel disease. Inflamm Bowel Dis. 2013;19:350–5.
57. Kunihiro M, Tanaka S, Sumii M, Ueno Y, Ito M, Kitadai Y, et al. Magnifying colonoscopic features of ulcerative colitis reflect histologic inflammation. Inflamm Bowel Dis. 2004;10:737–44.
58. Nishio Y, Ando T, Maeda O, Ishiquro K, Watanabe O, Ohmiya N, et al. Pit patterns in rectal mucosa assessed by magnifying colonoscope are predictive of relapse in patients with quiescent ulcerative colitis. Gut. 2006;55:1768–73.
59. Hurlstone DP, McAlindon ME, Sanders DS, Koegh R, Lobo AJ, Cross SS. Further validation of high-magnification chromoscopic-colonoscopy for the detection of intraepithelial neoplasia and colon cancer in ulcerative colitis. Gastroenterology. 2004;126:376–8.
60. Shin D, Protano MA, Polydorides AD, Dawsey SM, Pierce MC, Kim MK, et al. Quantitative analysis of high-resolution microendoscopic images for diagnosis of esophageal squamous cell carcinoma. Clin Gastroenterol Hepatol. 2015;13(2):272–9.

Chapter 2
Wide Angle Endoscopes and Accessory Devices to Improve the Field of View

Ioannis S. Papanikolaou and Peter D. Siersema

Introduction

Colonoscopy represents a widely established method for colorectal cancer (CRC) screening, given its ability to detect and remove precancerous lesions, namely adenomatous polyps [1, 2]. Interrupting adenoma-carcinoma sequence, increased colonoscopy utilization is possibly associated with the recently observed decline in the incidence of CRC and its earlier diagnosis [3, 4]. Despite the evidence regarding the effectiveness of colonoscopy, emerging data underline its imperfections. As shown in tandem colonoscopy studies, up to a quarter of polyps and adenomas are missed during colonoscopy, accounting for the development of interval cancer [5–7]. Several technical-, patient-, and endoscopist-related factors have been studied to explain variability in colonoscopy outcomes, which negatively influence the quality of the procedure [8–11].

It has been shown that important undetected lesions are often located in the right colon, on the proximal aspects of haustral folds, the area around the ileocecal valve and anatomical flexures. These sites are often hidden from the standard forward-viewing colonoscopes, which provide a 140–170° wide field of view, necessitating complex and time-consuming efforts for thorough mucosal examination.

I.S. Papanikolaou, M.D., Ph.D., F.E.B.G.H.
Hepatogastroenterology Unit, Second Department of Internal Medicine and Research Unit, "Attikon" University General Hospital, University of Athens, Athens, Greece

P.D. Siersema, M.D., Ph.D., F.A.S.G.E. (✉)
Department of Gastroenterology and Hepatology, University Medical Center Utrecht, Utrecht, The Netherlands

Department of Gastroenterology and Hepatology, Radboud University Medical Center, Geert Grooteplein Zuid 10, Nijmegen GA 6525, The Netherlands
e-mail: peter.siersema@radboudumc.nl

V.J.A. Konda, I. Waxman (eds.), *Endoscopic Imaging Techniques and Tools*,
DOI 10.1007/978-3-319-30053-5_2

Mounting evidence suggests that improving colonoscope technology may result in lower adenoma miss rates and increased diagnostic yield. In order to broaden the field of mucosal view, integrated devices, wide-angle colonoscopes as well as accessory devices are being implemented. The former include the Third Eye® Retroscope® (Avantis Medical Systems, Sunnyvale, CA, USA), the Fuse® Full Spectrum Endoscopy® colonoscopy platform (EndoChoice, Inc., Alpharetta, GA, USA), the G-EYE™ balloon colonoscope (SMART Medical Systems Ltd, Ra'anana, Israel), and the Extra-Wide-Angle-View colonoscope (Olympus, Tokyo, Japan). Accessory devices include transparent caps and the Endocuff that are attached to the distal tip of the colonoscope. This chapter aims to highlight the aforementioned techniques and discuss current data related to their clinical use.

Wide Angle Colonoscopes

Third Eye® Retroscope®

The Third Eye® Retroscope® (TER; Avantis Medical Systems, Sunnyvale, CA, USA) represents a through-the-scope device that intends to enhance visualization behind the proximal aspects of colonic folds and anatomical flexures. It consists of a video processor and a flexible single-use catheter with a miniaturized video camera located in its tip (Fig. 2.1a). By achieving a 180° retroflexion (Fig. 2.1b), it enables detailed examination of the colon during withdrawal (Fig. 2.1c). The efficacy of TER was initially assessed by Triadafilopoulos et al. in three colon models with simulated polyps, both "obvious" and "hidden" [12]. Based on the results of this randomized, blind study, standard colonoscopy detected 12 % of polyps located on the proximal aspects of folds, while TER identified 81 % of them. In a follow-up pilot study by the same author and colleagues, TER detected four additional polyps (three hyperplastic and one adenoma), resulting in an increase in diagnostic yield as high as 11.8 % [13]. Of note, no adverse event was reported.

Accordingly, the diagnostic yield of TER was evaluated in two prospective, multicenter studies by DeMarco et al. and Waye et al. [14, 15]. In the former study, 27 additional polyps were found with TER leading to an increase of 14.8 % and 16 % in polyp and adenoma detection, respectively. Similarly, increases reached 13.2 % and 11 %, respectively, in the latter study. All changes were of statistical significance.

The TERRACE study is the sole randomized, back-to-back, multicenter study with respect to TER [8]. The authors reported that TER yielded a net additional detection rate of 29.8 % for all polyps and 23.2 % for adenomas, in the per protocol analysis. TER underperformed in patients undergoing screening colonoscopy as compared to those undergoing colonoscopy for surveillance or symptomatic evaluation. However, criticism has been raised regarding this study due to significant higher withdrawal time with TER in comparison with standard procedure. Nevertheless, in a post-hoc analysis by Siersema et al., that difference was not associated with the risk of missing adenomas [16].

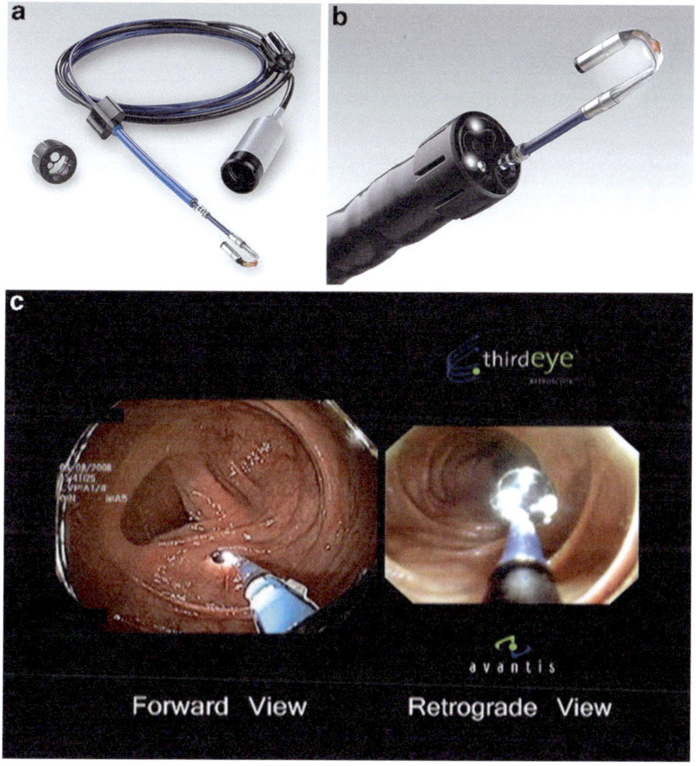

Fig. 2.1 Third Eye® Retroscope®: The devise (**a**), the devise through the endoscope; note its 180° retroflexion (**b**), and the endoscopic view (forward and retrograde) (**c**). With permission from Avantis Medical

Limitations of TER include an associated learning curve, significant cost, and blockage of the working channel preventing use of other devices unless removed. Obviously, a subsequent prolongation of the procedural time is expected.

The FUSE® System

The FUSE® system (EndoChoice, GA, USA) was recently developed as a new platform (Fig. 2.2a). It consists of a main control processor and a video colonoscope (168 cm working length, 12.8 mm outer diameter) with three imagers and LED groups located at the front and both sides of the flexible tip (Fig. 2.2b, c). Obtained images are displayed in three contiguous monitors (Fig. 2.2d), eventually achieving a 330° angle of colonic mucosa view (Fig. 2.2b). In that way, most of the "blind" areas of the colon become easily visualized.

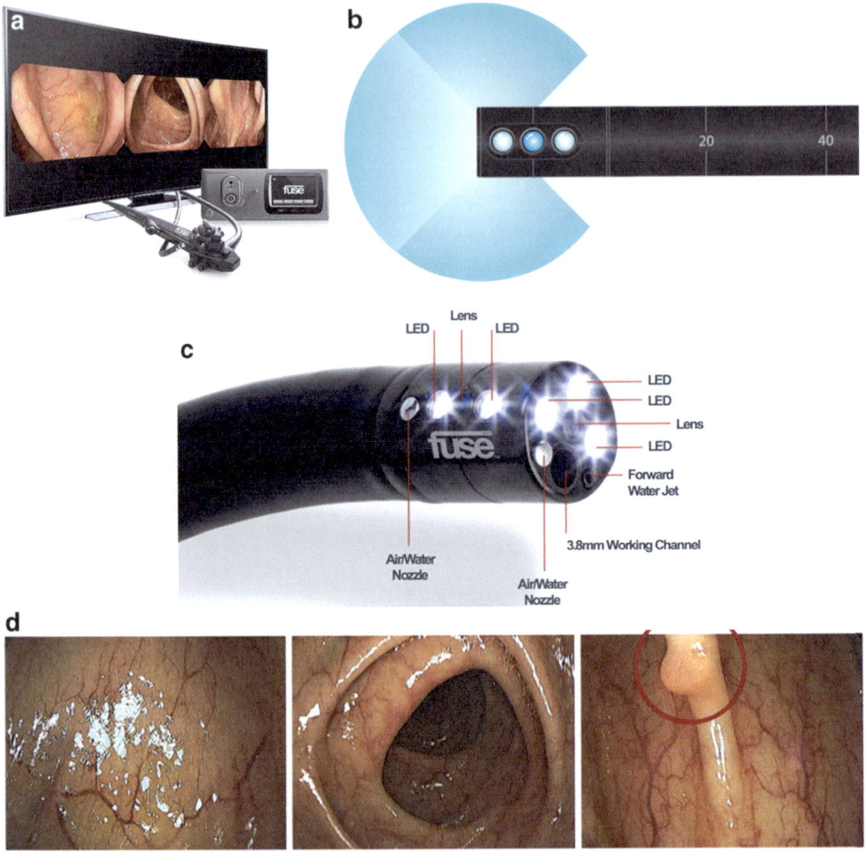

Fig. 2.2 The FUSE® system: Note, the system platform (including scope, processor, and monitor) (**a**), the system's three imagers, which provide a 330° angle view of the colonic mucosa (**b**), the LED groups at the front and sides of the scope's tip (**c**), and the endoscopic view on the three contiguous monitors (**d**). With permission from EndoChoice, Inc

Gralnek et al. reported in 2013 the first study that evaluated the FUSE® system [17]. It was a prospective, multicenter, non-randomized study in in vitro colon models with simulated polyps. As the results indicated, 85.7 % of the polyps were detected with the FUSE® platform compared to 52.9 % with the forward-viewing colonoscopy ($p<0.001$). Simulated polyp detection rates were significantly higher with the FUSE® system in all colon segments. Interestingly, FUSE® colonoscopy identified significantly more "hidden" behind flexures and folds polyps (81.9 % versus 31.9 %).

A subsequent prospective, single-center study aimed to assess feasibility, usability, and safety of this novel colonoscopy platform in 50 adult subjects [18]. Reported cecal intubation rate was 100 % and time to cecum (minutes, mean ± SD) was 3.1 ± 1.5 min. Withdrawal time was 12.7 ± 4.4 min and total procedure time was 15.3 ± 4.6 min. In 44 % of the cases, 26 interventions were performed: 19 (73.1 %) biopsies and 7 (26.9 %) polypectomies. No acute or delayed adverse events were noticed. Both patients' and endoscopists' satisfaction were high.

An international, multicentre, randomized, tandem colonoscopy trial compared the adenoma miss rates of FUSE® colonoscopy with standard forward-viewing colonoscopy [19]. One hundred and ninety seven individuals were initially randomly assigned (1:1) to which procedure was done first. Per-lesion analysis in 185 patients showed that the adenoma miss rate was significantly lower with FUSE® colonoscopy than in the standard forward-viewing procedure: 7 % versus 41 % of adenomas were missed with FUSE® and standard colonoscopy, respectively ($p < 0.0001$). Standard forward-viewing colonoscopy missed 20 adenomas in 15 patients, three (15 %) of those being advanced. Full-spectrum endoscopy missed five adenomas (non-advanced) in five patients in whom an adenoma had already been found with first-pass standard forward-viewing examination. Five minor adverse events were reported, including vomiting, diarrhea, cystitis, gastroenteritis, and bleeding. The authors concluded that the FUSE® colonoscopy may enhance the efficacy of colorectal cancer screening and surveillance.

Very recently, Hassan and Gralnek demonstrated in a population-based program that, compared to standard colonoscopy, full-spectrum endoscopy appears to be more cost-effective for colon cancer screening and surveillance [20].

G-EYE™ Balloon Colonoscope

The G-EYE™ includes the G-EYE™ balloon colonoscope combined with the NaviAid™ SPARK²C inflation system. The G-EYE™ colonoscope integrates a reusable and inflatable by the endoscopist balloon onto its flexible tip (Fig. 2.3). The balloon has three intermediate pressure levels with a maximal inflation diameter reaching 60 mbar. By inflating the balloon after cecum intubation, flattening of

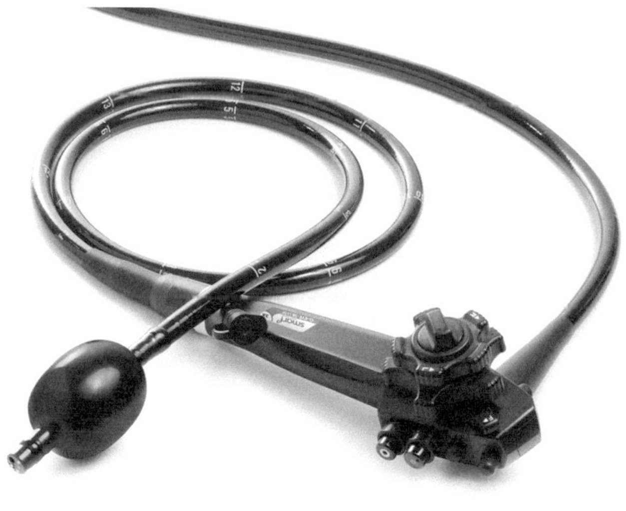

Fig. 2.3 G-EYE™ balloon colonoscope. With permission from Smart Medical Systems Ltd

haustral folds is achieved aiming to improve inspection and increase lesion detection. Additionally, it may also provide anchoring and stabilization of the colon during therapeutic interventions.

Hassan and colleagues compared the diagnostic yield of balloon-assisted colonoscopy versus that of standard colonoscopy in the detection of simulated polyps in a colon model [21]. G-EYE™ balloon colonoscope demonstrated significantly higher median polyp detection rate (91.7 % versus 45.8 %, $p<0.0001$). This result was evident both in non-obscured and in obscured polyps.

In 2014, Gralnek et al. aimed to establish the safety and feasibility of this novel balloon-colonoscope in 50 patients referred for colonoscopy [22]. According to the results, two patients experienced minor adverse events (diarrhea, abdominal pain). Cecal intubation was achieved in all cases and mean times to reach the cecum, to withdrawal, the scope, as well as the mean time of the total procedure were 4.3, 7.4, and 16.5 min, respectively. Polyp and adenoma detection rates reached 53.2 % and 44.7 %, respectively, although most (79.5 %) of the findings were of diminutive size. The authors concluded that the studied system appears safe and feasible to use.

A multicenter, randomized, prospective, controlled study in 126 patients undergoing colonoscopy for screening/surveillance or diagnostic evaluation has been very recently published [23]. The adenoma detection and miss rates were compared between the two procedures. The adenoma miss rate of G-EYE™ balloon colonoscopy was significantly lower than that of standard colonoscopy (7.5 % versus 44.7 %; $p=0.0002$). The detection of additional adenomas by balloon colonoscopy was also significant (81.0 %; $p=0.0002$). Interestingly, the number of adenomas detected in the ascending colon by balloon colonoscopy was 41 % versus 14 % for standard colonoscopy. Given the significantly higher adenoma detection rate as well as the lower miss rate, the investigators suggested that balloon colonoscopy may increase the effectiveness of colorectal cancer screening and surveillance.

Extra-Wide-Angle-View Colonoscope

The Extra-Wide-Angle-View colonoscope (Olympus, Tokyo, Japan) has a 13.9-mm-tip diameter and a 144–232° lateral-backward viewing lens in addition to a 140° forward-viewing lens at the tip of the scope. Obtained views are presented simultaneously on a video monitor as a single image. This system aims to provide more extensive inspection of the colonic mucosa without any specific manipulations. To assess its diagnostic yield, Uraoka et al. conducted a simulated pilot study of two anatomic colorectal models, each prepared with eight polyps positioned in obvious locations and eight polyps hidden behind folds. Thirty-two endoscopists performed examinations on models by using the extra-wide-angle-view colonoscope and a standard colonoscope. The results indicated that the mean detection rate for all simulated polyps with the extra-wide-angle-view colonoscope was significantly higher than that of the standard colonoscope (68 % versus 51 %; $p<0.0001$). In addition, the detection rate for "hidden" polyps was also significantly higher in the extra-wide-angle-view colonoscope than in the standard colonoscope (61.7 % versus 46.9 %; $p = 0.0009$) [24].

Similarly, the same investigators presented in 2013 during the Digestive Disease Week a randomized trial comparing this novel colonoscope with a standard one, on the basis of polyp/adenoma detection. Nevertheless, the results showed no significant differences regarding polyp/adenoma detection rates between the two types of colonoscope. As an exception, the Extra-Wide-Angle-View colonoscope performed significantly better with respect to adenoma detection rate in the sigmoid colon, as compared to the standard scope (mean ADR 0.4 versus 0.2, $p = 0.04$).

Accessory Devices

Endocuff-Assisted Colonoscopy

The Endocuff (EC) is a recently developed attachable endoscopic cuff, which is approved for medical use in humans in order to improve the feasibility of colon polypectomy as well as visualization of the mucosa. The EC is a 2 cm long, flexible cuff with two rows of flexible, hinged wings (Fig. 2.4a) that flatten mucosal folds during scope withdrawal (Fig. 2.4b–d). Its first use was reported in 2012 for

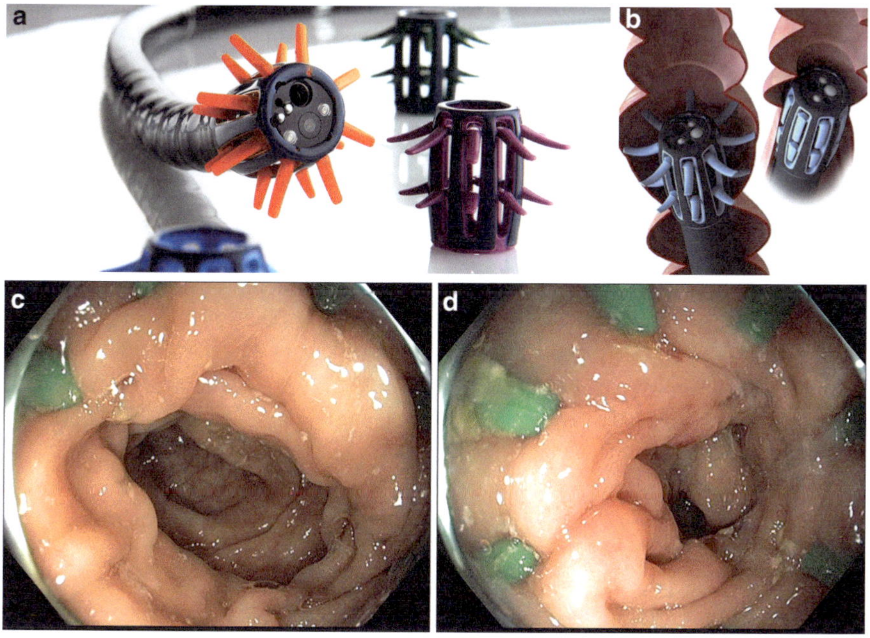

Fig. 2.4 Endocuff-assisted colonoscopy: Note, the device placed on the tip of the scope (**a**), the straightening of the colonic mucosal folds during scope withdrawal (**b**), and the endoscopic view with the device in place (**c**, **d**). With permission from Arc Medical Design Limited

complex polyp resections in the sigmoid colon [25]. Thereafter, a study in 50 patients assessed retrospectively the EC-assisted colonoscopy [26]. According to the results, the intubation rates of the cecum and terminal ileum were 98 % and 76 %, respectively. EC caused some minor superficial lesions in 30 % of the cases. In total, 80 polyps (36 adenomas, 9 advanced adenomas) were identified and the adenoma detection rate was 34 %, reaching 41 % in the screening group. Of note, 42 % of the adenomas were right-sided. The authors concluded that the EC is safe and may improve the adenoma detection rate and also facilitate polypectomy.

The first randomized controlled trial comparing EC-assisted versus standard colonoscopy (SC) was published in 2014 by Biecker and colleagues [27]. EC utilization did not influence the cecum or the ileum intubation rates. However, it did significantly increase the total procedure time. Polyp detection rates with EC-assisted and SC were 56 % and 42 %, respectively ($p=0.001$). EC superiority regarding polyp detection was significantly evident in the sigmoid colon and the cecum for polyps sized less than 1 cm. In the EC group, the number of adenomas per patient increased significantly by 86 % ($p=0.002$). No major complications were reported in both groups. As the investigators state, EC use is feasible and safe and leads to significantly higher polyp detection rates, especially for lesions located in the sigmoid colon. In that way, EC may improve the efficacy of colonoscopy and reduce the incidence of colorectal cancer.

Similarly, a recently published randomized prospective multicenter trial conducted at four academic units in Germany aimed to compare the adenoma detection rates (ADR) between EC-assisted and standard colonoscopy (SC) [28]. As indicated by the results, ADR significantly increased with EC (35.4 % versus 20.7 % $p<0.0001$). Additionally, EC identified significantly more sessile polyps. Overall procedure time and withdrawal time did not differ. Cecum and ileum intubation rates were similar. No major adverse events occurred in both groups. In multivariate analysis, age (odds ratio [OR] 1.03; 95 % [CI] 1.01–1.05), male sex (OR 1.74; 95 % CI 1.10–2.73), withdrawal time (OR 1.16; 95 % CI 1.05–1.30), procedure time (OR 1.07; 95 % CI 1.04–1.10), colon cleanliness (OR 0.60; 95 % CI 0.39–0.94), and use of EC (OR 2.09; 95 % CI 1.34–3.27) were independent predictors of adenoma detection rates. As concluded, EC increases the ADR by 14.7 % (95 % CI 6.9–22.5 %) and is safe, effective, and easy to handle. It is supposed that EC might reduce the incidence of colorectal interval cancers.

Cap-Assisted Colonoscopy

In cap-assisted colonoscopy (CAC), a transparent cap is attached to the distal tip of the colonoscope. Originally, caps were designed to assist endoscopic mucosal resections, but they can also depress colonic folds improving visualization behind them. Several studies support that CAC reduces cecal intubation time and improves cecal intubation rates for trainees [29–32]. Its beneficial effect may also account for cases in which standard colonoscopy (SC) was initially incomplete [33, 34].

Regarding CAC additive yield in terms of polyp/adenoma detection rates (PDR/ADR), available results are conflicting. In 2007, Kondo et al. found that PDR was significantly higher in the CAC group than in the no cap group (49.3 % versus 39.1 %, $p=0.04$) [30]. Similarly, in a randomized trial including 420 subjects, the proportion of subjects with at least one adenoma was higher with CAC compared to SC (69 % versus 56 %, $p=0.009$). CAC also detected a higher number of adenomas per subject (2.3 versus 1.4, $p<0.001$) [31]. Moreover, a post-hoc analysis revealed that CAC offers a higher detection rate of significant serrated polyps when compared to SC [35]. Moreover, patients undergoing initial CAC had a significantly lower miss rate for all adenomas compared with that of patients undergoing regular colonoscopy (21 % versus 33 %, $p=0.039$), according to a randomized tandem colonoscopy study published by Hewett and Rex [36].

On the other hand, several studies demonstrated that CAC does not increase PDR and ADR and thus has no efficacy [29, 33, 37, 38]. More detailed, a bi-centric randomized trial in 2012 demonstrated that CAC does not improve ADR, but does reduce cecal intubation time and the discomfort during the procedure [29]. The same outcomes were presented by Harada and colleagues, although more prominent in the expert endoscopists than in those with moderate experience [37]. In addition, Lee et al. reported that CAC should be reserved as a rescue method when cecal intubation fails, but it did not improve the initial cecal intubation rate and had a significantly lower ADR as compared to SC [33]. Finally, no significant differences in terms of cecal intubation time and PDR between CAC and SC were found in a 2010 single-center prospective randomized study [38].

Taking the above together, a meta-analysis by Ng and colleagues aimed to evaluate CAC with regard to cecum intubation time and PDR [39]. Accordingly, PDR with CAC was marginally higher than that of SC [relative risk (RR): 1.08; 95 % confidence interval (CI): 1.00–1.17]. In contrast, ADR showed no statistically significant difference. In subgroup analyses, a short cap (≤4 mm) was associated with improved PDR, whereas a long cap (≥7 mm) was associated with a shorter cecal intubation time. To sum up, CAC demonstrated incremental benefit over SC for polyp detection and shortened cecum intubation time. During the same year, a Cochrane meta-analysis suggested that cap utilization may give a marginally faster cecal intubation time compared with SC. It also proposed that there is an increased PDR and less pain with the cap. However, the authors feel that further randomized controlled trials in this area are needed to provide more clinically significant information regarding these issues [40].

A final remark regarding the new endoscopes and devices that were presented in this chapter has to do with their cost-effectiveness: One of the basic concerns whenever some new innovation is presented, should be if it can actually affect prognosis of patients [41]. As most of these new endoscopes and devices usually help us detect mostly small adenomas, their real-life clinical impact on patients' health should be always in focus. Thus, studies regarding change of patients' management, as well as the cost-effectiveness of such changes, should be especially welcome.

Conclusion

It is well-recognized that a considerable proportion of polyps and adenomas are missed during standard colonoscopy, especially when located in "hidden" aspects of the colonic surfaces. Recent tandem colonoscopy studies report miss rates reaching 25 % and even 40 % with standard and new endoscopic technologies, respectively. As a consequence, increasing cases of interval colorectal cancers appear, raising questions regarding the efficacy of colonoscopy as a protective means.

In this setting, several technological advances have been made in order to improve visualization of the colonic mucosa and therefore enhance colonoscopy's diagnostic yield. This goal is likely to be achieved by exciting emerging innovations, either directly concerning colonoscopes or related to accessories like those presented in this chapter. Although early results demonstrate the impressive potential of many of these endoscopic facilities, generalization of their use is still not recommended. Apart from their efficacy, concerns regarding costs and training demands should be taken into account. Undoubtedly, more well-designed studies assessing these issues are warranted, aiming to achieve evidence-based use of these technologies for early diagnosis and best management of colorectal neoplasia.

References

1. Rex DK, Johnson DA, Anderson JC, et al. American College of Gastroenterology guidelines for colorectal cancer screening 2009 [corrected]. Am J Gastroenterol. 2009;104:739–50.
2. Winawer SJ, Zauber AG, Ho MN, et al. Prevention of colorectal cancer by colonoscopic polypectomy. The National Polyp Study Workgroup. N Engl J Med. 1993;329:1977–81.
3. Gross CP, Andersen MS, Krumholz HM, et al. Relation between Medicare screening reimbursement and stage at diagnosis for older patients with colon cancer. JAMA. 2006;296:2815–22.
4. Rim SH, Seeff L, Ahmed F, et al. Colorectal cancer incidence in the United States, 1999–2004: an updated analysis of data from the National Program of Cancer Registries and the Surveillance, Epidemiology, and End Results Program. Cancer. 2009;115:1967–76.
5. van Rijn JC, Reitsma JB, Stoker J, et al. Polyp miss rate determined by tandem colonoscopy: a systematic review. Am J Gastroenterol. 2006;101:343–50.
6. Huang Y, Gong W, Su B, et al. Risk and cause of interval colorectal cancer after colonoscopic polypectomy. Digestion. 2012;86:148–54.
7. Laiyemo AO, Doubeni C, Sanderson II AK, et al. Likelihood of missed and recurrent adenomas in the proximal versus the distal colon. Gastrointest Endosc. 2011;74:253–61.
8. Leufkens AM, DeMarco DC, Rastogi A, et al. Effect of a retrograde-viewing device on adenoma detection rate during colonoscopy: the TERRACE study. Gastrointest Endosc. 2011;73:480–9.
9. Benson ME, Reichelderfer M, Said A, et al. Variation in colonoscopic technique and adenoma detection rates at an academic gastroenterology unit. Dig Dis Sci. 2010;55:166–71.
10. Long MD, Martin C, Sandler RS, et al. Reduced polyp detection as endoscopy shift progresses: experience with screening colonoscopy at a tertiary-care hospital. J Clin Gastroenterol. 2011;45:253–8.
11. Kilgore TW, Abdinoor AA, Szary NM, et al. Bowel preparation with split-dose polyethylene glycol before colonoscopy: a meta-analysis of randomized controlled trials. Gastrointest Endosc. 2011;73:1240–5.

12. Triadafilopoulos G, Watts HD, Higgins J, et al. A novel retrograde-viewing auxiliary imaging device (Third Eye Retroscope) improves the detection of simulated polyps in anatomic models of the colon. Gastrointest Endosc. 2007;65:139–44.
13. Triadafilopoulos G, Li J. A pilot study to assess the safety and efficacy of the Third Eye retrograde auxiliary imaging system during colonoscopy. Endoscopy. 2008;40:478–82.
14. DeMarco DC, Odstrcil E, Lara LF, et al. Impact of experience with a retrograde-viewing device on adenoma detection rates and withdrawal times during colonoscopy: the Third Eye Retroscope study group. Gastrointest Endosc. 2010;71:542–50.
15. Waye JD, Heigh RI, Fleischer DE, et al. A retrograde-viewing device improves detection of adenomas in the colon: a prospective efficacy evaluation (with videos). Gastrointest Endosc. 2010;71:551–6.
16. Siersema PD, Rastogi A, Leufkens AM, et al. Retrograde-viewing device improves adenoma detection rate in colonoscopies for surveillance and diagnostic workup. World J Gastroenterol. 2012;18:3400–8.
17. Gralnek IM, Carr-Locke DL, Segol O, et al. Comparison of standard forward-viewing mode versus ultrawide-viewing mode of a novel colonoscopy platform: a prospective, multicenter study in the detection of simulated polyps in an in vitro colon model (with video). Gastrointest Endosc. 2013;77:472–9.
18. Gralnek IM, Segol O, Suissa A, et al. A prospective cohort study evaluating a novel colonoscopy platform featuring full-spectrum endoscopy. Endoscopy. 2013;45:697–702.
19. Gralnek IM, Siersema PD, Halpern Z, et al. Standard forward-viewing colonoscopy versus full-spectrum endoscopy: an international, multicentre, randomised, tandem colonoscopy trial. Lancet Oncol. 2014;15:353–60.
20. Hassan C, Gralnek IM. Cost-effectiveness of "full spectrum endoscopy" colonoscopy for colorectal cancer screening. Dig Liver Dis. 2015;47(5):390–4.
21. Hasan N, Gross SA, Gralnek IM, et al. A novel balloon colonoscope detects significantly more simulated polyps than a standard colonoscope in a colon model. Gastrointest Endosc. 2014;80:1135–40.
22. Gralnek IM, Suissa A, Domanov S. Safety and efficacy of a novel balloon colonoscope: a prospective cohort study. Endoscopy. 2014;46:883–7.
23. Halpern Z, Gross SA, Gralnek IM, et al. Comparison of adenoma detection and miss rates between a novel balloon colonoscope and standard colonoscopy: a randomized tandem study. Endoscopy. 2015;47:238–44.
24. Uraoka T, Tanaka S, Matsumoto T, et al. A novel extra-wide-angle-view colonoscope: a simulated pilot study using anatomic colorectal models. Gastrointest Endosc. 2013;77:480–3.
25. Tsiamoulos ZP, Saunders BP. A new accessory, endoscopic cuff, improves colonoscopic access for complex polyp resection and scar assessment in the sigmoid colon (with video). Gastrointest Endosc. 2012;76:1242–5.
26. Lenze F, Beyna T, Lenz P, et al. Endocuff-assisted colonoscopy: a new accessory to improve adenoma detection rate? Technical aspects and first clinical experiences. Endoscopy. 2014;46:610–4.
27. Biecker E, Floer M, Heinecke A, et al. Novel endocuff-assisted colonoscopy significantly increases the polyp detection rate: a randomized controlled trial. J Clin Gastroenterol. 2015;49(5):413–8.
28. Floer M, Biecker E, Fitzlaff R, et al. Higher adenoma detection rates with endocuff-assisted colonoscopy—a randomized controlled multicenter trial. PLoS One. 2014;9, e114267.
29. de Wijkerslooth TR, Stoop EM, Bossuyt PM, et al. Adenoma detection with cap-assisted colonoscopy versus regular colonoscopy: a randomised controlled trial. Gut. 2012;61:1426–34.
30. Kondo S, Yamaji Y, Watabe H, et al. A randomized controlled trial evaluating the usefulness of a transparent hood attached to the tip of the colonoscope. Am J Gastroenterol. 2007;102:75–81.
31. Rastogi A, Bansal A, Rao DS, et al. Higher adenoma detection rates with cap-assisted colonoscopy: a randomised controlled trial. Gut. 2012;61:402–8.

32. Park SM, Lee SH, Shin KY, et al. The cap-assisted technique enhances colonoscopy training: prospective randomized study of six trainees. Surg Endosc. 2012;26:2939–43.
33. Lee YT, Lai LH, Hui AJ, et al. Efficacy of cap-assisted colonoscopy in comparison with regular colonoscopy: a randomized controlled trial. Am J Gastroenterol. 2009;104:41–6.
34. Lee YT, Hui AJ, Wong VW, et al. Improved colonoscopy success rate with a distally attached mucosectomy cap. Endoscopy. 2006;38:739–42.
35. Rzouq F, Gupta N, Wani S, et al. Cap assisted colonoscopy for the detection of serrated polyps: a post-hoc analysis. BMC Gastroenterol. 2015;15:11.
36. Hewett DG, Rex DK. Cap-fitted colonoscopy: a randomized, tandem colonoscopy study of adenoma miss rates. Gastrointest Endosc. 2010;72:775–81.
37. Harada Y, Hirasawa D, Fujita N, et al. Impact of a transparent hood on the performance of total colonoscopy: a randomized controlled trial. Gastrointest Endosc. 2009;69:637–44.
38. Tee HP, Corte C, Al-Ghamdi H, et al. Prospective randomized controlled trial evaluating cap-assisted colonoscopy vs standard colonoscopy. World J Gastroenterol. 2010;16:3905–10.
39. Ng SC, Tsoi KK, Hirai HW, et al. The efficacy of cap-assisted colonoscopy in polyp detection and cecal intubation: a meta-analysis of randomized controlled trials. Am J Gastroenterol. 2012;107:1165–73.
40. Morgan J, Thomas K, Lee-Robichaud H, et al. Transparent cap colonoscopy versus standard colonoscopy to improve caecal intubation. Cochrane Database Syst Rev. 2012;12:CD008211.
41. Ransohoff DF. What is the effect of more sensitive diagnostic technology? Lancet Oncol. 2014;15:256–7.

Chapter 3
Chromoendoscopy

Ammar O. Kheir, Roy Soetikno, and Tonya Kaltenbach

Introduction

Gastrointestinal cancers represent the leading cause of cancer-related death worldwide. The detection, diagnosis, and treatment of precursor and early gastrointestinal cancers are critical for improvements in morbidity and mortality. Often subtle in appearance, these pre- and early cancers can pose a challenge to endoscopic visualization with white light. Advancements in endoscopic techniques and technologies have aided endoscopists to better differentiate normal from dysplastic lesions [1]. Image enhancement using chromoendoscopy, for example, through the application of dye solutions, has been shown to facilitate mucosal visualization to improve endoscopic localization, characterization, and therapy. In this review, we will focus on the techniques and tools of chromoendoscopy available in the United States

---

Electronic supplementary material: The online version of this chapter (doi:10.1007/978-3-319-30053-5_3) contains supplementary material, which is available to authorized users. Videos can also be accessed at http://link.springer.com/chapter/10.1007/978-3-319-30053-5_3.

A.O. Kheir, M.B.B.S., M.R.C.P., F.R.A.C.P.
Department of Gastroenterology, Queen Elizabeth II Jubilee Hospital,
Brisbane, QLD, Australia

School of Medicine and Public Health, University of Newcastle, Newcastle, NSW, Australia

R. Soetikno, M.D., M.S.
Department of Gastroenterology and Hepatology, Singapore General Hospital,
Singapore, Singapore

National Cancer Center Singapore, Singapore, Singapore

Duke–National University Singapore Graduate Medical School, Singapore, Singapore

T. Kaltenbach, M.D., M.S. (✉)
Veteran Affairs Palo Alto Health Care System and Stanford University School of Medicine,
3801 Miranda Avenue, GI-111, Palo Alto, CA 94305, USA
e-mail: endoresection@me.com

V.J.A. Konda, I. Waxman (eds.), *Endoscopic Imaging Techniques and Tools*,
DOI 10.1007/978-3-319-30053-5_3

including Lugol's solution for squamous cell carcinoma of the esophagus, and indigo carmine and methylene blue for high-risk surveillance populations such as Barrett's esophagus, inflammatory bowel disease, and hereditary nonpolyposis colorectal cancer syndrome.

Technology Overview

High-definition (1080 system) endoscopy provides image signals of higher pixel density and sharpness than standard-definition (480 system) [2]. High-definition imaging, however, does not provide contrast to enhance subtle, often flat or depressed, neoplasia and early cancer. Image-enhanced endoscopy using dye spray onto the intestinal epithelial surface, also termed chromoendoscopy, does provide contrast of normal and abnormal mucosa. It improves visualization of epithelial surface detail and accentuates the changes in the surface topography of the gastro-intestinal tract to facilitate the recognition of subtle lesions, borders delineation, pathology interrogation, and real-time treatment. The endoscopic recognition of dysplastic lesions may have important implications for their surveillance and management. Expanding the practice of targeted detection and diagnosis of early lesions can provide patients curative minimally invasive endoscopic options such as endoscopic mucosal resection, endoscopic submucosal dissection, or radiofrequency ablation and ultimately reduce the morbidity and mortality associated with advanced cancer and surgery.

Classification of Stains

Chromoendoscopy dyes, though all transient, have different staining properties and are classified into (Table 3.1) [3, 4]:

- Absorptive stains (vital stains)
- Nonabsorptive stains (contrast stains)
- Reactive stains

Vital stains are absorbed into cells, in turn, highlighting mucosal surface details and pattern. Commonly used vital stains in chromoendoscopy are Lugol's iodine, methylene blue, and acetic acid. Cells do not absorb contrast stains such as indigo carmine. Indigo carmine, thus, enhances mucosal surface topography by accumulating in mucosal grooves and crevices. Reactive stains such as Congo red and phenol red stains react chemically to specific cellular components resulting in color change. They are not commonly used in endoscopy.

Table 3.1 Chromoendoscopy dyes

Stain class	Staining mechanism	Clinical indication
Vital (absorptive)		
Lugol's iodine	Uptake by intracellular glycogen containing in normal squamous epithelium	Esophageal squamous cell carcinoma and anal intraepithelial neoplasia
Methylene blue	Uptake by epithelial cells of small bowel, colon, and intestinal metaplasia	Barrett's esophagus dysplasia, gastric intestinal metaplasia and dysplasia, colorectal dysplasia
Contrast (nonabsorptive)		
Indigo carmine	Does not stain cells but rather accumulates in mucosal grooves and crevices	Colon, gastric, duodenal, and esophageal lesions. Also used in Barrett's esophagus

Key Clinical Indications

Chromoendoscopy augments the endoscopic detection, diagnosis, and therapy of gastrointestinal neoplasia and early cancer. We will focus on three key clinical indications:

1. Lugol's solution for esophageal squamous cell dysplasia or early cancer
2. Indigo carmine or methylene blue for Barrett's dysplasia
3. Indigo carmine or methylene blue for colorectal neoplasia

Esophageal Squamous Cell Carcinoma

The use of Lugol's solution has been shown to improve the endoscopic detection and delineation of high-grade dysplasia and squamous cell cancer of the anus and esophagus (Figs. 3.1 and 3.2) [5–8]. Lugol's solution increased the diagnostic yield for esophageal squamous cell high-grade dysplasia and cancer by 20 % in a study of 1095 high-risk patients, such as those with head and neck cancer, heavy tobacco use, history of lye ingestions, and heavy alcohol use [9]. Lugol's high sensitivity (up to 26 % of a cohort of 629 patients had unstained lesions) however is limited by its low specificity (only 3 % of the patients were diagnosed with cancer) [10]. The pink color sign, a dramatic color change after iodine staining whereby an initial whitish yellow color then transitions to pink 2–3 min later, has been associated with cancerous lesions and improves the specificity of Lugol's for early esophageal squamous cell carcinoma [11]. Narrow band imaging (NBI) has been studied as an alternative to Lugol's solution. NBI highlights the distorted intrapapillary capillary loops of early squamous cell lesions. In a multicenter, prospective, randomized controlled trial of 320 patients, NBI showed higher sensitivity and specificity for superficial cancers than white-light imaging of the hypopharynx and esophagus [12].

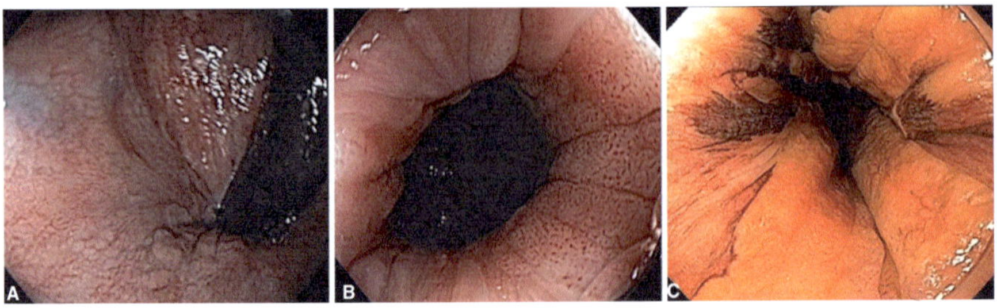

Fig. 3.1 Anal intraepithelial neoplasia. (**a**) Retroflexion view in the rectum shows slightly raised irregular mucosa at the dentate line, in the 6 o'clock position. (**b**) The lesion (from the 12 o'clock to 6 o'clock position) shows abnormal microvessels with dilatation, tortuosity, caliber change, and varied shapes—that are similar appearance to the intrapapillary capillary loop patterns seen in squamous cell carcinoma in situ of the esophagus. (**c**) With spraying of Lugol's solution, the normal squamous epithelium stains brown but the abnormal dysplastic tissue does not

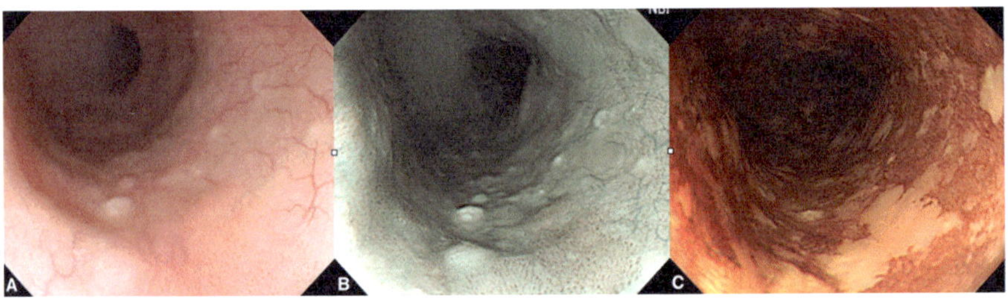

Fig. 3.2 Squamous cell high-grade dysplasia of the esophagus. (**a**) Multiple erythematous areas with irregular intracapillary papillary loops can be faintly seen using white light endoscopy. (**b**) Under narrow band imaging, the color contrast and intracapillary papillary loops of the lesion is more easily seen. (**c**) With spraying of Lugol's solution, the normal squamous epithelium stains brown but the abnormal dysplastic tissue does not stain and shows a pink color. This contrast allows the dysplastic areas to be demarcated and can be more easily demarcated

Barrett's Esophagus

Chromoendoscopy has been shown to improve dysplasia localization in Barrett's esophagus patients (Fig. 3.3) [13–15]. The nonpolypoid lesion is the most common shape of Barrett's early neoplasms. Pech et al. prospectively studied 380 Barrett's neoplastic lesions detected by high-resolution video endoscopy with four-quadrant biopsies and/or chromoendoscopy using methylene blue or acetic acid [16]. They showed 85 % appeared as flat, slightly elevated lesions. Furthermore, of the high-grade intraepithelial lesions, 70 % appeared completely flat. Random four quadrant biopsies every 2 cm is inadequate to detect Barrett's with early neoplasms. It is associated with significant sampling error and miss rates [17]. Chromoendoscopy is necessary to improve surveillance performance. Qumseya et al. reviewed and analyzed 14 studies (843 patients) comparing dye-based (indigo carmine and

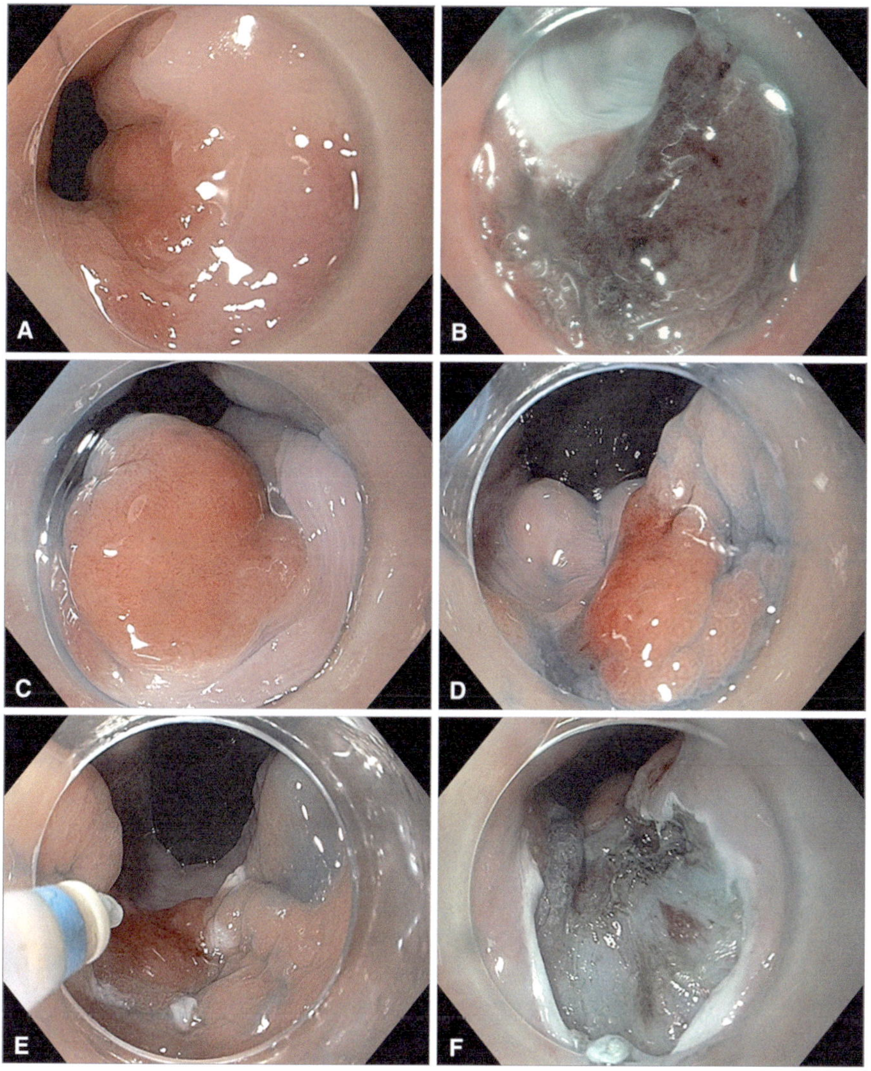

Fig. 3.3 Gastroesophageal junction early adenocarcinoma. (**a**) The distal attachment cap can be very useful to view the normally closed hiatus and to view the mucosa when there is a lot of contraction. A slightly raised erythematous area of gastroesophageal mucosa is seen in the 3–6 o'clock position. (**b**) The neoplasia appears to be brown on narrow band imaging. (**c**) Indigo carmine chromoendoscopy can also be useful to determine the lesion border. (**d**) After 1–2 min of spraying indigo carmine onto the surface the tumor appears to be less blue than the surrounding mucosa. (**e**) The periphery of the flat lesion is first marked in the retroflexion position prior to resection. (**f**) The mucosal defect is seen following enbloc endoscopic resection using endoscopic submucosal dissection technique. Pathology showed intramucosal adenocarcinoma

methylene blue) and equipment-based image-enhanced endoscopy with standard white-light endoscopy with random biopsies [18]. They showed that chromoendoscopy increases the diagnostic yield of dysplasia or cancer by 35 %, with similar benefit seen in dye-based and equipment-based methods.

Gastric Neoplasia

Dye-based image-enhanced endoscopy can be used in the diagnosis and treatment of early gastric cancer. Diluted indigo carmine or methylene blue can facilitate the evaluation of suspicious areas for early gastric cancer by highlighting the border and surface topography of lesions (Fig. 3.4).

Colorectal Neoplasia

Image-enhanced endoscopy (IEE) optimizes the colonoscopic detection, diagnosis, and removal of pre- or early colorectal cancers, and ultimately, improves advanced colorectal cancer prevention [19].

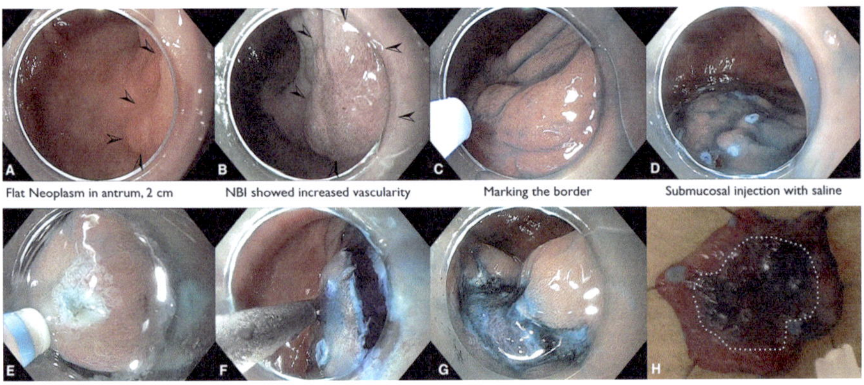

Fig. 3.4 Gastric high-grade dysplastic lesion. (**a**) A 2 cm flat lesion on the posterior wall of the antrum. (**b**) The lesion appears relatively brown using narrow band imaging. (**c**) Following indigo carmine surface spray, the periphery of the flat lesion is marked. (**d**) Using dynamic submucosal injection technique, the lesion is lifted with mixture of diluted indigo carmine and saline. (**e**) Circumferential incision is performed using an endoscopic submucosal dissection knife. (**f**) The lesion is then further lifted with large volume of injectant into the submucosa. (**g**) The circumferential incision has allowed the lesion to now be amenable to enbloc snare resection. (**h**) The resected enbloc specimen is oriented for pathologic evaluation. The lesion is outlined (white dots) with surrounding normal borders

High-Risk Screening

Inflammatory Bowel Disease

Chromoendoscopy with targeted biopsies has been shown to be more sensitive than white-light endoscopy with random biopsies in detecting dysplasia and neoplasia in patients with IBD [20] (Fig. 3.5). Data from randomized and prospective trials demonstrate increased efficacy in the detection of lesions with chromoendoscopy compared to white light; however, most studies have assessed its use with standard-definition (SD). In a meta-analysis of eight trials, chromoendoscopy with targeted biopsies was significantly superior to standard-definition white-light colonoscopy in the detection of patients with dysplasia (incremental yield = 6 % [95 % CI 2.8–9.2]; relative risk = 1.8 [95 % CI 1.2–2.6]) [21]. Additionally, chromoendoscopy detected significantly more patients with endoscopically visible dysplasia compared with SD white-light colonoscopy (incremental yield = 7 % [95% CI 3.0–10.0]; relative risk = 2.3 [95 % CI 1.4–3.7]). One prospective study using high-definition colonoscopy in 75 patients with IBD found a significantly higher rate of dysplasia identification with chromoendoscopy (21 %) vs white-light alone (9 %; P = 0.007) [22]. Recently, a prospective randomized controlled trial also showed significantly higher detection of dysplastic lesions with high definition plus chromoendoscopy compared to high-definition white-light colonoscopy alone: 0.26 vs. 0.12 lesions per patient [23].

Multiple gastrointestinal societies have recommended the use of chromoendoscopy in inflammatory bowel diseases surveillance [24–26]. The SCENIC International Consensus Statement on Surveillance and Management of

Additional resources on chromoendoscopy and targeted biopsy techniques

SCENIC Consensus	Laine L, Kaltenbach T, Barkun A, et al. SCENIC international consensus statement on surveillance and management of dysplasia in inflammatory bowel disease. *Gastrointest Endosc* 2015;81:489-501 e26. http://www.asge.org/uploadedFiles/Publications_(public)/Practice_guidelines/SCENIC_consensus_statement.pdf
Atlas	Soetikno R, Sanduleanu S, Kaltenbach T. An atlas of the nonpolypoid colorectal neoplasms in inflammatory bowel disease. *Gastrointest Endosc Clin N Am* 2014;24:483-520. http://www.sciencedirect.com/science/article/pii/S1052515714000415
Clinical Decision Support Tool	**Soetikno** R, Subramanian V, Kaltenbach T, Rouse RV, Sanduleanu S, Suzuki N, Tanaka S, **McQuaid** K. The detection of nonpolypoid (flat and depressed) colorectal neoplasms in patients with inflammatory bowel disease. Gastroenterology. 2013 Jun;144(7):1349-52.
Video	Kaltenbach T, McQuaid K, Sanchez-Yague A, McGill S and Soetikno R.Chromoendoscopy with targeted biopsy to detect nonpolypoid colorectal neoplasms in IBD. www.youtube.com/watch?v=OARkbgwlObI

Fig. 3.5 Resources on chromoendoscopy and targeted biopsy technique for colorectal dysplasia surveillance in patients with inflammatory bowel disease

Dysplasia in Inflammatory Bowel Disease (SCENIC) highlighted the importance of chromoendoscopy to detect, diagnose, and treat colorectal lesions [21]. SCENIC followed the prescribed processes for guideline development from the Institute of Medicine, including systematic reviews, full synthesis of evidence and deliberations by panelists, and incorporation of the GRADE methodology. The key summary recommendations from SCENIC for surveillance colonoscopy included (1) the use of high definition and the routine performance of chromoendoscopy for the detection of dysplasia, (2) the endoscopic removal of visible dysplasia, and (3) referral to an endoscopist with expertise in IBD surveillance using chromoendoscopy with high-definition colonoscopy for patients with endoscopically invisible dysplasia (confirmed by a GI pathologist).

Hereditary Nonpolyposis Colorectal Cancer

The application of chromoendoscopy significantly improves adenoma detection in patients with hereditary nonpolyposis colorectal cancer (HNPCC) syndrome [27, 28]. Studies showed the efficacy of indigo carmine for improved adenoma detection in the proximal colon in patients with HNPCC, and reported significantly higher diagnoses of flat lesions, increasing from 6 % before to 24 % after chromoendoscopy [27].

Additional Applications of Chromoendoscopy in the Colon

Average-Risk Screening

Pancolonic chromoendoscopy markedly enhances adenoma detection rates in an average-risk population [29]. In a prospective, randomized two-center trial, chromoendoscopy (with 0.4 % indigo carmine spraying during continuous extubation) was compared with standard colonoscopy in consecutive patients undergoing routine colonoscopy [30]. In over 1000 randomized patients, the proportion of patients with at least one adenoma was significantly higher in the chromoendoscopy group (46.2 %) than in the control group (36.3 %; $p<0.002$). Chromoendoscopy increased the overall detection rate for adenomas (0.95 vs. 0.66 per patient), flat adenomas (0.56 vs. 0.28 per patient), and serrated lesions (1.19 vs. 0.49 per patient) ($p<0.001$). This finding was confirmed by a Cochrane meta-analysis of five randomized controlled studies that found that chromoendoscopy detected significantly more patients with at least one neoplastic lesion (odds ratio [OR] 1.67) and significantly more patients with three or more neoplastic lesions (OR 2.55) [31].

Colorectal Neoplasia Differentiation and Complete Resection (Figs. 3.6, 3.7, 3.8, and 3.9)

Chromoendoscopy has been shown to facilitate accurate real-time histopathologic diagnosis of colon lesions [32–34]. Kudo described the characteristic pit-pattern morphology of normal, nonneoplastic, and neoplastic colon mucosa in detail, using indigo carmine coupled with high magnification colonoscopy in order to accurately diagnose colorectal lesions, and define its borders (Table 3.2) [35]. IEE with indigo carmine or methylene blue is commonly used to assess the lesion morphology and border to precisely direct endoscopic therapy [36–38]. Immediately following mucosectomy, it is suggested to analyze the pattern of the tissue at the resection margins with chromoendoscopy to assure completeness of resection. If residual neoplasm is

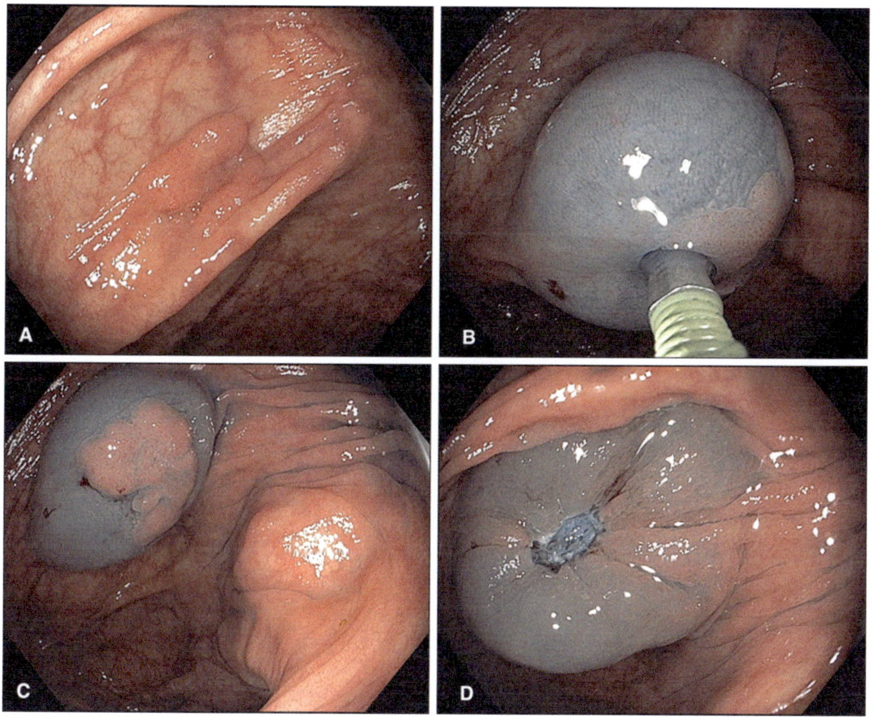

Fig. 3.6 Dynamic submucosal injection technique for a nonpolypoid colorectal neoplasm. (**a**) We first plan the flight path based on the lesion shape and location. In this case, we plan to inject by directing the injection up and to the right. (**b**) We engage the catheter probe of the injection needle at the intended lesion site and expose the needle by instructing our assistant needle out. While instructing the assist to inject the mixture of diluted indigo carmine and saline in a rapid and steady fashion, while we simultaneously make subtle maneuvers to produce a localized submucosal bleb (e.g., we adjust the catheter position further in or out of the accessory channel according to the plane, we suction the lumen in order for the submucosal injectant to form a large bleb, and we angulate the tip of the endoscope up. (**c**) A local submucosal bleb is created after about 20 mL of submucosal injection. (**d**) A stiff snare was used to capture and resect the lesion enbloc

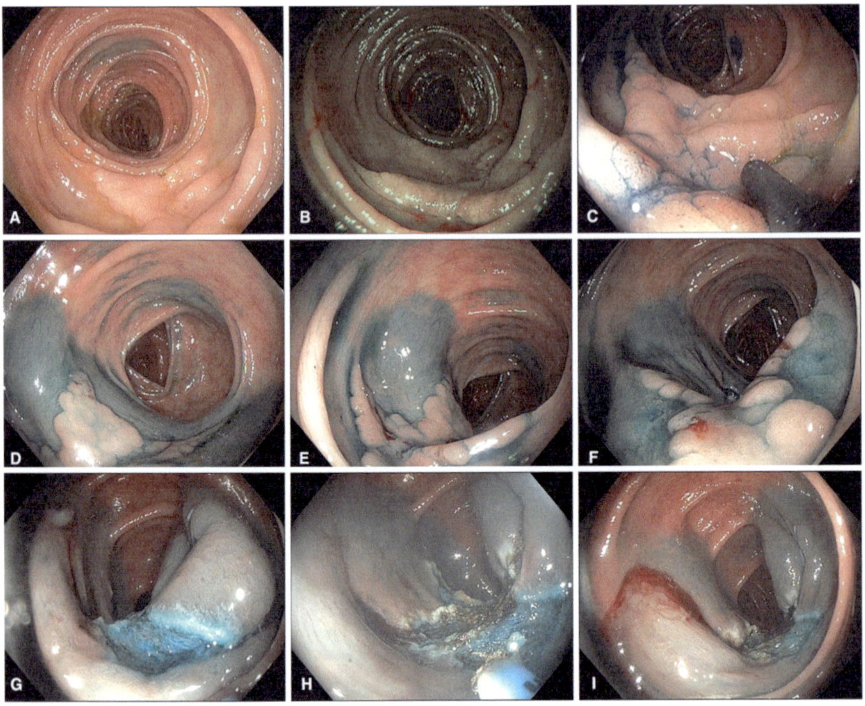

Fig. 3.7 Complete removal of large flat lateral spreading tumor in transverse colon. (**a**) A flat lateral spreading nongranular lesion is seen in white light. Its appearance is subtle making it difficult to distinguish from the surrounding folds. (**b**) The lesion appears dark in narrow band imaging view. (**c**) Chromoendoscopy with indigo carmine enhances the lesion surface pattern and borders. (**d**)–(**f**) The lesion was injected with saline tinged with indigo carmine. Dynamic submucosal injection was performed and the lesion extends over several folds. (**g**) The lesion was resected piecemeal using a stiff snare until no further neoplastic tissue can be seen. (**h**) and (**i**) Argon plasma coagulation is then applied to ablate superficial vessels and microscopic residual neoplastic tissue

present, further resection or ablative techniques can be directly applied. Using the application of diluted indigo carmine or methylene blue onto the surface of the lesion as well as a mixture in the submucosal injectant enables higher complete resection and lower local recurrence rates [39].

Techniques

Stains and applicators, such as syringes, foot pumps, or spraying catheters, are needed in addition to standard endoscopic equipment [1, 3]. Spraying catheters provide controlled and accurate spraying of the targeted mucosa. For surface chromoendoscopy, application of dye using a syringe through the working channel. For pancolonic chromoendoscopy using indigo carmine or methylene, many experts use the scope's foot pedal pump to directly apply the dye (Fig. 3.10, Video 3.1).

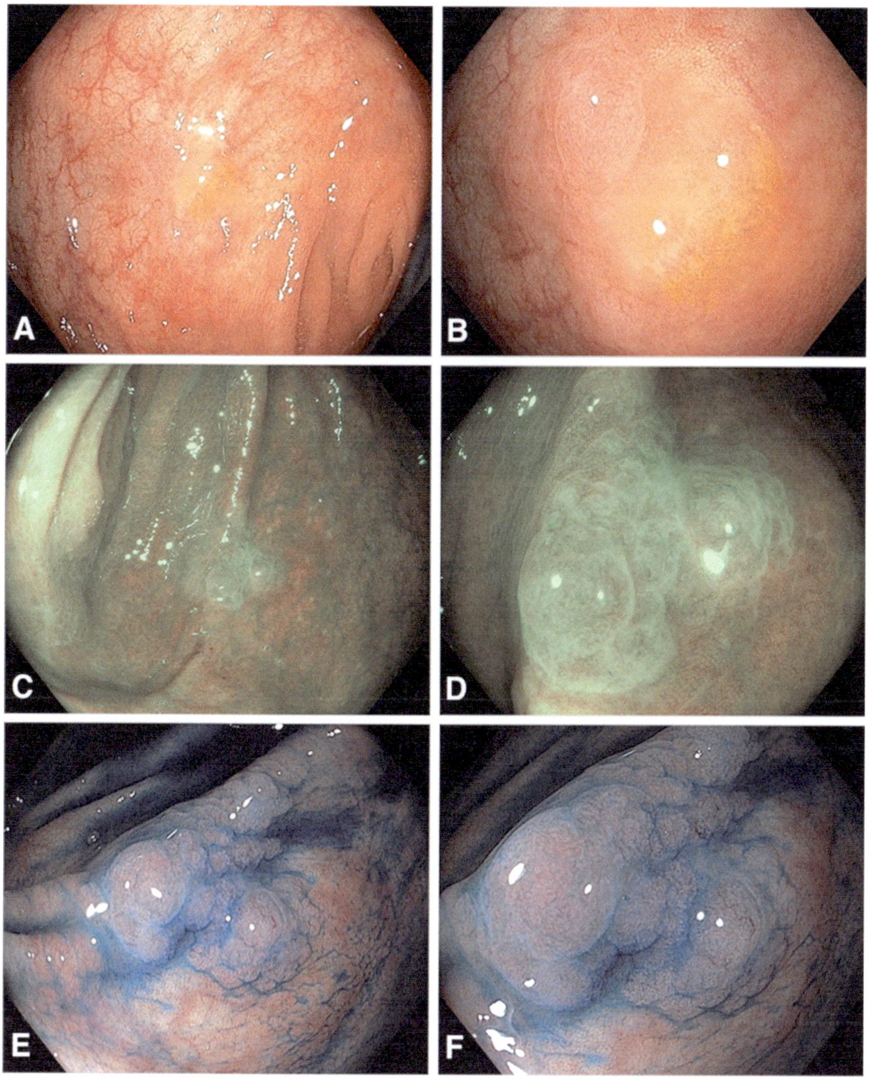

Fig. 3.8 Sessile serrated polyp/adenoma with local recurrence. The patient had standard polypectomy of cecal serrated lesion 1-year prior at an outside facility and was referred for reevaluation as the lesion could not be appreciated in its entirety on the initial surveillance. (**a**) The scar site can be seen with features of sessile serrated polyp/adenoma, including mucus cap, cloud-like surface, and indistinct borders. (**b**) The features of the lesion are seen in more detailed in a closer view. (**c**) Narrow band imaging in a long view shows a relatively pale lesion compared to the surrounding mucosa. (**d**) Closer view shows lacy vessels and open pits, and highlight the indistinct borders. (**e**) and (**f**) Methylene blue chromoendoscopy enhance the lesion borders to facilitate complete resection

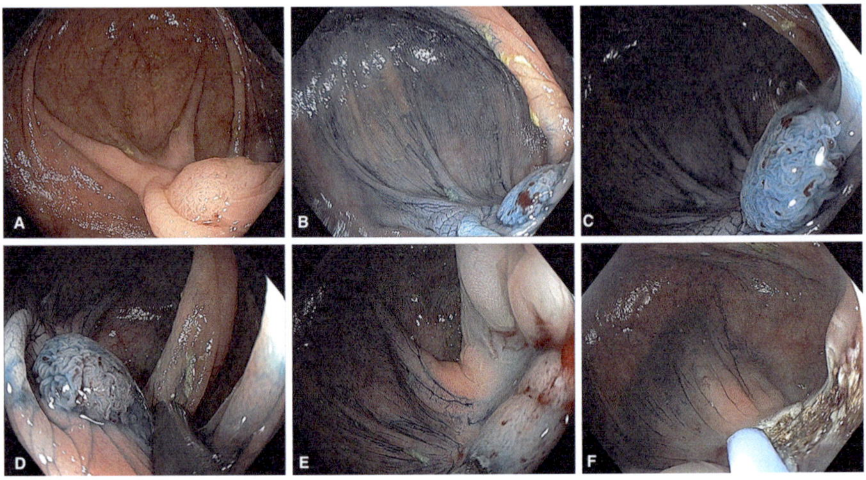

Fig. 3.9 Assessment and treatment of local recurrence using methylene blue following index piecemeal polypectomy and ablation. Repeat endoscopic resection of an incomplete prior resection is very difficult. Immediately following mucosectomy, it is suggested to analyze the pattern of the tissue at the resection margins with chromoendoscopy to assure completeness of resection. In this case, the patient was referred following polypectomy 6 months prior. The scar is shown under (**a**) white light and (**b**) after methylene blue spray, and (**c**) under magnified view, the gyrus pattern (Kudo Type V) of the villous lesion is seen. (**d**) and (**e**) The lesion lifts partially and could not be fully captured enbloc with a snare. (**f**) Following snaring, argon plasma coagulation was performed to ablate residual neoplastic tissue

Table 3.2 The characteristic pit-pattern morphology of normal, nonneoplastic, and neoplastic colon mucosa described by Kudo

Kudo type	Features	Likely diagnosis
Type I	Round	Normal
Type II	Stellar/papillary	Hyperplastic
Type III_S	Small tubular/small round	Adenoma
Type III_L	Large tubular/large round	Adenoma
Type IV	Gyrus-like	Villous adenoma
Type V	Amorphous/nonstructural	Submucosal cancer

General Techniques

Excess water and debris should be suctioned prior to dye application. The stain is applied onto target mucosa via syringe, spray catheter, or pump. Spraying catheters are inserted through the biopsy (working) channel, and the catheter tip is aimed at the target mucosa or lesion.

Lugol's iodine solution is an absorptive dye composed of water iodine and potassium iodide. Methylene blue is an absorptive dye that stains normal intestinal epithelium. It is not taken up by inflamed or neoplastic cells. Indigo carmine is water soluble, inexpensive, and easy to prepare. It is nonabsorbable and improves visualization and surface topography by filling surface grooves and crevices.

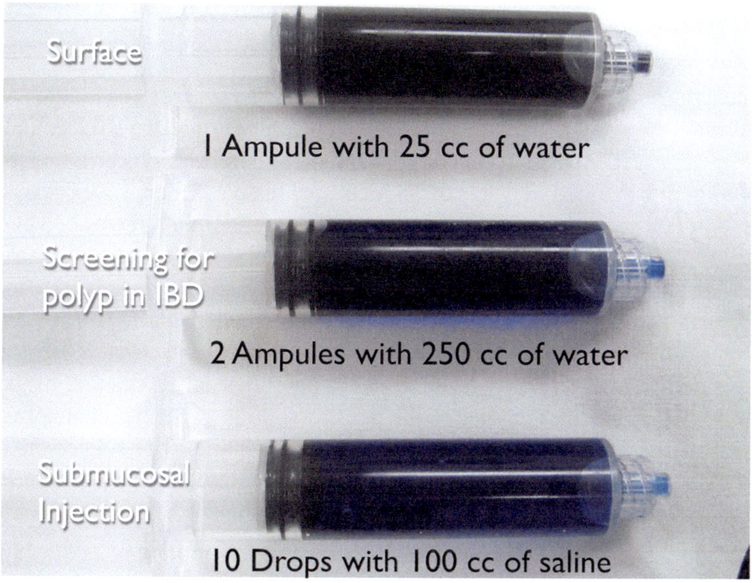

Fig. 3.10 Dilutions of methylene blue and indigo carmine for chromoendoscopy applications

Disease-Specific Techniques

Esophageal Squamous Cell Dysplasia and Anal Intraepithelial Neoplasia

Dye-based chromoendoscopy using Lugol's iodine solution is most commonly used in staining esophageal and anal squamous mucosa. The diluted solution (0.5–3.0 %) is sprayed on the mucosa via a spray catheter or syringe and is absorbed by glycogen-containing cells to produce a dark greenish-brown stain. Normal mucosa will stain intensively for about 5–8 min, whereas dysplastic and neoplastic areas will not stain. The initial whitish yellow color then transitions to pink 2–3 min later. The pink color sign has high specificity for early esophageal squamous cell carcinoma [11].

Barrett's Esophagus

Optimal methylene blue or indigo carmine staining for evaluation of Barrett's dysplasia may require the removal of surface mucus with a mucolytic agent, such as 10 % acetylcysteine solution, before its application [1]. The technique involves the use of approximately 10 mL of acetylcysteine and 20 mL of methylene blue or indigo carmine dye for every 5 cm of circumferential columnar lined epithelium.

Colon Neoplasia

Chromoendoscopy, using a dye solution of either methylene blue or indigo carmine applied onto the colonic mucosa to enhance contrast during surveillance colonoscopy, is performed either in a pancolonic fashion to detect lesions or targeted fashion to allow for detailed viewing of an identified lesion (Video 3.2). Clean bowel preparation is a prerequisite. Small amounts of debris or fluid are washed and suctioned during insertion. Once the cecum is reached and the mucosa is cleaned, the application of either diluted indigo carmine or methylene blue dyes is initiated. We spray a total of approximately 250 mL of diluted dye (indigo carmine 0.03–0.1 % or methylene blue 0.04–0.1 %) circumferentially throughout the colon either through the water jet channel by using a pump or through the biopsy channel by using a spray catheter. Efficient spraying of the dye through the water jet channel is typically performed by directing the stream of dye to the antigravity side of the colon. When a spray catheter is used, the spray catheter is inserted through the biopsy channel until its tip protrudes 2–3 cm, and dye is sprayed throughout the mucosa while the colonoscope is being withdrawn. During inspection, by using the pan-chromoendoscopy technique, the endoscopist looks for areas that appear to be different from the surrounding background in color, pattern, or level. Nonpolypoid lesions may appear discolored (uneven redness), nodular or villous, slightly elevated or depressed, friable, or have an obscure vascular pattern. Polypoid lesions are easier to detect, but the dye can help delineate the lesion's border. Once a suspicious lesion is identified, we selectively spray approximately 30 mL of a more concentrated dye (indigo carmine 0.13 % or methylene blue 0.2 %) directly from a 60-mL syringe through the biopsy channel. With targeted chromoendoscopy, the darker blue dye can be helpful to further enhance the border and surface topography of a lesion. In inflammatory bowel disease surveillance, colonoscopy should be performed when the disease is in remission in order to minimize potential misdiagnosis between inflammatory changes and dysplasia (Table 3.3).

Safety and Cost Considerations

The dyes and equipment used for chromoendoscopy are generally safe and affordable [1, 3].

Chromoendoscopy agents are biologically inert and transient. This is in contrast to the dyes used for tattooing, which contain carbon particles that remain in the submucosal injection site permanently and cause fibrosis. Different side effects can be expected based on the type of stain used. Lugol's iodine solution can cause retrosternal discomfort, pain, and nausea due to mucosal irritation [40]. Chemical esophagitis and gastritis have been described after spraying Lugol's iodine. However, spraying 20 mL of 5 % sodium thiosulfate solution, which is a water soluble compound, has been shown to be helpful in reversing staining and reducing

Table 3.3 Techniques of chromendoscopy

Technique	Method	Dilution	Color
Pan- and targeted chromoendoscopy for esophageal squamous cell dysplasia or anal intraepithelial neoplasia	Spray onto esophageal or anal surface using a spraying catheter or syringe	Prepare 20 mL of 2 % Lugol's iodine by mixing 8 mL of 5 % solution with 12 mL of water	The initial whitish yellow unstained color then transitions to pink 2–3 min later
			Normal squamous mucosa stain dark-brown green for up to 8 min; and repeated spraying might be required
			Dysplastic and neoplastic tissue remains unstained
Panchromoendoscopy for lesion detection	Apply segmentally with water jet channel using auxillary foot pump or biopsy channel using spray catheter	Methylene blue (1 %,10 mL ampule): Prepare 1 ampule + 240 mL water (0.04 %)	Methylene blue uptake occurs within 2–3 min and is subsequently resistant to washing
		Prepare 0.03 % indigo carmine by mixing 10 mL 0.8 % indigo carmine (2 ampules) in 250 mL of water	Indigo carmine is nonabsorbable and water soluble, and immediate provides contrast color by filling surface grooves and crevices
Targeted chromoendoscopy for lesion interrogation	Spray onto mucosal surface using a syringe or spraying catheter	Methylene blue (1 %,10 mL ampule): Prepare 1 ampule + 40 mL water (0.2 %)	
		Prepare 0.13 % indigo carmine by mixing 5 mL of 0.8 % indigo carmine (1 ampule) with 25 mL of water	

retrosternal discomfort [40]. Lugol's iodine should also be avoided in patients with thyroid disease to prevent hyperthyroidism. Methylene blue can cause transient urinary and fecal blue discoloration when used in large quantities but this has no clinical significance. Methylene blue application has been shown in a small study to be associated with oxidative DNA damage in Barrett's esophagus when exposed to white light photosensitization during endoscopy [41, 42]. The clinical importance of this finding is not known. Furthermore, injectable methylene blue in patients with glucose-6-phosphate dehydrogenase (G6PD) deficiency can precipitate hemolysis and even paradoxical methemoglobinemia [43–45]. No such complications have been reported with chromoendoscopy using diluted methylene blue. Nonetheless, its use is cautioned in patients with G6PD deficiency or in untested patients with family history of G6PD deficiency or methemoglobinemia. Indigo carmine is quite safe and adverse events have not been described. Green urinary discoloration can transiently occur if large quantities of indigo carmine are used.

Recently, indigo carmine supply has been limited in the United States due to manufacturing issues. Endoscopists have been therefore required to use methylene blue, but costs of this dye are now relatively higher. Given the lack of physician or facility reimbursement for chromoendoscopy, the expense may become prohibitive for many centers.

Conclusion and Future Directions

Improvements in the endoscopic recognition of dysplastic gastrointestinal lesions using image-enhanced endoscopy, such as chromoendsocopy, could have important implications for the detection, diagnosis, and management of dysplasia. Uniformity of guidelines and teaching will foster practice towards targeted sampling and resection of visible lesions and away from the random biopsy technique for diagnosis and from colectomy for management. Linking reimbursement to quality of performance will also likely encourage its wider adoption.

Helpful Hints

Esophageal and Anal Squamous Cell Carcinoma (Lugol's Solution)

- Dysplastic and neoplastic areas remains unstained
  - Look for the "pink color" sign which is specific for high-grade dysplasia and carcinoma

Barrett's Chromoendoscopy (Methylene Blue)

- Use a mucolytic prewash
  - Spray methylene blue, wait for 2 min, then wash excess dye with water
  - Intestinal metaplasia stains blue
  - Dysplastic cells do not uptake blue stain

Colonic Chromoendoscopy

- Use high-definition scope and ensure excellent bowel preparation
  - Use two concentrations of dye

    Dilute for detection
    More concentrated for differentiation
  - Irrigate well and clean mucus and debris on insertion
  - Suction residual water prior to dye application
  - Apply the dilute dye segmentally on withdrawal, starting from the cecum
  - Start dye spraying on non dependent colonic wall to facilitate dye pooling
  - Apply the more concentrated dye onto detected abnormalities for differentiation and border delineation

What to Look for During IBD Chromoendoscopy?

- Hypervascularity or obscure vascular pattern
  - Mucosal friability
  - Irregular nodularity
  - Uneven mucosal surface
  - Mucosal discoloration

References

1. Kaltenbach T, Sano Y, Friedland S, Soetikno R, American Gastroenterological Association. American Gastroenterological Association (AGA) Institute technology assessment on image-enhanced endoscopy. Gastroenterology. 2008;134(1):327–40.
2. Subramanian V, Ragunath K. Advanced endoscopic imaging: a review of commercially available technologies. Clin Gastroenterol Hepatol. 2014;12(3):368–76. e1.
3. Committee AT, Wong Kee Song LM, Adler DG, Chand B, Conway JD, Croffie JM, et al. Chromoendoscopy. Gastrointest Endosc. 2007;66(4):639–49.

4. Trivedi PJ, Braden B. Indications, stains and techniques in chromoendoscopy. QJM. 2013;106(2):117–31.
5. Shiozaki H, Tahara H, Kobayashi K, Yano H, Tamura S, Imamoto H, et al. Endoscopic screening of early esophageal cancer with the Lugol dye method in patients with head and neck cancers. Cancer. 1990;66(10):2068–71.
6. Meyer V, Burtin P, Bour B, Blanchi A, Cales P, Oberti F, et al. Endoscopic detection of early esophageal cancer in a high-risk population: does Lugol staining improve videoendoscopy? Gastrointest Endosc. 1997;45(6):480–4.
7. Hashimoto CL, Iriya K, Baba ER, Navarro-Rodriguez T, Zerbini MC, Eisig JN, et al. Lugol's dye spray chromoendoscopy establishes early diagnosis of esophageal cancer in patients with primary head and neck cancer. Am J Gastroenterol. 2005;100(2):275–82.
8. Fagundes RB, de Barros SG, Putten AC, Mello ES, Wagner M, Bassi LA, et al. Occult dysplasia is disclosed by Lugol chromoendoscopy in alcoholics at high risk for squamous cell carcinoma of the esophagus. Endoscopy. 1999;31(4):281–5.
9. Dubuc J, Legoux JL, Winnock M, Seyrig JA, Barbier JP, Barrioz T, et al. Endoscopic screening for esophageal squamous-cell carcinoma in high-risk patients: a prospective study conducted in 62 french endoscopy centers. Endoscopy. 2006;38(7):690–5.
10. Yokoyama A, Ohmori T, Makuuchi H, Maruyama K, Okuyama K, Takahashi H, et al. Successful screening for early esophageal cancer in alcoholics using endoscopy and mucosa iodine staining. Cancer. 1995;76(6):928–34.
11. Shimizu Y, Omori T, Yokoyama A, Yoshida T, Hirota J, Ono Y, et al. Endoscopic diagnosis of early squamous neoplasia of the esophagus with iodine staining: high-grade intra-epithelial neoplasia turns pink within a few minutes. J Gastroenterol Hepatol. 2008;23(4):546–50.
12. Muto M, Minashi K, Yano T, Saito Y, Oda I, Nonaka S, et al. Early detection of superficial squamous cell carcinoma in the head and neck region and esophagus by narrow band imaging: a multicenter randomized controlled trial. J Clin Oncol. 2010;28(9):1566–72.
13. Sharma P, Weston AP, Topalovski M, Cherian R, Bhattacharyya A, Sampliner RE. Magnification chromoendoscopy for the detection of intestinal metaplasia and dysplasia in Barrett's oesophagus. Gut. 2003;52:24–7.
14. Connor MJ, Sharma P. Chromoendoscopy and magnification endoscopy for diagnosing esophageal cancer and dysplasia. Thorac Surg Clin. 2004;14(1):87–94.
15. Sturm MB, Wang TD. Emerging optical methods for surveillance of Barrett's oesophagus. Gut. 2015;64(11):1816–23.
16. Pech O, Gossner L, Manner H, May A, Rabenstein T, Behrens A, et al. Prospective evaluation of the macroscopic types and location of early Barrett's neoplasia in 380 lesions. Endoscopy. 2007;39(7):588–93.
17. Sharma P, Falk GW, Weston AP, Reker D, Johnston M, Sampliner RE. Dysplasia and cancer in a large multicenter cohort of patients with Barrett's esophagus. Clin Gastroenterol Hepatol. 2006;4(5):566–72.
18. Qumseya BJ, Wang H, Badie N, Uzomba RN, Parasa S, White DL, et al. Advanced imaging technologies increase detection of dysplasia and neoplasia in patients with Barrett's esophagus: a meta-analysis and systematic review. Clin Gastroenterol Hepatol. 2013;11(12):1562–70. e1–2.
19. Kaltenbach T, Soetikno R. Image-enhanced endoscopy is critical in the detection, diagnosis, and treatment of non-polypoid colorectal neoplasms. Gastrointest Endosc Clin N Am. 2010;20(3):471–85.
20. Soetikno R, Subramanian V, Kaltenbach T, Rouse RV, Sanduleanu S, Suzuki N, et al. The detection of nonpolypoid (flat and depressed) colorectal neoplasms in patients with inflammatory bowel disease. Gastroenterology. 2013;144(7):1349–52. e1–6.
21. Laine L, Kaltenbach T, Barkun A, McQuaid KR, Subramanian V, Soetikno R, et al. SCENIC international consensus statement on surveillance and management of dysplasia in inflammatory bowel disease. Gastroenterology. 2015;148(3):639–51. e28.
22. Picco MF, Pasha S, Leighton JA, et al. Procedure time and the determination of polypoid abnormalities with experience: implementation of a chromoendoscopy program for surveillance colonoscopy for ulcerative colitis. Inflamm Bowel Dis. 2013;19:1913–20.

23. Mohammed N, Kant P, Abid F, Rotimi O, Prasad P, Hamlin J, et al. High definition white light endoscopy (Hdwle) versus high definition with chromoendoscopy (Hdce) in the detection of dysplasia in long standing ulcerative colitis: a randomized controlled trial. Gastrointest Endosc. 2015;81(5):AB148.
24. Committee ASP, Shergill AK, Lightdale JR, Bruining DH, Acosta RD, Chandrasekhara V, et al. The role of endoscopy in inflammatory bowel disease. Gastrointest Endosc. 2015;81(5):1101–21. e1-13.
25. Cairns SR, Scholefield JH, Steele RJ, Dunlop MG, Thomas HJ, Evans GD, et al. Guidelines for colorectal cancer screening and surveillance in moderate and high risk groups (update from 2002). Gut. 2010;59(5):666–89.
26. Annese V, Daperno M, Rutter MD, Amiot A, Bossuyt P, East J, et al. European evidence based consensus for endoscopy in inflammatory bowel disease. J Crohn's Colitis. 2013;7(12):982–1018.
27. Lecomte T, Cellier C, Meatchi T, Barbier JP, Cugnenc PH, Jian R, et al. Chromoendoscopic colonoscopy for detecting preneoplastic lesions in hereditary nonpolyposis colorectal cancer syndrome. Clin Gastroenterol Hepatol. 2005;3(9):897–902.
28. Huneburg R, Lammert F, Rabe C, Rahner N, Kahl P, Buttner R, et al. Chromocolonoscopy detects more adenomas than white light colonoscopy or narrow band imaging colonoscopy in hereditary nonpolyposis colorectal cancer screening. Endoscopy. 2009;41(4):316–22.
29. Bartel MJ, Picco MF, Wallace MB. Chromocolonoscopy. Gastrointest Endosc Clin N Am. 2015;25(2):243–60.
30. Pohl J, Schneider A, Vogell H, Mayer G, Kaiser G, Ell C. Pancolonic chromoendoscopy with indigo carmine versus standard colonoscopy for detection of neoplastic lesions: a randomised two-centre trial. Gut. 2011;60(4):485–90.
31. Brown SR, Baraza W. Chromoscopy versus conventional endoscopy for the detection of polyps in the colon and rectum. Cochrane Database Syst Rev. 2010;10:CD006439.
32. Fry S, Fleischer DE, Axelrad AM, et al. High-resolution chromoendoscopy: an affordable and accurate non-biopsy technique for predicting histology of colorectal polyps. Gastrointest Endosc. 1996;43:365.
33. Eisen GM, Kim CY, Fleischer DE, Kozarek RA, Carr-Locke DL, Li TCM, et al. High-resolution chromoendoscopy for classifying colonic polyps: a multicenter study. Gastrointest Endosc. 2002;55(6):687–94.
34. Longcroft-Wheaton G, Brown J, Cowlishaw D, Higgins B, Bhandari P. High-definition vs. standard-definition endoscopy with indigo carmine for the in vivo diagnosis of colonic polyps. United European Gastroenterol J. 2013;1(6):425–9.
35. Kudo S, Tamura S, Nakajima T, et al. Diagnosis of colorectal tumorous lesions by magnifying endoscopy. Gastrointest Endosc. 1996;44:8–14.
36. Fu KI, Sano Y, Kato S, Fujii T, Nagashima F, Yoshino T, et al. Chromoendoscopy using indigo carmine dye spraying with magnifying observation is the most reliable method for differential diagnosis between non-neoplastic and neoplastic colorectal lesions: a prospective study. Endoscopy. 2004;36(12):1089–93.
37. Axelrad AM, Fleischer DE, Geller AJ, Nguyen CC, Lewis JH, Al-Kawas FH, et al. High-resolution chromoendoscopy for the diagnosis of diminutive colon polyps: implications for colon cancer screening. Gastroenterology. 1996;110(4):1253–8.
38. Monkemuller K, Wilcox CM. Interventional chromoendoscopy. Gastrointest Endosc. 2013;78(2):346–50.
39. Holt BA, Jayasekeran V, Sonson R, Bourke MJ. Topical submucosal chromoendoscopy defines the level of resection in colonic EMR and may improve procedural safety (with video). Gastrointest Endosc. 2013;77(6):949–53.
40. Kondo H, Fukuda H, Ono H, Gotoda T, Saito D, Takahiro K, et al. Sodium thiosulfate solution spray for relief of irritation caused by Lugol's stain in chromoendoscopy. Gastrointest Endosc. 2001;53(2):199–202.
41. Olliver JR, Wild CP, Sahay P, Dexter S, Hardie LJ. Chromoendoscopy with methylene blue and associated DNA damage in Barrett's oesophagus. Lancet. 2003;362(9381):373–4.

42. Davies J, Burke D, Olliver JR, Hardie LJ, Wild CP, Routledge MN. Methylene blue but not indigo carmine causes DNA damage to colonocytes in vitro and in vivo at concentrations used in clinical chromoendoscopy. Gut. 2007;56(1):155–6.
43. Rosen PJ, Johnson C, McGehee WG, Beutler E. Failure of methylene blue treatment in toxic methemoglobinemia. Association with glucose-6-phosphate dehydrogenase deficiency. Ann Intern Med. 1971;75(1):83–6.
44. Ginimuge PR, Jyothi SD. Methylene blue: revisited. J Anaesthesiol Clin Pharmacol. 2010;26(4):517–20.
45. Rehman UR. Methemoglobinemia. West J Med. 2001;175:193–6.

Chapter 4
Virtual Chromoendoscopy

Dileep Mangira, Stephanie Wong, Prateek Sharma, and Rajvinder Singh

Introduction

Novel endoscopic imaging techniques have been developed in recent times as an alternative to dye-based chromoendoscopy to enhance visualization of mucosal surface architecture and capillary patterns. These techniques have been termed virtual chromoendoscopy and encompass built-in endoscopic image enhancement technologies that alter the white-light image with a push of a button on the endoscope [1]. Terms such as digital, electronic, optical or dye-less chromoendoscopy have been used to describe virtual chromoendoscopy.

Most of the interest in virtual chromoendoscopy revolves around early detection and characterization of gastrointestinal lesions based on the architecture of their mucosal surface. If lesions can be confidently identified and histology predicted, pathological testing could potentially be avoided thus reducing cost as well as complications related to tissue sampling.

There are currently three systems available. They are Narrow Band Imaging (NBI), Flexible Spectral Imaging Colour Enhancement (FICE) and i-Scan. Here, we present the technological aspects and published evidence to date for each technology in the gastrointestinal tract.

D. Mangira, M.B.B.S. (F.R.A.C.P.) • S. Wong, M.B.B.S. • P. Sharma, M.D.
R. Singh, F.R.A.C.P., A.M., F.R.C.P. (✉)
The Lyell McEwin Hospital and The University of Adelaide,
Haydown Road, Elizabeth Vale, SA 5112, Australia
e-mail: rajvinder.singh@sa.gov.au

V.J.A. Konda, I. Waxman (eds.), *Endoscopic Imaging Techniques and Tools*,
DOI 10.1007/978-3-319-30053-5_4

Narrow Band Imaging

Technological Aspects

Narrow Band Imaging (NBI) utilizes narrow-band filters to produce short wavelengths of light, which penetrate into superficial layers of the mucosa to highlight abnormal mucosal and vascular patterns. NBI relies on the penetration properties of light, which is directly proportional to the wavelength [2]. Shorter wavelengths can only penetrate superficial layers of the mucosa whereas longer wavelengths can penetrate into deeper layers of the tissue. A white-light source filter located directly in front of a xenon arc lamp produces two narrow bands of light with specific wavelengths (415 and 540 nm). These two wavelengths correspond to the primary and secondary light absorption peaks of haemoglobin, respectively [3]. Capillaries in the superficial mucosa appear brown when highlighted by the shorter wavelength light (415 nm) and deeper mucosa and submucosa appear blue-green when highlighted by the longer wavelength light (540 nm). Two different NBI systems are commercially available in the market, each of which having their own distinct advantages. The 290 series system uses a red-green-blue (RGB) filter, which produces high-resolution images whereas its counterpart, the 190 series uses a charge-coupled device (CCD) chip, which produces better quality videos. The video image processor has a built-in adjustable 'structural enhancement' and 'colour enhancement' image-processing feature. Structural enhancement has two image modes: A and B modes. In the A mode, vessel architecture and surface structures are enhanced which appear as thickened linear objects. In the B mode, enhancement is obtained by contrasting the outline, which gives an image a sharper edge. The colour enhancement feature of the processor enables the endoscopist to change the gain ratio of the blue and green colour tones in the displayed image.

Oesophagus

Gastro-Oesophageal Reflux Disease vs. Non-erosive Reflux Disease

More than half of patients with typical reflux symptoms have a normal standard endoscopy and are often labelled as suffering from non-erosive reflux disease (NERD) [4]. Typical changes of gastro-oesophageal reflux disease (GERD) may take several years to appear. NBI can detect microvascular changes in oesophageal mucosa that can aid in early diagnosis and treatment of NERD. These changes include micro erosions, increased vascularity, increased number and dilatation of intra papillary capillary loops (IPCL) which results in an inverted fern tree appearance and loss of vascular palisade pattern and triangular indentation of the squamo-columnar junction above the Z-line [5, 6]. The presence of increased number of

IPCLs are the best predictors for the diagnosis of GERD (odds ratio [OR], 5.5) and dilatation (OR, 11.3) [6]. Fock et al. [7] in a prospective case–control study established that NBI detected a significantly higher prevalence of micro erosions (gastro-oesophageal reflux disease 100 %, non-erosive reflux disease 52.8 % and controls 23 %) and increased vascularity (gastro-oesophageal reflux disease 95 %, non-erosive reflux disease 91.7 % and controls 36.7 %) but a lower prevalence of round pit patterns (gastro-oesophageal reflux disease 4.9 %, non-erosive reflux disease 5.6 % and controls 70 %) in patients with GERD. Hence, certain features of NBI can improve the detection of subtle lesions in patients with NERD who could effectively be treated which in turn may prevent long-term complications related to the disease.

Barrett's Oesophagus and Oesophageal Adenocarcinoma

In Barrett's oesophagus (BE), regular squamous epithelium is replaced by columnar epithelium with or without intestinal metaplasia, which can develop into oesophageal adenocarcinoma. Current surveillance guidelines mandate performing four quadrant biopsies every 2 cm of a Barrett's segment [8]. This process is labour intensive and maybe less effective for detecting dysplasia or early cancer in BE [9]. NBI may enable endoscopists to make an in vivo diagnosis and aid treatment strategy [10–12].

Several studies have defined the spectrum of Barrett's-related changes that can be seen with NBI ranging from intestinal metaplasia to dysplasia by proposing various classification systems based on the mucosal surface and vascular pattern [13–15]. Although available results from these studies are promising, it is important to note that most groups developed their own classification system. As a consequence, there is no validated and standardized classification system for the use of NBI in BE. Because of these limitations, future directions should focus on validation of these classification systems and to determine the effectiveness of NBI by comparing it with conventional While Light Endoscopy (WLE) and chromoendoscopy.

Stomach

NBI with magnification demonstrates characteristic features that are contrasting in different parts of stomach. The normal mucosa of the gastric fundus and body demonstrates honeycomb-like subepithelial capillary network (SECN) with collecting venules (CVs) that usually surround oval-shaped gastric pits. However, collecting venules are rarely seen in the gastric antrum; the mucosa here, displaying ridges that are separated by narrow sulci with elongated SECN in the centre [16, 17].

Helicobacter infection leads to chronic atrophic gastritis and intestinal metaplasia, which is a major risk factor of gastric cancer [18]. A recent study demonstrated the advantage of NBI over conventional WLE in identifying specific mucosal changes of gastric atrophy characterized by complete loss of mucosal pit pattern and SECN with irregular arrangement of CVs with high sensitivity (90 %) and specificity (96 %) [19].

Light blue crest (LBC) is a fine white blue-white line seen on the crest of epithelial surface. When identified with magnifying NBI, this specific feature is a highly accurate indicator for intestinal metaplasia with a sensitivity, specificity and accuracy of 72.1 %, 96.0 % and 84.9 %, respectively [20]. Lipid droplets that accumulate in the superficial epithelial neoplastic tissue of the gastric mucosa appear as a white opaque substance (WOS). The presence of an irregularly arranged WOS is a strong predictor of malignant transformation [21].

Early malignant features of gastric cancer such as amorphous pit pattern, irregular size and distortion or complete loss of pits along with abnormal microvascular pattern can be identified with NBI and high magnification [22, 23]. However, these discrete features are altered by other coexisting conditions such as chronic inflammation, ulceration, atrophy and Helicobacter infection which make the diagnosis challenging [23]. Considering these limitations, a consensus of expert endoscopists in the Asia-Pacific region concluded that NBI is not useful for detection of early gastric cancers. However, NBI may be able to characterize lesions well and aids in distinguishing tumour margins from surrounding normal mucosa compared to conventional WLE. NBI has a poor predictive value in assessing the depth of tumour invasion as the narrow band of light can only penetrate into the superficial mucosa [24].

Duodenum

NBI may be effective in identifying villous atrophy, which is a characteristic feature of celiac disease with an overall sensitivity, specificity, positive predictive value and negative predictive values of 100 %, 91 %, 83 % and 100 %, respectively [25]. Considering the patchy distribution of coeliac disease, Benerjee et al. [26] suggested that NBI could be a potential adjunctive tool to aid the endoscopists in performing targeted biopsies. Singh et al. [27] further proposed a simplified classification system to assess villous morphology. They also demonstrated high sensitivity and specificity rates along with good inter and intra-observer agreement among endoscopists with no previous NBI exposure in discriminating the various villous patterns seen in the patients with Coeliac Disease [28].

Colon

The role of NBI has been extensively investigated in detecting and characterising colonic polyps. A meta-analysis of eight randomized trials compared standard or high definition (HD) WLE with NBI. This study demonstrated no statistically significant difference between WLE (standard and HD) and NBI for the detection of patients with colorectal polyps (six trials, relative risk [RR] 0.97), colorectal adenomas (eight trials, RR 0.94) or colorectal hyperplastic polyps (two trials, RR 0.87) [29]. Similar to this review, other meta-analyses demonstrated no significant difference between HD-NBI and HD-WLE in the detection of colonic polyps [30–32]. In contrast to the above results, one meta-analysis demonstrated that NBI was superior to SD-WLE in the detection of flat adenomas with a pooled RR of 1.96. Another interesting finding of this study was that overall withdrawal time increased with the use of NBI (pooled weighted mean difference, 0.90) [33]. Most of the above studies were based on earlier generation endoscopes with limited technological advancement in relation to NBI. Newer generation colonoscopes have incorporated multiple improvements in the definition, contrast as well as in the brightness. A recent randomized trial with tandem colonoscopy compared the new generation NBI (190 series) system, which is twice as bright as the previous version with HD-WLE. This study demonstrated that both the adenoma and polyp detection rates were significantly higher in the 190-NBI group compared with the HD-WL group (adenoma: 48.3 % vs. 34.4 %, $P=0.01$; polyps: 61.1 % vs. 48.3 %, $P=0.02$) [34]. This evolving information demonstrates that newer generation colonoscopes with advanced technology and brighter images may have the potential to improve adenoma detection rate. However, further large randomized studies are needed before routine clinical use can be considered. Until more consistent results are obtained demonstrating efficacy of NBI, there is no good substitute for excellent bowel preparation and meticulous withdrawal techniques for careful interrogation of mucosal folds to improve adenoma detection.

NBI in Polyp Characterization

In vivo characterization has been proposed as a part of the 'resect and discard' strategy where diminutive (≤5 mm) adenomatous polyps are resected without any pathological evaluation and non-adenomatous polyps in the recto-sigmoid region are left in situ. This strategy could confer substantial cost savings by avoiding pathology and major colonoscopy-related complications.

Multiple classifications (Sano, Hiroshima and more recently the NICE classification) have been proposed to describe polyp histology using NBI [35–37], Figs. 4.1, 4.2, 4.3 and 4.4 demonstrates various morphological features of polyps according to Sano and NICE classification. These classification systems are primarily based on the microvascular architecture of the polyps. Wu et al. assessed the accuracy of NBI for polyp characterization in a meta-analysis, which included 11 relevant studies [38]. The overall sensitivity and specificity and the AUC (area under the curve) for NBI was 0.92, 0.83 and 0.95, respectively. This study concluded that NBI with or without magnification was accurate in identifying adenomas based on visualization. Another meta-analysis by McGill et al. reviewed the real-time diagnostic operating characteristics of NBI during colonoscopy. Based on 28 studies involving 6280

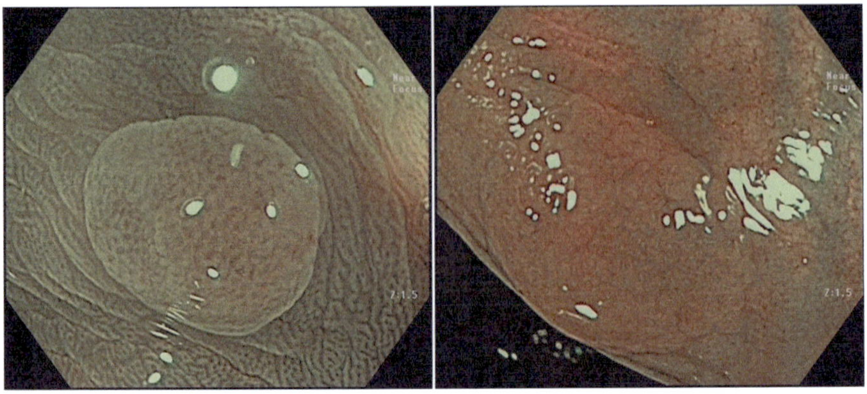

Fig. 4.1 Polyps with Sano Class I and NICE class I features. Hyperplastic polyp (*Left*) Modified Sano I: Meshed capillary vessels; (*Right*) NICE I: Similar colour compared to background, no vessels with uniform white spots

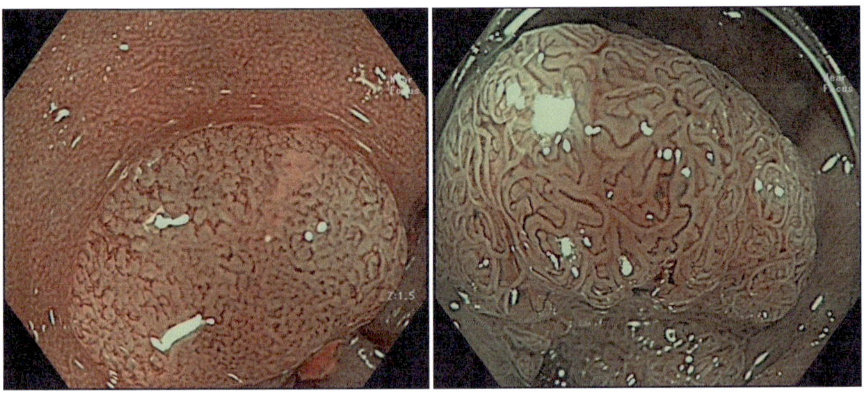

Fig. 4.2 Polyps with Sano II/NICE II features (*Left*) Modified Sano II - Brown capillary vessels surrounding white pits/mucosal glands (Tubular Adenoma) (*Right*) NICE II - Browner than background and brown vessels surrounding branched white structures (Tubular Adenoma)

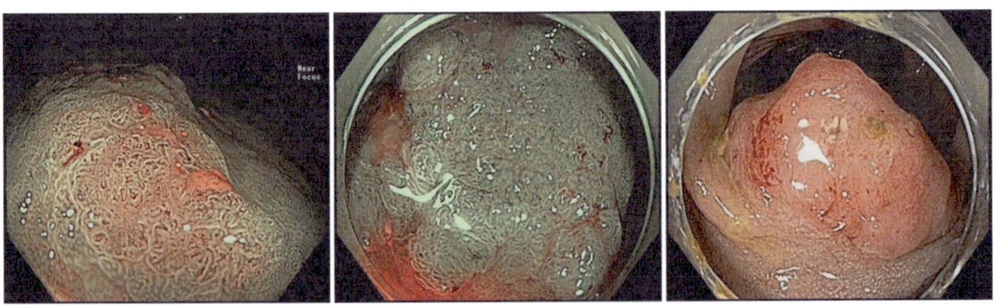

Fig. 4.3 Polyps with Sano IIIa/IIIb features (*Left*) Modified Sano IIIa - Increased capillary density with villous and cerebreform appearing pits (Tubular Villous Adenoma) (*Middle and Right*) Modified Sano IIIb: loss of vasculature (Invasive Cancer)

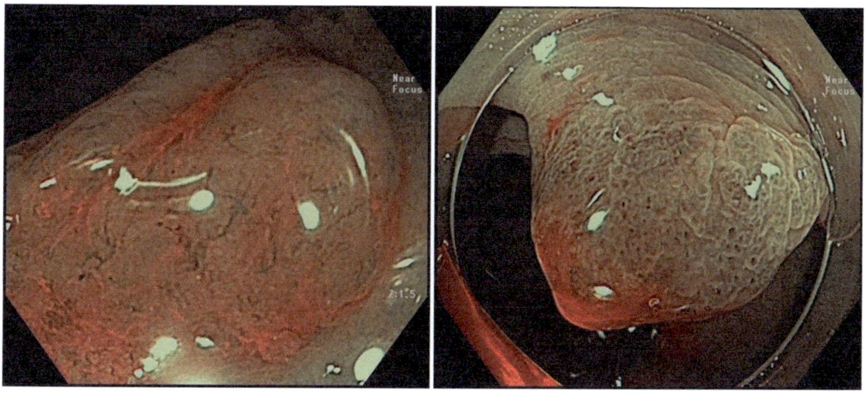

Fig. 4.4 Polyp with Sano II_o features Modified Sano II_o - Pink mucous cap with brown 'open' pits (noticeable on the *right* image) (Sessile Serrated Adenoma)

polyps, the real-time endoscopic diagnosis of colonic polyps was highly accurate with an area under the receiver operator curve exceeding 0.90. Surveillance intervals directed by endoscopic diagnosis were in agreement with pathology-directed surveillance intervals for more than 90 % of patients [39]. Although evidence for polyp characterization with NBI is promising, one major limitation is its generalizability. Most of the studies were performed at tertiary care centres by expert endoscopists using various different classification systems. So far, there is limited evidence available regarding non-expert endoscopists' learning curve in using NBI to assess colonic polyps [40]. In a prospective study by Rogart et al. ($n=131$), three of four endoscopists significantly improved their accuracy of diagnosing adenomas in the second half of the study compared with the first from 74 % to 87 %, respectively. All endoscopists received feedback every 2 weeks on their diagnostic accuracy. This study suggests that with frequent feedback, significant improvement in the accuracy can be obtained in a relatively short period of time [41]. Presently, NBI is effective in differentiating neoplastic from non-neoplastic colonic polyps with high sensitivity and specificity in expert hands. Future research should focus on defining learning curves and validation in the non-expert centres.

Flexible Spectral Imaging Colour Enhancement and i-Scan

Due to the limited data available, Flexible Spectral Imaging Colour Enhancement (FICE) and i-Scan will be discussed together.

Technological Aspects

FICE is produced by Fujifilm, Tokyo, Japan. It enhances vascular and surface patterns using a spectral-estimation technology that processes images at different wavelengths based on white-light images and displays them in real time [42, 43]. FICE has ten preset wavelength patterns and therefore does not have standardized settings making comparison in studies difficult [42].

i-Scan is a product of Pentax, Tokyo, Japan. i-Scan works to emphasize changes of the mucosal surface by applying a digital colour filter to images [44]. Unlike FICE, uniform settings have been recommended by an international consensus allowing better comparability in future studies. Three different algorithms, surface enhancement (SE), contrast enhancement (CE) and tone enhancement (TE), are used to process reflected light. SE allows for the assessment of mucosal surface and lesions borders by emphasizing luminance and contrast of the edges. CE enhances vessels by recognizing areas that are lower in luminance intensity compared with surrounding pixels and refines the image with a slight suppression of red and green frequencies. This results in the staining of dark areas in a slightly bluish colour. With TE, the reflected white light is divided into three colours (red, green and blue) followed by selective modification of each frequency and subsequently real-time image construction. i-Scan algorithm 1 which uses only SE is for detection of lesions. i-Scan 2 which combines SE and TE is used for characterization of lesions. i-Scan 3 uses all three algorithms for demarcation of lesions [45].

Oesophagus

A study comparing FICE and WLE to distinguish between BE and gastric mucosa revealed that the FICE images had a significantly higher median colour contrast compared to that of WLE [46]. Another study evaluating the difference between FICE and chromoendoscopy with acetic acid in the detection of high-grade BE showed that they both had a sensitivity of 87 %. Although the sensitivity of directed biopsies for FICE was higher at 92 % compared to 83 % in the chromoendoscopy with acetic acid group, this was apparently not statistically significant [47].

In the only randomized controlled trial with i-Scan to evaluate oesophagitis, the diagnostic yield was higher in the i-Scan compared to WLE (30.1 % vs. 21.6 %, $p=0.034$) [48].

Gastric Neoplasia

In a study comparing FICE and WLE in patients with depressed-type early gastric cancers, FICE images had a statistically significant greater median colour difference between the malignant lesions and the surrounding mucosa leading the authors to believe that FICE could be used to facilitate diagnosis of this cancer [49].

Another study evaluated the feasibility of a new magnified i-Scan system in the diagnosis of gastric neoplasia in comparison with magnified HD-WLE. The authors concluded that although magnified i-Scan improved image quality, its value in improving diagnostic yield was limited [50].

Colon

The overall sensitivity, specificity and negative predictive value for FICE in the diagnosis of colonic polyps were reported to be 91.8 %, 83.5 % and 83.7 %, respectively [51]. The use of FICE with high magnification has been shown to significantly improve the accuracy of diagnosis, particularly for polyps 5 mm or less [52]. FICE, however is inferior to dye-based chromoendoscopy in this area [43].

A recent randomized controlled study comparing the adenoma detection rates and diagnostic efficacy between FICE and WLE revealed no difference between the two systems [53]. This is conflicting with previous non-randomized studies showing that FICE was superior to WLE in detecting colonic polyps [42–44, 54].

In regard to detection of colorectal polyps with i-Scan, it has been shown to have a similar sensitivity and specificity to NBI [43]. A meta-analysis on the performance of i-Scan in this area established an overall sensitivity, specificity and negative predictive value to be 89.3 %, 88.2 % and 86.5 %, respectively [51].

Compared to WLE, i-Scan is superior in the prediction of adenomas as well as assessing disease activity and extent in inflammatory bowel disease [43, 45].

Conclusion

Virtual chromoendoscopy appear to have a huge impact in characterizing lesions in the gastrointestinal tract. Further studies are needed to address issues such as standardization of classifications and development of validated teaching modules before widespread clinical use can be recommended.

References

1. Kamiński M, Hassan C, Bisschops R, Pohl J, Pellisé M, Dekker E, et al. Advanced imaging for detection and differentiation of colorectal neoplasia: European Society of Gastrointestinal Endoscopy (ESGE) guideline. Endoscopy. 2014;46(05):435–57.
2. Gono K, Obi T, Yamaguchi M, Ohyama N, Machida H, Sano Y, et al. Appearance of enhanced tissue features in narrow-band endoscopic imaging. J Biomed Opt. 2004;9(3):568.
3. Kuznetsov K, Lambert R, Rey J. Narrow-band imaging: potential and limitations. Endoscopy. 2006;38(01):76–81.
4. Hershcovici T, Fass R. Nonerosive reflux disease (NERD)—an update. J Neurogastroenterol Motility. 2010;16(1):8–21.

5. Tseng P, Chen C, Chiu H, Liao W, Wu M, Lin J, et al. Performance of narrow band imaging and magnification endoscopy in the prediction of therapeutic response in patients with gastroesophageal reflux disease. J Clin Gastroenterol. 2011;45(6):501–6.
6. Sharma P, Wani S, Bansal A, Hall S, Puli S, Mathur S, et al. A feasibility trial of narrow band imaging endoscopy in patients with gastroesophageal reflux disease. Gastroenterology. 2007;133(2):454–64.
7. Fock K, Teo E, Ang T, Tan J, Law N. The utility of narrow band imaging in improving the endoscopic diagnosis of gastroesophageal reflux disease. Clin Gastroenterol Hepatol. 2009;7(1):54–9.
8. Evans J, Early D, Fukami N, Ben-Menachem T, Chandrasekhara V, Chathadi K, et al. The role of endoscopy in Barrett's esophagus and other premalignant conditions of the esophagus. Gastrointest Endosc. 2012;76(6):1087–94.
9. Booth C, Thompson K. Barrett's esophagus: a review of diagnostic criteria, clinical surveillance practices and new developments. J Gastroenterol Oncol. 2012;3(3):232–42.
10. Singh R, Karageorgiou H, Owen V, Garsed K, Fortun P, Fogden E, et al. Comparison of high-resolution magnification narrow-band imaging and white-light endoscopy in the prediction of histology in Barrett's oesophagus. Scand J Gastroenterol. 2009;44(1):85–92.
11. Wolfsen H, Crook J, Krishna M, Achem S, Devault K, Bouras E, et al. Prospective, controlled tandem endoscopy study of narrow band imaging for dysplasia detection in Barrett's esophagus. Gastroenterology. 2008;135(1):24–31.
12. Spechler S, Goyal R. The columnar-lined esophagus, intestinal metaplasia, and Norman Barrett. Gastroenterology. 1996;110(2):614–21.
13. Kara M, Ennahachi M, Fockens P, ten Kate F, Bergman J. Detection and classification of the mucosal and vascular patterns (mucosal morphology) in Barrett's esophagus by using narrow band imaging. Gastrointest Endosc. 2006;64(2):155–66.
14. Sharma P, Bansal A, Rastogi A, Cherian R, McGregor D, Higbee A, et al. The utility of a novel narrow band imaging (NBI) endoscopy system in patients with Barrett's esophagus (BE). Gastrointest Endosc. 2005;61(5):AB240.
15. Singh R, Anagnostopoulos G, Yao K, Karageorgiou H, Fortun P, Shonde A, et al. Narrow-band imaging with magnification in Barrett's esophagus: validation of a simplified grading system of mucosal morphology patterns against histology. Endoscopy. 2008;40(6):457–63.
16. Yao K, Takaki Y, Matsui T, Iwashita A, Anagnostopoulos G, Kaye P, et al. Clinical application of magnification endoscopy and narrow-band imaging in the upper gastrointestinal tract: new imaging techniques for detecting and characterizing gastrointestinal neoplasia. Gastrointest Endosc Clin N Am. 2008;18(3):415–33.
17. Yagi K, Nakamura A, Sekine A. Characteristic endoscopic and magnified endoscopic findings in the normal stomach without Helicobacter pylori infection. J Gastroenterol Hepatol. 2002;17(1):39–45.
18. Muto M, Horimatsu T, Ezoe Y, Hori K, Yukawa Y, Morita S, et al. Narrow-band imaging of the gastrointestinal tract. J Gastroenterol. 2009;44(1):13–25.
19. Banerjee R, Reddy N. A primer on narrow band imaging. India: Paras; 2009.
20. An J, Song G, Kim G, Park D, Shin N, Lee B, et al. Marginal turbid band and light blue crest, signs observed in magnifying narrow-band imaging endoscopy, are indicative of gastric intestinal metaplasia. BMC Gastroenterol. 2012;12(1):169.
21. Ueyama H, Matsumoto K, Nagahara A, Gushima R, Hayashi T, Yao T, et al. A white opaque substance-positive gastric hyperplastic polyp with dysplasia. World J Gastroenterol. 2013;19(26):4262–6.
22. Yao K, Anagnostopoulos G, Ragunath K. Magnifying endoscopy for diagnosing and delineating early gastric cancer. Endoscopy. 2009;41(5):462–7.
23. Tsuji Y, Ohata K, Sekiguchi M, Ohno A, Ito T, Chiba H, et al. Magnifying endoscopy with narrow-band imaging helps determine the management of gastric adenomas. Gastric Cancer. 2012;15(4):414–8.
24. Uedo N, Fujishiro M, Goda K, Hirasawa D, Kawahara Y, Lee J, et al. Role of narrow band imaging for diagnosis of early-stage esophagogastric cancer: current consensus of experienced endoscopists in Asia-Pacific region. Digest Endosc. 2011;23:58–71.

25. Cammarota G, Pirozzi G, Martino A, Zuccalà G, Cianci R, Cuoco L, et al. Reliability of the "immersion technique" during routine upper endoscopy for detection of abnormalities of duodenal villi in patients with dyspepsia. Gastrointest Endosc. 2004;60(2):223–8.
26. Banerjee R, Reddy D. High-resolution narrow-band imaging can identify patchy atrophy in celiac disease: targeted biopsy can increase diagnostic yield. Gastrointest Endosc. 2009;69(4):984–5.
27. Singh R, Nind G, Tucker G, Nguyen N, Holloway R, Bate J, et al. Narrow-band imaging in the evaluation of villous morphology: a feasibility study assessing a simplified classification and observer agreement. Endoscopy. 2010;42(11):889–94.
28. Singh R, Chen Y, Mei S, Jayanna M, Ruszkiewicz A. Gastrointestinal: patchy distribution of Coeliac Disease diagnosed with narrow band imaging and optical magnification. J Gastroenterol Hepatol. 2013;28(3):584.
29. Nagorni A, Bjelakovic G, Petrovic B. Narrow band imaging versus conventional white light colonoscopy for the detection of colorectal polyps (Review). The Cochrane Collaboration. 2012;(1):1–43.
30. Pasha S, Leighton J, Das A, Harrison M, Gurudu S, Ramirez F, et al. Comparison of the yield and miss rate of narrow band imaging and white light endoscopy in patients undergoing screening or surveillance colonoscopy: a meta-analysis. Am J Gastroenterol. 2011;107(3):363–70.
31. Sabbagh L, Reveiz L, Aponte D, de Aguiar S. Narrow-band imaging does not improve detection of colorectal polyps when compared to conventional colonoscopy: a randomized controlled trial and meta-analysis of published studies. BMC Gastroenterol. 2011;11(1):100.
32. Dinesen L, Chua T, Kaffes A. Meta-analysis of narrow-band imaging versus conventional colonoscopy for adenoma detection. Gastrointest Endosc. 2012;75(3):604–11.
33. Jin X, Chai T, Shi J, Yang X, Sun Q. Meta-analysis for evaluating the accuracy of endoscopy with narrow band imaging in detecting colorectal adenomas. J Gastroenterol Hepatol. 2012;27(5):882–7.
34. Leung WK, Lo OS, Liu KS, et al. Detection of colorectal adenoma by narrow band imaging (HQ190) vs. high-definition white light colonoscopy: a randomized controlled trial. Am J Gastroenterol. 2014;109(6):855–63.
35. Oba S, et al. Current status of narrow-band imaging magnifying colonoscopy for colorectal neoplasia in Japan. Digestion. 2011;83(3):167–72.
36. Uraoka T, et al. 'Sano's capillary pattern classification for narrow-band imaging of early colorectal lesions. Digest Endosc. 2011;23:112–5.
37. Hewett DG, et al. Validation of a simple classification system for endoscopic diagnosis of small colorectal polyps using narrow-band imaging. Gastroenterology. 2012;143(3):599–607. e1.
38. Wu L, Li Y, Li Z, Cao Y, Gao F. Diagnostic accuracy of narrow-band imaging for the differentiation of neoplastic from non-neoplastic colorectal polyps: a meta-analysis. Colorectal Dis. 2012;15(1):3–11.
39. McGill SK, et al. Narrow band imaging to differentiate neoplastic and non-neoplastic colorectal polyps in real time: a meta-analysis of diagnostic operating characteristics. Gut. 2013;62(12):1704–13.
40. Higashi R, Uraoka T, Kato J, Kuwaki K, Ishikawa S, Saito Y, et al. Diagnostic accuracy of narrow-band imaging and pit pattern analysis significantly improved for less-experienced endoscopists after an expanded training program. Gastrointest Endosc. 2010;72(1):127–35.
41. Rogart J, Siddiqui U, Jain D, Oren T, Lim J, Jamidar P, et al. Narrow band imaging without high magnification to differentiate polyps during real-time colonoscopy: improvement with experience. Gastrointest Endosc. 2008;67(5):AB101.
42. Longcroft-Wheaton G, Higgins B, Bhandari P. Flexible spectral imaging color enhancement and indigo carmine in neoplasia diagnosis during colonoscopy. Eur J Gastroenterol Hepatol. 2011;23(10):903–11.
43. Yoshida N, Naito Y, Inada Y, Kugai M, Inoue K, Uchiyama K, et al. The detection of surface patterns by flexible spectral imaging color enhancement without magnification for diagnosis of colorectal polyps. Int J Colorectal Dis. 2011;27(5):605–11.

44. Koo J. Equipment-based image-enhanced endoscopy for differentiating colorectal polyps. Clin Endosc. 2014;47(4):330.
45. Tontini G, Vecchi M, Neurath M, Neumann H. Review article: newer optical and digital chromoendoscopy techniques vs. dye-based chromoendoscopy for diagnosis and surveillance in inflammatory bowel disease. Aliment Pharmacol Ther. 2013;38(10):1198–208.
46. Osawa H, Yamamoto H, Yamada N, Yoshizawa M, Sunada K, Kita H, et al. Diagnosis of endoscopic Barrett's esophagus by transnasal flexible spectral imaging color enhancement. J Gastroenterol. 2009;44(11):1125–32.
47. Pohl J, May A, Rabenstein T, Pech O, Nguyen-Tat M, Fissler-Eckhoff A, et al. Comparison of computed virtual chromoendoscopy and conventional chromoendoscopy with acetic acid for detection of neoplasia in Barrett's esophagus. Endoscopy. 2007;39(7):594–8.
48. Kang HS, et al. The efficacy of I-SCAN for detecting reflux esophagitis: a prospective randomized controlled trial. Dis Esophagus. 2012;26(2):204–11.
49. Osawa H, Yamamoto H, Miura Y, Ajibe H, Shinhata H, Yoshizawa M, et al. Diagnosis of depressed-type early gastric cancer using small-caliber endoscopy with flexible spectral imaging color enhancement. Digest Endosc. 2011;24(4):231–6.
50. Li C, Li Y, Zuo XL, Ji R, Gu XM, Yu T, et al. Magnified and enhanced computed virtual chromoendoscopy in gastric neoplasia: a feasibility study. WJG. 2013;19(26):4221.
51. Wanders L, East J, Uitentuis S, Leeflang M, Dekker E. Diagnostic performance of narrowed spectrum endoscopy, autofluorescence imaging, and confocal laser endomicroscopy for optical diagnosis of colonic polyps: a meta-analysis. Lancet Oncol. 2013;14(13):1337–47.
52. Kim Y, Kim D, Chung S, Park M, Shin C, Cho S, et al. Differentiating small polyp histologies using real-time screening colonoscopy with Fuji intelligent color enhancement. Clin Gastroenterol Hepatol. 2011;9(9):744–9. e1.
53. Chung S, Kim D, Song J, Kang H, Chung G, Choi J, et al. Comparison of detection and miss rates of narrow band imaging, flexible spectral imaging chromoendoscopy and white light at screening colonoscopy: a randomised controlled back-to-back study. Gut. 2013;63(5):785–91.
54. Kiriyama S, Matsuda T, Nakajima T, Sakamoto T, Saito Y, Kuwano H. Detectability of colon polyp using computed virtual chromoendoscopy with flexible spectral imaging color enhancement. Diagn Therapeut Endosc. 2012;2012:1–6.

Chapter 5
Autofluorescence Imaging

Massimiliano di Pietro and Krish Ragunath

Introduction

Over the last 20 years, the field of endoscopy has been revolutionized by two major technological advancements. On the one hand, there has been a rapid development of high-resolution endoscopic techniques leading to improved knowledge about morphology, endoscopic classification and significance of early neoplastic lesions. On the other hand, the introduction of endoluminal therapy has allowed endoscopists to offer minimally invasive modalities for the treatment of early neoplasia and prevention of gastrointestinal (GI) cancers. With a positive feedback loop, this has posed the challenging task to detect early neoplasia before it becomes visible by conventional endoscopic modalities. For example, low- and high-grade dysplasia in Barrett's oesophagus is often inconspicuous at white-light endoscopy, but it is associated to significant risk of cancer progression at routine surveillance interval if missed by random biopsy sampling. Similarly, colonic adenoma can be flat, and it is often overlooked at standard screening colonoscopy. Hence, research in GI endoscopy has pursued the holy grail of red-flag imaging techniques to reveal inconspicuous neoplasia. Autofluorescence imaging (AFI) is one such technique as it is based

---

Electronic supplementary material: The online version of this chapter (doi:10.1007/978-3-319-30053-5_5) contains supplementary material, which is available to authorized users. Videos can also be accessed at http://link.springer.com/chapter/10.1007/978-3-319-30053-5_5.

M. di Pietro, M.D.
MRC Cancer Unit, University of Cambridge, Cambridge Biomedical Campus, Cambridge CB2 0XZ, UK
e-mail: K.Ragunath@nottingham.ac.uk

K. Ragunath, M.D., F.R.C.P., F.A.S.G.E. (✉)
NIHR Biomedical Research Unit in Gastrointestinal and Liver Diseases at Nottingham University Hospitals NHS Trust and the University of Nottingham, Queens Medical Centre Campus, Nottingham NG7 2UH, UK
e-mail: K.Ragunath@nottingham.ac.uk

V.J.A. Konda, I. Waxman (eds.), *Endoscopic Imaging Techniques and Tools*,
DOI 10.1007/978-3-319-30053-5_5

on a radically different imaging algorithm compared to white-light endoscopy. AFI exploits the different fluorescent properties of GI neoplasia compared to healthy mucosa and has the potential to unmask lesions otherwise not visible on conventional imaging. In this chapter, we will discuss the technological background of AFI and the current evidence supporting its application in different GI tracts for the detection and demarcation of premalignant and early malignant conditions.

Technology Overview

Autofluorescence (AF) imaging is a type of spectroscopic technique aimed to improve detection of early cancer in luminal organs. Spectroscopy is the study of the interaction of tissue with any type of incident light. The incident light on a tissue plane can be reflected after interaction with tissue particles (scattering), can be absorbed by specific molecules or can be absorbed and then re-emitted at a longer wavelength (fluorescence). There are two main types of spectroscopic techniques applied to the endoscopy field (Table 5.1) [1, 2]. Scattering spectroscopy refers to the study of reflected light after scattering events, which can be single or multiple within the tissue. In scattering spectroscopy, the reflected light is measured at the same wavelength as the incident light, (elastic scattering spectroscopy) or alternatively as wavelength shift, i.e. inelastic (Raman) spectroscopy. In both cases, the principle is that normal and diseased tissues present different types of scattering events. The second type of spectroscopy relates to absorption and emission of light at higher wavelength (fluorescent spectroscopy). This is further divided in photodynamic technologies, which use fluorescent drugs (i.e. porfimer sodium or aminolevulinic acid) administered topically or systemically that are excited to emit fluorescence by various wavelengths, and autofluorescence imaging, which exploits the natural fluorescence of the tissue upon excitation by specific wavelength without the use of photosensitizers. This chapter focuses on the use of autofluorescence imaging in the gastrointestinal (GI) tract.

Autofluorescence imaging (AFI) is based on the principle that certain endogenous substances naturally occurring in the mucosa and submucosa of the GI tract

Table 5.1 Spectroscopic techniques and their characteristics

Technique	Principle	Use of dye	Incident light	Characteristics of detected light
Elastic spectroscopy	Scattering	No	White light	Same wavelength
Inelastic spectroscopy	Scattering	No	Near-infrared	Minor wavelength shift
Autofluorescence	Fluorescence (endogenous fluorophores)	No	Monochromatic (blue)	Longer wavelength
Photodynamic imaging	Fluorescence (exogenous fluorophores)	Yes	Monochromatic (typically blue)	Longer wavelength

(fluorophores) can be excited by short wavelengths of light to emit longer wavelengths in the form of green fluorescence. When an incoming photon excites an electron of these fluorophores to a higher energy state, the electron will subsequently relax back to its ground state and emit a photon of lower energy, hence of longer wavelength. Different fluorophores are present in human tissues, including nicotinamide adenine dinucleotide (NADH), flavins, such as flavin adenine dinucleotide (FAD), porphyrins and collagen. Conversely, haemoglobin has an absorption effect in the green spectrum. Different fluorophores have specific emission range of wavelengths as a function of the excitation wavelength. This range is known as fluorescent spectrum. It has been shown that the main mechanism whereby early neoplastic lesions have different autofluorescence patterns compared to healthy tissue is the thickening of the mucosal layer, which creates a masking effect to the autofluorescence originating from the submucosal collagen [3]. Other proposed mechanisms that explain the reduced autofluorescence in diseased GI tissue are: (a) Increased nucleo-cytoplasmic ratio, due to the fact that most of the cellular NADH is localized in the mitochondria within the cytoplasm; (b) neovascularization accompanying cancerous degeneration, which causes absorption of induced autofluorescence by haemoglobin [4].

Techniques

Two clinical technologies have been used to capture autofluorescence in the GI tract. Early in 1990s, the light-induced fluorescence endoscopy (LIFE) system has been studied for detection of early GI neoplasia. In the LIFE system, a mercury lamp is used to emit light and a blue excitation filter allows selection of a 437 nm blue light to illuminate the mucosa. The system, which uses a fibre-endoscope, has a high sensitivity coupled-charged device (CCD) at the distal end to amplify the autofluorescence signal and two built-in high sensitivity imaging elements that capture green (490–560 nm) and red (>630 nm) wavelengths. The images are then processed real time by a processor and displayed in pseudo-colour on the monitor. In the LIFE endoscopy system, normal tissue appears in light blue/green and cancer is shown as red. The inconvenience of the fibre-endoscopic system as well as a heavy image-intensifying camera made this system incompatible with clinical use in the video-endoscopy era of late 1990s and early 2000s. In addition, the LIFE system failed to provide good quality image and suitable manoeuvrability. These factors led to the development of a new autofluorescence system (AFI, Olympus Medical System Co), which has been made available since 2001. The AFI endoscope appears as a conventional endoscope and is equipped with a button-switch to select either the standard Red-Green-Blue (RGB) light or the illumination light for AFI. The two incorporated imaging systems are detected by two separate CCDs mounted within the distal end of the endoscope that is therefore 2 mm thicker than a conventional high-resolution endoscope. The light source has a rotational filter that sequentially select the blue excitation light (395–475 nm) and a narrow-band green (G′-) light (550 nm) for recording reflection images (Fig. 5.1). The CCD has

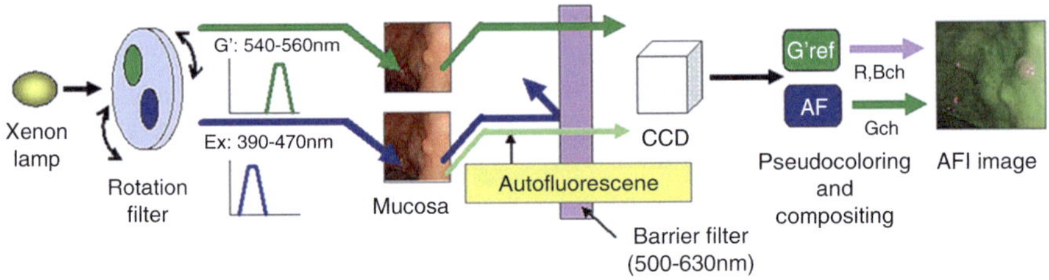

Fig. 5.1 Schematic description of AFI technology. A rotational filter (left) alternatively selects high frequency *blue* light for excitation at 390–470 nm and *green* light for recording reflection images at 540–560 nm. Normal tissue emits *green* fluorescence, whereas in early malignancy there is reduction of *green* fluorescence. The fluorescence is captured by a high-sensitivity CCD (middle). The autofluorescence patterns is reconstructed by the imagining processor in pseudo-colour images, where normal tissue appears as *green* signal and early cancer is appears as *magenta* colour (right). Courtesy Dr., Takahisa Matsuda, National Cancer Centre, Tokyo, Japan, with permission

high sensitivity and has a filter to select only wavelengths in the 490–625 range. The image processor displays a pseudo-colour image which results from the composition of the autofluorescence and green reflectance images. The wavelength of G′-light is determined by absorption features of haemoglobin. As haemoglobin absorbs both autofluorescence and green reflectance, areas of high vascularization appears as dark green. Normal mucosa appears bright green, due to the high level of emission of autofluorescence. Since areas of neoplasia absorb autofluorescence well, they look magenta in colour. Importantly, the AFI endoscope is equipped with the same high-definition CCD as conventional high-resolution systems; therefore, the autofluorescence image is assisted by a high-quality white-light image, for enhanced detection on both imaging modalities. The latest generation EVIS LUCERA ELITE Xenon Light Source CLV-290SL has an increased frame rate in AFI mode. This results in decreased noise in images and a higher resolution of the AFI, which enables more accurate observation of mucosal conditions.

Scientific Evidence and Clinical Indications

Light-Induced Fluorescence Endoscopy

The Light-Induced Fluorescence Endoscopy Gastrointestinal (LIFE-GI) system (Xillix Technologies, Vancouver, Canada) captures autofluorescence signals induced by blue light at a wavelength of 437 nm. In this fibreoptic system, two image intensifier cameras attached to the endoscope external to the body are used to detect autofluorescence in the green and red spectral ranges, which are fused to create a real-time "red-green" image. Generally, there is less green fluorescence in neoplastic tissue than in normal tissue, while red fluorescence is stronger in

Table 5.2 Performance of autofluorescence imaging system in different areas of the GI tract

Technology	Organ	Sensitivity (range) (%)	Specificity (range) (%)
LIFE	Oesophagus[a]	62–97	95
	Stomach	94–96	49–86
	Colon[b]	91	90
AFI	Oesophagus[c]	89–100	N/A
	Stomach	68–90[d]	44–100[d]
	Colon	90–97	37–56

[a]Data refer to both early adenocarcinoma and squamous cell carcinoma
[b]Data are based on one small study
[c]Data refer to Barrett's related neoplasia
[d]Higher figures of sensitivity and specificity refer to the addition of NBI magnification

neoplastic tissue than in normal tissue. The bulky clinical operating characteristics of this system have been substantially improved in a second version (LIFE II), which however, is still based on fibreoptic endoscopes. A summary of the results of the LIFE system in the detection of the GI neoplasia is presented in Table 5.2.

Oesophagus

An initial study from Mayinger and colleagues in a small cohort of four patients with oesophageal adenocarcinoma and nine with squamous cell carcinoma showed that cancer tissue has different light-induced autofluorescence spectra compared to normal oesophageal mucosa [5]. In this study, a fibreoptic probe was used to deliver violet-blue light and the signal was analysed by a spectrograph using a mathematical algorithm. This system has a sensitivity and a specificity for oesophageal carcinoma of 97 % and 95 %, respectively. This initial data generated significant enthusiasm, especially in the field of Barrett's oesophagus, where dysplasia and early neoplasia can be completely inconspicuous on standard white-light endoscopy. Disappointing results were obtained in a cross-over study where fifty patients received LIFE endoscopy and standard gastroscopy by different endoscopists in a randomized order at 4–6 weeks interval [6]. In this study, targeted biopsies based on the autofluorescence pattern had a slightly lower sensitivity for high-grade dysplasia (HGD) and early cancer than biopsies directed by standard endoscopy (69 % vs. 85 %, $p=0.69$). The false positive rate was high and the positive predictive value only 13 %. This study overall demonstrated the limited value of LIFE technology for the detection of early oesophageal glandular neoplasia.

Stomach

Early studies with the LIFE system in 50 ex vivo resected stomach showed that LIFE can differentiate cancer tissue from healthy mucosa based on the colour pattern, with most of the cancers appearing dark red [7]. However, the detection rate for early mucosal cancer was only 57 % and increased to 74 and 88 %, for tumours invading the submucosa and muscularis propria, respectively. In addition, this study showed that the detection rate for well-differentiated cancer was higher than undifferentiated caner (82 % vs. 61 %). A subsequent in vivo study in 52 patients with 54 lesions (33 early cancer and 21 benign lesions) confirmed that malignant lesions appeared mostly as dark red, as opposed to benign lesions which had the same background light blue colour of normal mucosa [8]. In this study, the sensitivity and specificity for a diagnosis of cancer were 94 % and 86 %, respectively. Interestingly, an analysis of over 300 spectra form 15 patients with gastric adenocarcinoma and 16 patients with signet-ring cells showed poor detection rate of signet-ring cell lesion with a sensitivity of only 55 %, as compared with 84 % for intestinal-type adenocarcinoma [9]. These differences are explained with the unique sub-mucosal growth pattern of signet-ring cells carcinoma, with high enrichment of collagen fibres and no significant thickening of the underlying mucosa, with little or no masking effect of the autofluorescence signal. In a larger retrospective study on 79 patients with a total of 109 gastric lesions, three independent endoscopists with different degree of experience in interpretation of AF images scored the LIFE images. Even though the agreement was good, with a value of 0.71 and the overall sensitivity for cancer was high at 96.4 %, the authors found a high false-positive rate which led to a specificity of 49.1 %, indicating a limited clinical utility in routine practice [10].

Colon

Limited data are available for LIFE in the lower GI tract. Only a small cohort study by Brand and co-workers has looked at the diagnostic accuracy of LIFE for colonic adenoma [11]. In this study, 20 patients with previous history of previous malignant (colon cancer) or premalignant conditions (adenomas or inflammatory bowel disease) were recruited and a total of 42 mucosal abnormalities were detected or which 22 had conformed histopathological dysplasia. The lesions were classified as suspicious or non-suspicious based on the appearances on white-light endoscopy and LIFE-positive or LIFE-negative based on whether they appeared red or green on LIFE imaging, respectively. In this study, all the dysplastic lesions were considered abnormal on WLE, but two of them were judged negative by LIFE. Hence, the sensitivity and specificity were 100 and 80 %, respectively, for WLE and 91 and 90 %, respectively, for LIFE.

The evidence suggest that even though LIFE can detect different AF spectra in malignant and non-malignant tissue the value in the clinical setting is only limited. Overall, the studies that have investigated this technology for the detection of GI neoplasia are small and do not have a robust design with very few exceptions. However, these studies and the use of this technology have been instrumental to the further development of autofluorescence-based systems.

AFI

Three generations video AFI systems have been evaluated so far. The first-generation autofluorescence endoscope (XGIF-Q240FY, Olympus Medical Systems) represented a major advancement compared to the fibreoptic-based LIFE technology, as it had AFI incorporated in a single endoscope with high-resolution white-light video-endoscopy (HR-WLE) [12]. This allows enhanced detection of subtle mucosal changes both in AFI and conventional imaging. The AFI mode of the endoscope uses a combination of blue-light excitation for autofluorescence, green and red reflectance and high-resolution CCD. However, despite the improved image quality compared to LIFE, as discussed in the following paragraphs, this system is limited by high false-positive rate, and the HR-WLE view often does not allow to discriminate false positives from true positives. In a second-generation endoscope (GIF-FQ260Z, Olympus Medical Systems), the AFI has been incorporated into an endoscopic trimodal imaging (ETMI) system with HR-WLE and narrow band imaging (NBI) with magnification (Video 5.1). The advantage of this system is the possibility to perform magnification endoscopy on AFI-positive areas to predict histology based on the pattern of mucosal pit and vascular net. A button switch allows interchanging in real time the three imaging modalities for a dynamic inspection of the GI mucosa. As mentioned, the main tissue determinant of AFI positivity is the thickness of the mucosal layer which can mask autofluorescence signal coming from the submucosal layer. This implies that non-neoplastic processes of the mucosal architecture, such extensive inflammation, can alter the AFI signal [13]. Indeed, the commonest cause of false AFI positivity is tissue inflammation. A third-generation AFI system (AFI III-prototype) has been developed to address this issue, based on the principle that combining different excitation wavelengths and acquiring multiple fluorescent spectra it is possible to target specifically fluorophores in malignant cells rather than global tissue architecture [14]. AFI III induces fluorescence with a dual narrow wavelength excitation, F_{380ex} ($\lambda = 380$–390 nm) and F_{405ex} ($\lambda = 400$–420 nm) combined with green reflectance. A summary of the results of the AFI system in the detection of the GI neoplasia is presented in Table 5.2.

Oesophagus

Oesophageal squamous cell carcinoma (OSCC) is the most prevalent oesophageal malignancy world-wide with higher incidence compared to the adenocarcinoma in Asia, developing world and several European Countries [15]. The precursor lesion to OSCC is squamous dysplasia, which is often completely inconspicuous on conventional WLE, but can be detected by advanced imaging modalities, such as NBI and Lugol's chromoendoscopy [16]. The first report on the use of the AFI for detection of superficial OSCC described a small cohort of five patients where the lesion was demarcated with the use of WLE, AFI and Lugol's chromoendoscopy (LCE) [12]. The extent of the lesion was correctly delineated only in 2/5 cases by WLE endoscopy, but in 5/5 by both AFI and chromoendoscopy. The AFI showed the typical well-contrasted red/magenta image on a green background in all five cases. Two studies have compared AFI and NBI for the visualization of early OSCC [17, 18]. Both studies showed that early OSCC can be subtle and hard to characterize on WLE. In this context, NBI appears to be more useful than AFI in delineating the area of interest. In the first study, 25 endoscopists evaluated 20 sets of WLE, NBI, AFI and LCE images from 16 patients. NBI and LCE scored higher than AFI and WLE, and AFI outperformed WLE only for flat/elevated lesions or those larger than 2 cm. In the second study, three endoscopists evaluated images from 31 superficial OSCC (patient $n=24$). Image quality scores were higher for NBI than AFI ($p<0.05$) and so was the interobserver agreement ($\kappa=0.42$ for NBI and 0.35 for AFI). Figure 5.2 shows a case of superficial OSCC which is poorly delineated by WLE, but AFI, LCE

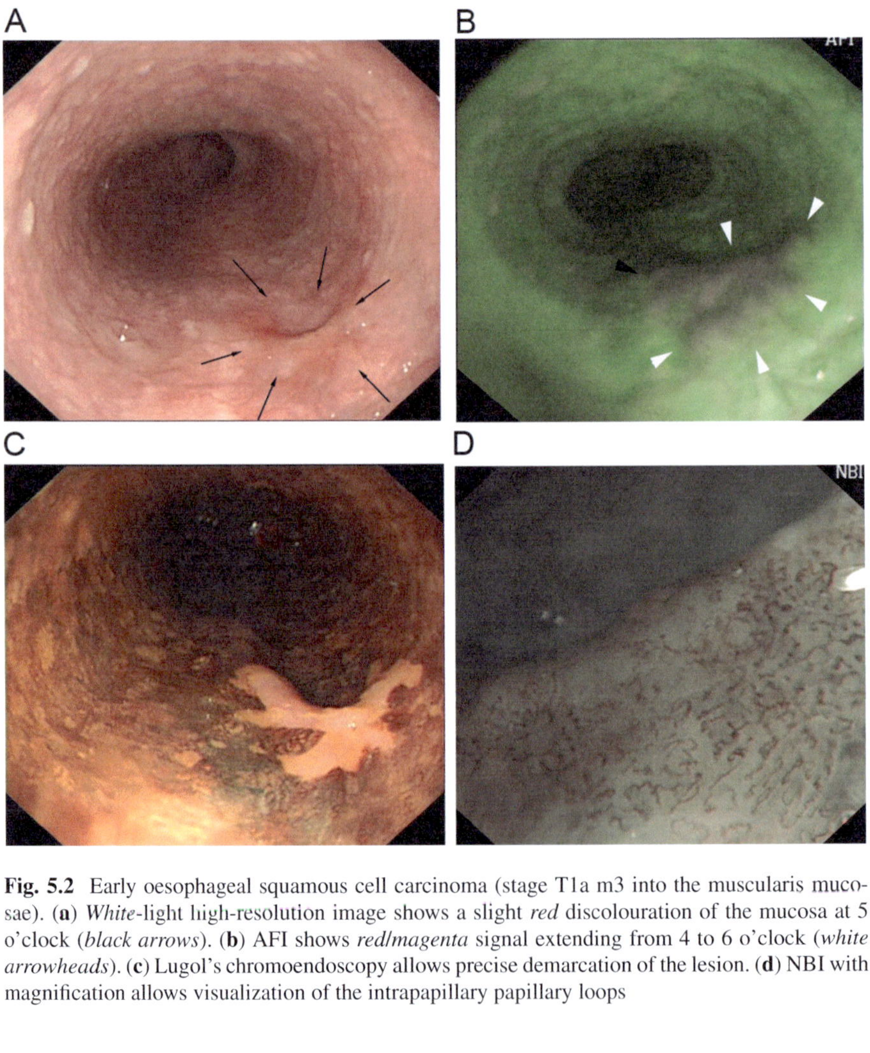

Fig. 5.2 Early oesophageal squamous cell carcinoma (stage T1a m3 into the muscularis mucosae). (**a**) *White*-light high-resolution image shows a slight *red* discolouration of the mucosa at 5 o'clock (*black arrows*). (**b**) AFI shows *red/magenta* signal extending from 4 to 6 o'clock (*white arrowheads*). (**c**) Lugol's chromoendoscopy allows precise demarcation of the lesion. (**d**) NBI with magnification allows visualization of the intrapapillary papillary loops

and NBI help significantly in the endoscopic characterization. Even though the lesion is well demarcated by AFI, definition of margins is best achieved with LCE, while NBI magnification is particularly useful in the assessment of the vascular pattern, which in this case suggest deep mucosal/early submucosal invasion based on the type V-3 pattern of the intrapapillary capillary loops [19]. Endoscopic resection specimen confirmed invasive OSCC into the muscularis mucosae with no signs of lymph-vascular invasion.

AFI has been extensively investigated for the detection of glandular oesophageal dysplasia and early cancer in Barrett's oesophagus (BO). The rising incidence of oesophageal adenocarcinoma (OAC), the high prevalence of BO in Western populations, the fact that endoscopic surveillance is currently recommended by all major endoscopic societies and the inconspicuous nature of dysplasia and often early adenocarcinoma have prompted enormous amount of research in the last 20 years to pursue novel endoscopic detection modalities for BO dysplasia. Figure 5.3 shows three cases of BE-associated neoplasia where AFI unmask or help demarcation of the endoscopic lesion. The first report on the use of AFI to detect BO-related high-grade dysplasia (HGD) and early OAC showed promising results [20]. In this study, a cohort of 60 patients was evaluated with WLE first and then imaged on AFI mode, followed by random quadratic biopsies according to the Seattle protocol. Of the 22 patients with HGD/early OAC, six were detected by AFI only and only one was missed by AFI and diagnosed on random biopsies only. In this study, AFI had a false-positive rate of 51 %. In order to reduce the false positive rate of AFI, this has been integrated with HR-WLE and NBI magnification into a single endoscopic tri-modal imaging (ETMI) endoscope. This second-generation AFI endoscope has provided the endoscopists with a powerful tool to combine a red-flag technique with high-resolution modalities to discard false-positive signal. ETMI has been evaluated in three subsequent studies led by the group of J. Bergman in Amsterdam. In the first cross-sectional multicentre cohort study ($n=84$), HR-WLE, AFI and AFI-targeted NBI magnification were performed sequentially in the same endoscopy, followed by random biopsies [21]. In total, 30 patients had a final diagnosis of HGD/early EAC, of which 11 were detected by AFI only and missed by HR-WLE and three were diagnosed on random biopsies only (missed by both AFI and HR-WLE). AFI had an 81 % false positive rate, which could be reduced by NBI magnification to 26 %. These encouraging results led to a multicentre trial in tertiary referral centres. This second study with cross-over design, recruited 87 patients referred for workup of inconspicuous HGD. Patients underwent both ETMI endoscopy and standard HR-WLE in a randomized fashion at 6–12 weeks interval [22]. In this study the authors could not demonstrate that AFI within ETMI had a clinical advantage on a per-patient analysis compared to standard HR-WLE with random biopsies, although the yield of HGD and OAC was increased in the biopsies targeted by AFI compared to those targeted by WLE. Finally, the AFI had a false-positive rate 71 %, which could be reduced to 48 % by NBI magnification. In a third study with similar design but based in community hospitals, the authors confirmed the results of the previous cross-over study in that ETMI could not replace the role of random biopsies since 7 of 24 patients with HGD/early OAC were only diagnosed

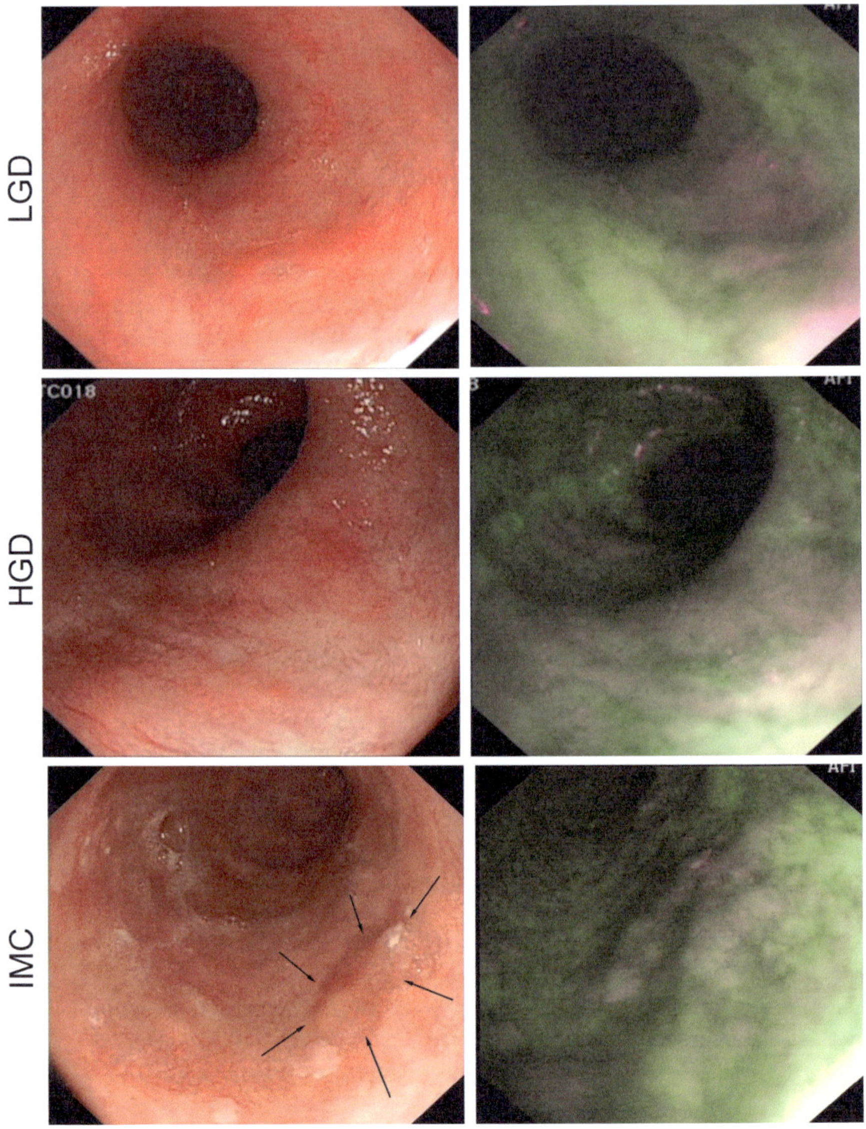

Fig. 5.3 AFI for detection of Barrett's dysplasia. The pictures at the *top* show a case of low-grade dysplasia (LGD) barely visible on *white*-light endoscopy and remarkably un-masked by AFI. Often, however, LGD has *green* signal on AFI. High-grade dysplasia (HGD) can be often difficult to visualize and delineate on conventional *white*-light endoscopy and generally better seen on AFI mode (*middle*). The bottom pictures show and example of intramucosal carcinoma (IMC) at the 4 o'clock position which is well demarcated by AFI

based on the quadratic biopsies [23]. A subsequent retrospective study looked at outcome and treatment modalities of the 371 patients were included in the aforementioned studies [24]. This study showed that AFI has little diagnostic value in that it changed the final diagnosis only in 2 % of patients and informed the selection of therapeutic modality in a similar percentage of cases (2 %). One of the limiting factors of AFI in BO is the high false-positive rate, which can be as high as 80 %. It has been proposed that inflammation might explain a proportion of the AFI false-positive signal. Indeed there is evidence that in the context of gastro-oesophageal reflux disease streaks of AFI-positive signal >1 cm in close proximity with the gastro-oesophageal junction correlate with pathological acid exposure with an overall accuracy of 67 % [25]. Since AFI positivity in superficial neoplasia is also explained by the increased nucleo-cytoplasmic ratio, which in turn at least in part relate to increased nuclear DNA content and mutations at tumour suppressor genes, it has been looked at whether areas of AFI positivity correlate with molecular abnormalities in BO. In a prospective cross-sectional multicentre study that recruited over 200 patients with BO, biopsies taken from areas with AFI positive and negative signal were assessed for a large panel of nine molecular biomarkers commonly associated with dysplasia, including gross DNA abnormalities, loss of tumor suppressor genes, methylation and immunohistochemistry markers [26]. The yield of molecular biomarkers was significantly higher in biopsies from AFI-positive endoscopic locations, which was independent of the presence of histologic dysplasia (Table 5.3). The question is whether a molecular diagnosis assisted by AFI technology can replace the intensive Seattle biopsies protocol, which represents the clinical standard in routine practice. In this study, it was found that a small biomarker panel made of aneuploidy, immunohistochemistry for p53 and cyclin A, on a minimal number of AFI-targeted biopsies has 96 % sensitivity and 89 % specificity for an overall diagnosis of HGD/early OAC. This study demonstrated for the first time that AFI signal is associated to enrichment of molecular biomarkers and has set the precedent for an algorithm were advanced imaging is assisted by molecular diagnosis. In a following cross-sectional study on 55 patients enriched for dysplasia, probe-based confocal laser endomicroscopy (pCLE) was performed on areas of AFI positive signal to achieve a real-time diagnosis of dysplasia [27]. AFI-positive endoscopic locations showed endomicroscopic evidence of dysplasia regardless of the presence of histologic dysplasia. In this cohort, the combination of AFI and pCLE had 96 % sensitivity and 74 % specificity for any grade of dysplasia. These data sug-

Table 5.3 Correlation between AFI signal in BE and molecular biomarkers

	Number of abnormal biomarkers				
AFI appearance	0	1	2	3	*P* value
AFI negative	17 (42.7 %)	12 (31.6 %)	6 (15.8 %)	3 (7.9 %)	0.001
AFI positive	12 (17.9 %)	11 (16.4 %)	24 (35.8 %)	20 (29.9 %)	

The biomarkers showed here represent the three biomarker panel with the best correlation with dysplasia (aneuploidy plus p53 and cyclin A immunohistochemistry)
Data extrapolated from di Pietro et al. [26]

gest that AFI positive signal not associated to dysplasia on targeted biopsies not necessarily is clinically insignificant, since may have a role to direct sampling for molecular tests. In addition, there is a possibility of sampling error on large AFI positive areas which may be better inspected with a narrow field imaging technique such as pCLE to unmask areas of focal dysplasia.

Stomach

The first report on the use of AFI to diagnose neoplasia of the stomach described a cohort of 21 patients with early gastric cancer [12]. It was observed that early intestinal-type gastric cancer arising in the context of gastric atrophy appears as purple magenta signal in a green background, while diffuse type gastric cancer are seen as green signal on a purple background (Fig. 5.4). In this cohort of patients, the diagnostic accuracy of AFI (68 %, 95 % CI 49–88) was superior to WLE (36 %, 95 % CI 16–56), but inferior to conventional chromoendoscopy (91 %, 95 % CI 79–100). Less often early gastric cancer appears as green signal on green

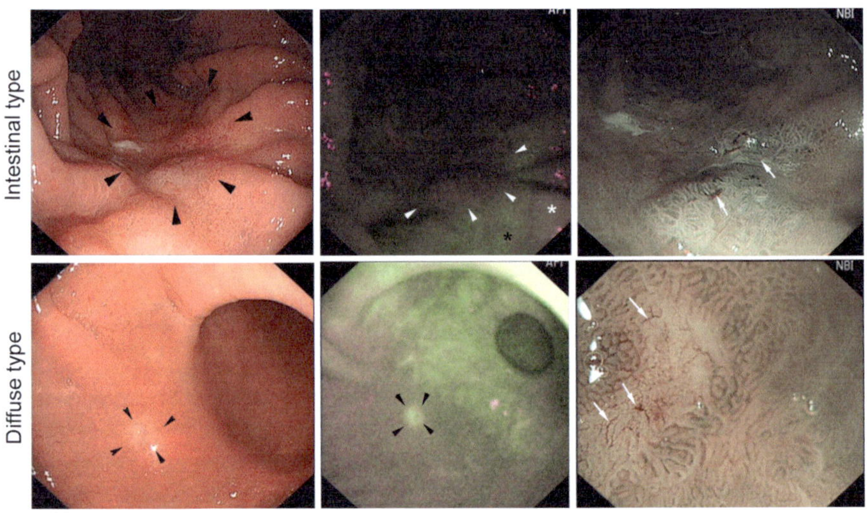

Fig. 5.4 AFI appearance of gastric cancer. A case of intestinal type gastric cancer (*top*) and diffuse gastric cancer (*bottom*) are shown. This intestinal adenocarcinoma appeared as flat/depressed lesion on *white*-light (*left—black arrowheads*). On AFI, the lesion appeared as *red/magenta* signal (*white small arrowheads*) within the *green* background of atrophic gastritis (*black asterisk*). Adjacent to that the healthy mucosa had *red/magenta* colour (*white asterisk*). NBI showed distortion of mucosal pit (*right—white arrows*). Biopsies confirmed poorly differentiated adenocarcinoma. This early diffuse-type gastric cancer appeared as pale area on *white*-light imaging (*left—black arrowheads*) and as *green* in *red* background on AFI (*middle—black arrowheads*). NBI magnification showed irregular neo-vessel formation (*right—white arrows*) with loss of mucosal pit. Endoscopic resection specimen showed a poorly differentiated intramucosal cancer into the muscularis mucosae

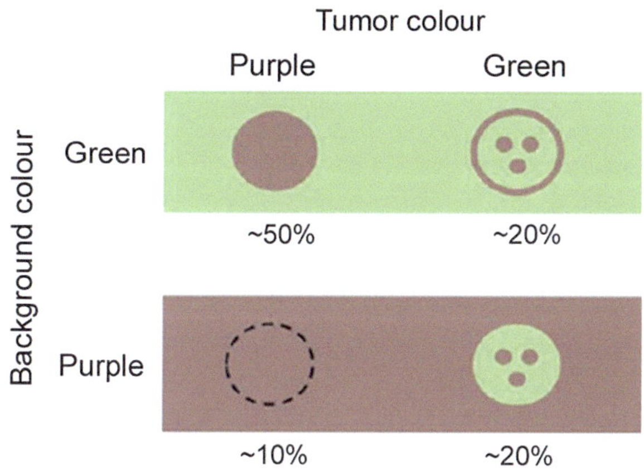

Fig. 5.5 Schematic representation of the different types of AFI appearance of early gastric cancer with the corresponding percentage distribution. *Purple/magenta* tumour within *green* background is the most common finding. Less commonly the tumour has *green* colour with purple spots within, surrounded by *green* or *purple* background. Rarely, the tumour has purple colour and is indistinguishable from the surrounding mucosa. Adapted with permission from Kato M et al. © International Gastric Cancer Association and the Japanese Gastric Cancer Association, 2009 [28]

background, generally demarcated by a rim of purple colour or rarely as purple on a purple background as shown in Fig. 5.5. Other factors can influence the colour of the tumour on AFI, in particular macroscopic features of the lesions and grade of differentiation. Clinical features associated with green appearance are depressed macroscopic type, undifferentiated histological type and purple colour of the background mucosa [28]. In general, AFI does not help demarcate flat/isochromatic lesions already ill-defined by WLE and can be heavily affected by the background inflammation, which could lead to overestimation of the extent of the lesion [12, 29, 30]. On the other hand, the possibility to enhance the contrast at the level of the tumour margin, compared to WLE may help less experienced endoscopists to identify and demarcate subtle or truly inconspicuous lesions. There is evidence that AFI improves diagnostic accuracy from 65 to 80 % and interobserver variability ($\kappa=0.29$ for WLE vs. 0.52 for AFI) for an endoscopic diagnosis of gastric neoplasia by less experienced endoscopists but not expert endoscopists [30]. It has also been suggested that an AFI index derived from the ratio between the green and red band of the AFI endoscopic image can help assess the depth of penetration of the tumour [31]. In this study, autofluorescence images from post-operative cases where split into three bands (green, red and blue) and the ration between the two was calculated. The data showed that higher the ratio to less likely the lesion is to have advanced T stage. This index however has not been replicated in in vivo endoscopic data and currently AFI cannot be utilized in endoscopic practice to estimate the depth of penetration. The second-generation AFI endoscope (ETMI) has also been evaluated in the field of gastric cancer. However, the only study that has addressed the diagnostic gain compared to WLE is a feasibility study on 62 patients at a single academic centre [32]. In this study, AFI alone had 68 % sensitivity and 44 % specificity for the detection and correct characterization of gastric neoplasia. The addition of NBI magnification over WLE and AFI alone improved the diagnostic accuracy both on a per-lesion and per-patient analyses. In particular, ETMI increased the per-patient sensitivity from 68 % for AFI alone to 91 % and the specificity from 44 % for AFI alone to 100 %. Formal cross-over studies however are missing to conclude whether ETMI offers a clinical utility in this setting. AFI can also inform on the presence of pre-neoplastic lesions like inflammation, intestinal metaplasia and gastric atrophy. Differently from other GI tracts, the proximal stomach normally has a purple colour on AFI due to the thickness of the gastric mucosa. The reduction of the thickness of the proximal gastric mucosa in gastric atrophy is associated to a colour switch from purple to green. The presence of a 'green' gastric body has a diagnostic accuracy of 88 % and 81 % for intestinal metaplasia and gastric atrophy, respectively [33]. A classification of the atrophic fundal gastritis has been proposed based on the extent of the green signal in the proximal stomach, whether it does not involve the cardia region (closed-type) or whether it extends to the cardia with different involvement of the corpus (open-type) (Fig. 5.6). The presence of an open-type atrophic fundal gastritis associates with an odds ratio of 4.88 (95 % CI 1.3–18.2) for metachronous gastric cancer, even after eradication of H. pylori. However, this classification can be rather complex to reproduce in endoscopy practice. More practical is targeting biopsies to areas of green colour in the proximal stomach. AFI-targeted histology has a diagnostic accuracy for atrophy and intestinal metaplasia of 88 and 81 %, respectively. A cross-over study evaluated the usefulness of ETMI to diagnose IM in a middle age Chinese cohort of patient ($n=65$) referred for dyspepsia. The use of ETMI had improved the sensitivity of conventional WLE from 34 to 65 % [34].

Colon

The main determinant for differential AF signal in normal vs. neoplastic colon resides in submucosal collagen, while no difference has been found in flavin and NADPH content. As discussed for the upper GI tract, also in the colon thickening of the mucosal layer in adenomatous and malignant lesions exerts a screening effect to the autofluorescence signal from the submucosal collagen. It has been hypothesized that the replacement of collagen by cancer cells could also play a role in reduced autofluorescence of neoplastic lesions [3]. Adenomatous polyps have reduced autofluorescence and appear as purple/magenta on a green background (Video 5.2), whereas hyperplastic polyps have normal AFI signal that has homogeneous green signal similar to the surrounding mucosa (Fig. 5.7) [35, 36]. However, in a cohort of patients with hyperplastic polyposis AFI had only a 65 % diagnostic accuracy for differentiating hyperplastic polyps, sessile serrated adenomas and adenomatous polyps suggesting that assessment of pit pattern and vascular morphology is necessary to assist the differential diagnosis [37]. Studies have showed conflicting results on the usefulness of AFI to improve adenoma detection rate. In a back-to-back study at

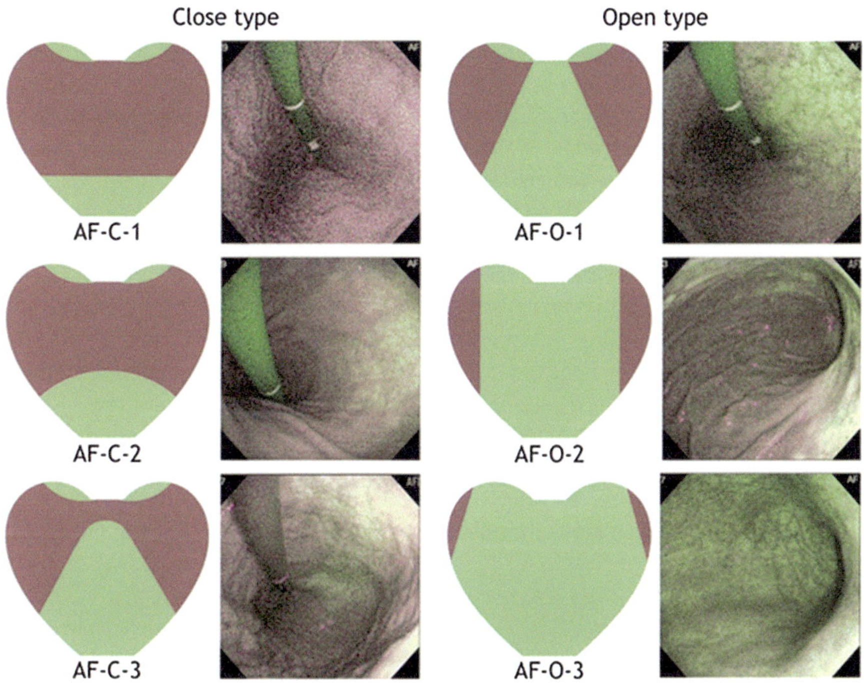

Fig. 5.6 AFI classification of atrophic fundal gastritis. Only the open type extends to the cardia. Three different close-types of atrophic gastritis are described, depending on whether the proximal stomach appears all purple (AF-C-1) or has green colour along the *lower* part of the lesser curve (AF-C-2) or *upper* part of the lesser curve (AF-C-3). Three different open-types are also described, depending on whether the *green* colour extends from the lesser curve to the anterior wall (AF-O-1), to the greater curve (AF-O-2), or extends to the entire proximal stomach (AF-O-3). The open-type on the right associates with increased of metachronous gastric cancer. Adapted with permission from Inoue et al. © Springer, 2009. [33]

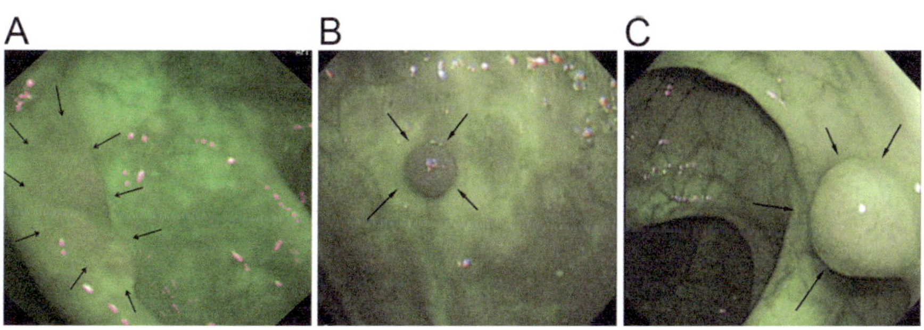

Fig. 5.7 AFI appearance of adenomatous and hyperplastic polyps. Adenomatous polyps generally appear as *red* on a *green* background, regardless of whether they are flat (**a**) or sessile (**b**). Hyperplastic lesions have green signal similar to that of the surrounding mucosa (**c**). Adapted with permission from Song et al. © American Society for Gastrointestinal Endoscopy, 2011 [35]

a single institution 167 patients underwent colonoscopy in a randomized fashion, whereby they received the first endoscopy with either AFI or WLE by a single endoscopist followed by the alternative technique [38]. In this study, AFI led to an increased number of total polyps detected and to a lower miss rate compared to WLE (30 % vs. 49 %, respectively). A second single centre study with similar design looked at the whole colon adenoma detection rate and miss rate by AFI and WLE. In contrast with the previous report, in this study no difference in the adenoma miss-rate was found (20 % for AFI and 29 % for WLE; $p = 0.351$) and the overall accuracy of AFI for a diagnosis of colonic adenoma was only 63 % [39]. Assessment of still images by AFI appears to help non-experienced endoscopist to classify endoscopic lesions, but not experienced endoscopists indicating that AFI is easier to use for polyp characterization in a non-experienced setting. However, a multicentre study in non-academic centres did not confirm that AFI improves the detection rate [40]. In this study, 234 patients were randomized to undergo tandem endoscopies with either ETMI or WLE. In the ETMI group the first colonoscopy was performed with HR-WLE followed by ETMI, whereas in the second group both examinations were performed using SVE. A similar number of additional polyps were found during the second colonoscopy, regardless of whether this was performed by ETMI or SVE, and hence the adenoma miss-rate was similar between the two.

AFI has also been investigated in the setting of ulcerative colitis (UC). In keeping with the evidence in the upper GI tract that inflammation can cause false AFI positivity, in UC there is a progressive decrease in the green signal with increasing severity of the inflammation (Fig. 5.8). AFI may be useful in the identification of inflammation compared to a healthy mucosa based on the progressive decrease of green signal; however, the differentiation of mild from moderate and moderate from

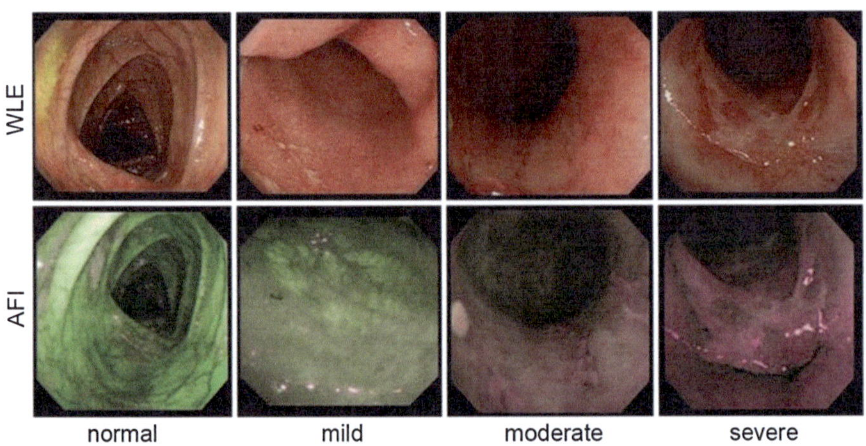

Fig. 5.8 AFI endoscopic appearance of ulcerative colitis with different degree of severity. The AFI view (*bottom*) is compared with the *white*-light endoscopy (WLE) picture (*top*). In ulcerative colitis with increasing degree of inflammation, there is progressive loss of *green* signal. Adapted with permission from Osada et al. [41]. © Baishideng Publishing Group, Inc., 2015

severe colitis is difficult purely based on the AFI appearance (Fig. 5.8) [41]. Perhaps more interesting is the role of AFI in the detection of neoplasia in patients with UC. In a single centre study with tandem design, 50 patients underwent a back to back colonoscopy and were randomized to receive either an AFI or WLE as first inspection technique at each colonic segment [42]. The results were striking: (a) the sensitivity of AFI for UC-associated dysplasia was 100 %; (b) the second inspection by AFI identified three additional neoplastic lesions, while the second WLE look none; (c) the neoplasia miss-rate was 0 % for AFI and 50 % for WLE. Although promising, the results of this study need to be confirmed in multicentre large studies and currently there is not sufficient data to conclude on the usefulness of AFI in routine surveillance of patients with UC. One of the drawbacks of AFI is that while it correctly identifies protruding neoplasia, flat dysplasia is more difficult to detect as it can be characterized by normal AF signal [43].

Safety and Cost Considerations

Similarly to other electronic chromoendoscopic techniques, AFI has an excellent safety profile. This stems from the fact that AFI does not involve harmful radiations and does not require administration of topic or intravenous dyes. Current ETMI endoscopes have the AFI system integrated in a single apparatus together with HRE and magnified NBI, hence AFI can be interchanged with two other imaging technologies without the need of additional intubations. In addition, the button switch makes the transition among these imaging modalities quick and easy to control by the endoscopist without added time related to topic spray of dye. In keeping with these features, available literature did not show any safety issues related to the use of AFI in screening and workup of GI neoplasia.

AFI endoscopes on average are 20 % more expensive than conventional high-resolution endoscopes but are compatible with standard Olympus video processors. This implies that no significantly increased capital costs investment is required to equip endoscopy units with the AFI technology provided that geographic location allows availability of the Lucera platform, which currently is only marketed in Japan and United Kingdom. This has clearly important implications in terms of accessibility to the technology in a world-wide perspective. There are no proper cost-effectiveness studies that have been conducted. Perhaps, the most robust literature available concerns the use of AFI in dysplasia detection in Barrett's oesophagus; hence, it is easier to evaluate potential economic issues within this context. As extensively discussed in the relevant section, despite early enthusiasm on the increased detection of dysplasia in BO, the pooled analysis published by Boerwinkel et al. has showed that the use of AFI-targeted biopsies in comparison with the Seattle protocol biopsies has a limited clinical value of 2 % only [24]. On the basis of this evidence, it is unlikely that the routine use of AFI in BO surveillance will prove to be cost-effective. The multicentre cross-sectional study on the combined used of AFI and biomarkers on a BO population enriched for dysplasia [26] suggested that the use of AFI in combination with molecular tests, while it did not improve the diagnostic value compared to white-light endoscopy with random biopsies, it may potentially increase cost-effectiveness as there was a fourfold reduction in the number of biopsies required. However, the cost implications of the added tissue biomarkers were not evaluated in this study; therefore, further studies are required to address this issue.

Conclusion and Future Directions

The available literature does not provide definite evidence that AFI increases detection rate of premalignant and early malignant lesions in the GI tract. Therefore, AFI cannot be recommended in routine endoscopy practice. However, research studies support the use of AFI as imaging adjunct to refine visualization and demarcation of neoplastic lesions.

In Barrett's oesophagus, AFI allows detection of a higher number of lesions with HGD/early cancer, but the per-patient diagnostic gain is limited especially in unselected populations [24]. In addition, the high false-positive rate remains the main issue, as it may significantly increase the number of targeted biopsies reducing cost-effectiveness of surveillance. For this reason, AFI requires an additional modality to help discard the false-positive areas. NBI magnification can be used within the ETMI for this purpose; however, even after detailed inspection with optical zoom and NBI the false-positive rate remains high (~40 %) [23]. Furthermore, NBI magnification still misclassifies as normal some HGD areas and a significant proportion of lesions with LGD. Probe-based confocal laser endomicroscopy (pCLE) can be an alternative modality to characterize AFI-positive signal, and there is evidence that pCLE has better sensitivity than magnification NBI especially for LGD [27]. In the future, multimodal imaging is likely to be the most effective approach; however, the best combination of endoscopic techniques remains to be established. Larger studies testing the combination of AFI and pCLE are required.

In the stomach, AFI can be a useful adjunct to help characterize the cancer field effect and the risk related to the background mucosa. In the field of atrophic gastritis, a wide-spread green signal in the proximal stomach can be used as screening tool to prompt biopsies [33]. Most of the data available come from Asian studies; hence, the applicability of this imaging approach to the Western populations remains to be assessed. In terms of detection of early neoplasia despite encouraging preliminary results for ETMI, the evidence is scarce and overall a step behind if compared to the studies in Barrett's neoplasia, as only a small series on an enriched population is available [32]. However, as in the oesophagus, AFI can be a useful imaging adjunct to demarcate gastric early cancer and inform endoscopic resections.

In the colon, the evidence does not support routine use of AFI to reduce the adenoma miss rate. Interesting preliminary results would encourage more research in the field of ulcerative colitis, where AFI could be a useful tool to reveal mild inflammation and to assist detection of dysplasia.

At the moment, there are two promising research avenues. First, there is initial evidence that AFI may help enrich the yield of molecular biomarkers in BO [26]. This is an area that needs further investigation in the oesophagus as well as in other GI pathologies such as atrophic gastritis and UC. Even though it is accepted that AFI has high false-positive rate, a possibility exists that a proportion of false positive signal based on histological assessment may carry useful molecular information, which could be used to aid the overall diagnosis. A second fertile ground of research is the use of AFI within a molecular imaging approach. In the context of BO, AFI has been tested ex vivo in conjunction with a fluorescent probe to unmask areas of inconspicuous neoplasia [44]. In this study, wheat germ agglutinin (WGA) linked to a fluorescent dye was sprayed on the mucosal surface of resected oesophagi and imaged with an AFI endoscope. Since WGA loses affinity in the dysplasia to adenocarcinoma sequence, a reduction of the AFI signal was seen in neoplastic tissue in keeping with reduced binding of WGA onto the abnormal mucosal surface. One limitation here is that the oesophagus has high autofluorescence, which can hamper in vivo the detection of specific fluorescence. In organs or conditions with reduced background fluorescence, like inflamed colon in UC and proximal stomach, the AFI-based molecular imaging approach could still prove a viable solution and worth further investigation.

References

1. Tajiri H. Autofluorescence endoscopy for the gastrointestinal tract. Proc Jpn Acad Ser B Phys Biol Sci. 2007;83(8):248–55.
2. Konda V, et al. Enhanced imaging in the GI tract: spectroscopy and optical coherence tomography. Gastrointest Endosc. 2013;78(4):568–73.
3. Izuishi K, Tajiri H, Fujii T, Boku N, Ohtsu A, Ohnishi T, et al. The histological basis of detection of adenoma and cancer in the colon by autofluorescence endoscopic imaging. Endoscopy. 1999;31(7):511–6.
4. Ragunath K. Autofluorescence endoscopy—not much gain after all? Endoscopy. 2007;39(11): 1021–2.
5. Mayinger B, Horner P, Jordan M, Gerlach C, Horbach T, Hohenberger W, et al. Light-induced autofluorescence spectroscopy for the endoscopic detection of esophageal cancer. Gastrointest Endosc. 2001;54(2):195–201.
6. Kara MA, Smits ME, Rosmolen WD, Bultje AC, Ten Kate FJ, Fockens P, et al. A randomized crossover study comparing light-induced fluorescence endoscopy with standard videoendoscopy for the detection of early neoplasia in Barrett's esophagus. Gastrointest Endosc. 2005;61(6):671–8.
7. Abe S, Izuishi K, Tajiri H, Kinoshita T, Matsuoka T. Correlation of in vitro autofluorescence endoscopy images with histopathologic findings in stomach cancer. Endoscopy. 2000;32(4): 281–6.
8. Kobayashi M, Tajiri H, Seike E, Shitaya M, Tounou S, Mine M, et al. Detection of early gastric cancer by a real-time autofluorescence imaging system. Cancer Lett. 2001;165(2):155–9.
9. Mayinger B, Jordan M, Horbach T, Horner P, Gerlach C, Mueller S, et al. Evaluation of in vivo endoscopic autofluorescence spectroscopy in gastric cancer. Gastrointest Endosc. 2004;59(2): 191–8.

10. Ohkawa A, Miwa H, Namihisa A, Kobayashi O, Nakaniwa N, Ohkusa T, et al. Diagnostic performance of light-induced fluorescence endoscopy for gastric neoplasms. Endoscopy. 2004;36(6):515–21.
11. Brand S, Stepp H, Ochsenkuhn T, Baumgartner R, Baretton G, Holl J, et al. Detection of colonic dysplasia by light-induced fluorescence endoscopy: a pilot study. Int J Colorectal Dis. 1999;14(1):63–8.
12. Uedo N, Iishi H, Tatsuta M, Yamada T, Ogiyama H, Imanaka K, et al. A novel videoendoscopy system by using autofluorescence and reflectance imaging for diagnosis of esophagogastric cancers. Gastrointest Endosc. 2005;62(4):521–8.
13. Tschanz ER. Do 40% of patients resected for Barrett esophagus with high-grade dysplasia have unsuspected adenocarcinoma? Arch Pathol Lab Med. 2005;129(2):177–80.
14. Imaizumi K, Harada Y, Wakabayashi N, Yamaoka Y, Konishi H, Dai P, et al. Dual-wavelength excitation of mucosal autofluorescence for precise detection of diminutive colonic adenomas. Gastrointest Endosc. 2012;75(1):110–7.
15. Arnold M, Soerjomataram I, Ferlay J, Forman D. Global incidence of oesophageal cancer by histological subtype in 2012. Gut. 2015;64(3):381–7.
16. Nagami Y, Tominaga K, Machida H, Nakatani M, Kameda N, Sugimori S, et al. Usefulness of non-magnifying narrow-band imaging in screening of early esophageal squamous cell carcinoma: a prospective comparative study using propensity score matching. Am J Gastroenterol. 2014;109(6):845–54.
17. Yoshida Y, Goda K, Tajiri H, Urashima M, Yoshimura N, Kato T. Assessment of novel endoscopic techniques for visualizing superficial esophageal squamous cell carcinoma: autofluorescence and narrow-band imaging. Dis Esophagus. 2009;22(5):439–46.
18. Suzuki H, Saito Y, Oda I, Kikuchi T, Kiriyama S, Fukunaga S. Comparison of narrowband imaging with autofluorescence imaging for endoscopic visualization of superficial squamous cell carcinoma lesions of the esophagus. Diagn Ther Endosc. 2012;2012:507597.
19. Inoue H, Kaga M, Ikeda H, Sato C, Sato H, Minami H, et al. Magnification endoscopy in esophageal squamous cell carcinoma: a review of the intrapapillary capillary loop classification. Ann Gastroenterol. 2015;28(1):41–8.
20. Kara MA, Peters FP, Ten Kate FJ, Van Deventer SJ, Fockens P, Bergman JJ. Endoscopic video autofluorescence imaging may improve the detection of early neoplasia in patients with Barrett's esophagus. Gastrointest Endosc. 2005;61(6):679–85.
21. Curvers WL, Singh R, Song LM, Wolfsen HC, Ragunath K, Wang K, et al. Endoscopic trimodal imaging for detection of early neoplasia in Barrett's oesophagus: a multi-centre feasibility study using high-resolution endoscopy, autofluorescence imaging and narrow band imaging incorporated in one endoscopy system. Gut. 2008;57(2):167–72.
22. Curvers WL, Herrero LA, Wallace MB, Wong Kee Song LM, Ragunath K, Wolfsen HC, et al. Endoscopic tri-modal imaging is more effective than standard endoscopy in identifying early-stage neoplasia in Barrett's esophagus. Gastroenterology. 2010;139(4):1106–14.
23. Curvers WL, van Vilsteren FG, Baak LC, Bohmer C, Mallant-Hent RC, Naber AH, et al. Endoscopic trimodal imaging versus standard video endoscopy for detection of early Barrett's neoplasia: a multicenter, randomized, crossover study in general practice. Gastrointest Endosc. 2011;73(2):195–203.
24. Boerwinkel DF, Holz JA, Kara MA, Meijer SL, Wallace MB, Wong Kee Song LM, et al. Effects of autofluorescence imaging on detection and treatment of early neoplasia in patients with Barrett's esophagus. Clin Gastroenterol Hepatol. 2014;12(5):774–81.
25. Wang W, Uedo N, Yang Y, Peng L, Bai D, Lu Z, et al. Autofluorescence imaging endoscopy for predicting acid reflux in patients with gastroesophageal reflux disease. J Gastroenterol Hepatol. 2014;29(7):1442–8.
26. di Pietro M, Boerwinkel DF, Shariff MK, Liu X, Telakis E, Lao-Sirieix P, et al. The combination of autofluorescence endoscopy and molecular biomarkers is a novel diagnostic tool for dysplasia in Barrett's oesophagus. Gut. 2015;64(1):49–56.
27. di Pietro M, Bird-Lieberman EL, Liu X, Nuckcheddy-Grant T, Bertani H, O'Donovan M, et al. Autofluorescence-directed confocal endomicroscopy in combination with a 3-biomarker panel

can inform management decisions in Barrett's esophagus. Am J Gastroenterol. 2015;110(11):1549–58.
28. Kato M, Uedo N, Ishihara R, Kizu T, Chatani R, Inoue T, et al. Analysis of the color patterns of early gastric cancer using an autofluorescence imaging video endoscopy system. Gastric Cancer. 2009;12(4):219–24.
29. Lee JH, Cho JY, Choi MG, Kim JS, Choi KD, Lee YC, et al. Usefulness of autofluorescence imaging for estimating the extent of gastric neoplastic lesions: a prospective multicenter study. Gut Liver. 2008;2(3):174–9.
30. Tada K, Oda I, Yokoi C, Taniguchi T, Sakamoto T, Suzuki H, et al. Pilot study on clinical effectiveness of autofluorescence imaging for early gastric cancer diagnosis by less experienced endoscopists. Diagn Ther Endosc. 2011;2011:419136.
31. Otani A, Amano Y, Koshino K, Takahashi Y, Mishima Y, Imaoka H, et al. Is autofluorescence imaging endoscopy useful for determining the depth of invasion in gastric cancer? Digestion. 2010;81(2):96–103.
32. Kato M, Kaise M, Yonezawa J, Goda K, Toyoizumi H, Yoshimura N, et al. Trimodal imaging endoscopy may improve diagnostic accuracy of early gastric neoplasia: a feasibility study. Gastrointest Endosc. 2009;70(5):899–906.
33. Inoue T, Uedo N, Ishihara R, Kawaguchi T, Kawada N, Chatani R, et al. Autofluorescence imaging videoendoscopy in the diagnosis of chronic atrophic fundal gastritis. J Gastroenterol. 2010;45(1):45–51.
34. So J, Rajnakova A, Chan YH, Tay A, Shah N, Salto-Tellez M, et al. Endoscopic tri-modal imaging improves detection of gastric intestinal metaplasia among a high-risk patient population in Singapore. Dig Dis Sci. 2013;58(12):3566–75.
35. Song LM, Banerjee S, Desilets D, Diehl DL, Farraye FA, Kaul V, et al. Autofluorescence imaging. Gastrointest Endosc. 2011;73(4):647–50.
36. Wang TD, Crawford JM, Feld MS, Wang Y, Itzkan I, Van Dam J. In vivo identification of colonic dysplasia using fluorescence endoscopic imaging. Gastrointest Endosc. 1999;49(4 Pt 1): 447–55.
37. Boparai KS, van den Broek FJ, van Eeden S, Fockens P, Dekker E. Hyperplastic polyposis syndrome: a pilot study for the differentiation of polyps by using high-resolution endoscopy, autofluorescence imaging, and narrow-band imaging. Gastrointest Endosc. 2009;70(5): 947–55.
38. Matsuda T, Saito Y, Fu KI, Uraoka T, Kobayashi N, Nakajima T, et al. Does autofluorescence imaging videoendoscopy system improve the colonoscopic polyp detection rate?—a pilot study. Am J Gastroenterol. 2008;103(8):1926–32.
39. van den Broek FJ, van Soest EJ, Naber AH, van Oijen AH, Mallant-Hent R, Bohmer CJ, et al. Combining autofluorescence imaging and narrow-band imaging for the differentiation of adenomas from non-neoplastic colonic polyps among experienced and non-experienced endoscopists. Am J Gastroenterol. 2009;104(6):1498–507.
40. Kuiper T, van den Broek FJ, Naber AH, van Soest EJ, Scholten P, Mallant-Hent R, et al. Endoscopic trimodal imaging detects colonic neoplasia as well as standard video endoscopy. Gastroenterology. 2011;140(7):1887–94.
41. Osada T, Arakawa A, Sakamoto N, Ueyama H, Shibuya T, Ogihara T, et al. Autofluorescence imaging endoscopy for identification and assessment of inflammatory ulcerative colitis. World J Gastroenterol. 2011;17(46):5110–6.
42. van den Broek FJ, Fockens P, van Eeden S, Reitsma JB, Hardwick JC, Stokkers PC, et al. Endoscopic tri-modal imaging for surveillance in ulcerative colitis: randomised comparison of high-resolution endoscopy and autofluorescence imaging for neoplasia detection; and evaluation of narrow-band imaging for classification of lesions. Gut. 2008;57(8):1083–9.
43. Matsumoto T, Nakamura S, Moriyama T, Hirahashi M, Iida M. Autofluorescence imaging colonoscopy for the detection of dysplastic lesions in ulcerative colitis: a pilot study. Colorectal Dis. 2010;12(10 Online):e291–7.
44. Bird-Lieberman EL, Neves AA, Lao-Sirieix P, O'Donovan M, Novelli M, Lovat LB, et al. Molecular imaging using fluorescent lectins permits rapid endoscopic identification of dysplasia in Barrett's esophagus. Nat Med. 2012;18(2):315–21.

Chapter 6
Luminal Confocal Laser Endomicroscopy

Christopher D. Atkinson and Satish K. Singh

Technology Overview

Confocal laser endomicroscopy (CLE) is a real-time, in vivo optical imaging modality that can be used to supplement standard as well as image-enhanced endoscopy. Guided by widefield views, CLE can help to identify and characterize living tissues in situ at the microscopic level, within the mucosa of the luminal gastrointestinal tract during endoscopic procedures.

Micro-scale images are obtained by passing a 488 nm collimated laser beam through a focusing lens into the mucosa to excite endogenous and/or exogenous fluorophores. Typically, mucosal background autofluorescence is weak in the gastrointestinal tract due to a low content of the most common endogenous fluorophores at this wavelength, i.e., collagen, elastin, NADPH, flavins, and lipofuscin. As such, performing CLE requires the administration of an exogenous fluorescent contrast dye, most commonly sodium fluorescein. Anionic fluorescein is a phthalic dye molecule with a molecular weight of 332.31 g/mol and a fluorescence excitation peak of 488 nm with emission detectable between 505 and 750 nm [1].

C.D. Atkinson, M.D.
Section of Gastroenterology & Hepatology, Department of Medicine
VA Boston Healthcare System, 150 South Huntington Avenue, GI-111,
Boston, MA 02130, USA

S.K. Singh, M.D., A.G.A.F. (✉)
Section of Gastroenterology and Hepatology, Department of Medicine,
VA Boston Healthcare System, 150 South Huntington Avenue,
GI-111, Boston, MA 02130, USA

Section of Gastroenterology, Department of Medicine, Boston University
School of Medicine and Department of Biomedical Engineering,
Boston University College of Engineering, Suite 504,
650 Albany Street, Boston, MA 02118, USA
e-mail: singhsk@bu.edu; Satish.singh@va.gov

V.J.A. Konda, I. Waxman (eds.), *Endoscopic Imaging Techniques and Tools*,
DOI 10.1007/978-3-319-30053-5_6

Because it is highly water-soluble, intravenously administered fluorescein concentrations are highest within blood vessels, intercellular spaces, and the cytoplasm—but not the nuclei—of epithelial cells.

Upon excitation of the contrast, fluorescently emitted photons are scattered in all directions. However, using the principle of pinhole-limited-rejection, photons travelling in the reverse path to the incident laser beam are returned through a small aperture. The pinhole serves to filter or "reject" photons scattered in all other directions, thus serving to remove out-of-focus light. The laser is systematically scanned in two dimensions over a region of tissue, and light that returns from fluorescence emission through the pinhole is detected. Consequently, an image, represented by a monochromatic intensity map, is derived from a single focal plane within the tissue. The use of a miniaturized water-immersion microscope objective permits a near 1000-fold magnification of mucosal structures in an *en face* orientation (i.e., parallel to the muscularis) at a depth determined by the fixed or variable working distance of a miniaturized microscope objective. Based on the relative distribution of fluorescein contrast, tissue architecture at the cellular and subcellular level can be seen within the field of view of the objective. In other words, microscopic structures themselves are not visualized by CLE, per se, but rather are inferred from the distribution of fluorescein among structural compartments. Fluorescence CLE has proven particularly useful for identifying neoplastic, vascular, and inflammatory changes in the luminal GI tract. In particular, CLE has found emerging roles in the detection and classification of esophageal, gastric, and colorectal neoplasia as well as in the assessment of inflammatory bowel disease.

Features of CLE Systems

At present, there are two variants of CLE used clinically: endoscope-based confocal laser endomicroscopy (eCLE) and probe-based confocal endomicroscopy (pCLE). As seen in Fig. 6.1, the eCLE system incorporates a laser scanning confocal microscope objective into the distal tip of a familiar dedicated video endoscope, thus enabling dual functionality as a traditional endoscope and as a fluorescence endomicroscope (EC3870K; Pentax, Tokyo, Japan). By employing micromechanical devices within the microscope objective, much like a benchtop confocal microscope, eCLE is capable of rendering two-dimensional images in a single focal plane (x and y axes) at variable depths (z-axis) within the mucosa. A contrast agent is required which is excited by 488 nm laser light. Because a water-immersion objective is used, microscope mode requires that the objective come into direct contact with the mucosa. To do this, the terminal face of the endoscope is placed directly against the tissue in question, thus temporarily obscuring widefield endoscopic views. As such, tandem—but not simultaneous—widefield endoscopy and fluorescence endomicroscopy are enabled. Suction via the scope's accessory channel is applied to affix the scope to the mucosa transiently to dampen motion artifacts. A 475×475 μm image, with a lateral resolution of 0.7 μm, is obtained with an

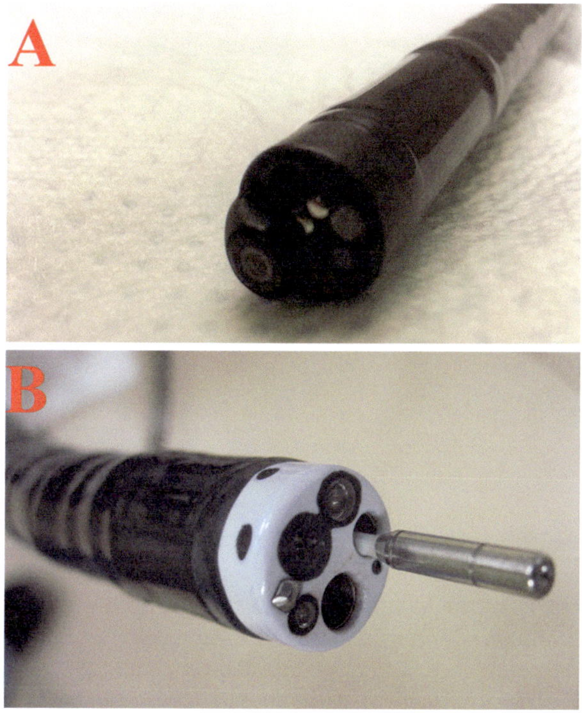

Fig. 6.1 (**a**) With endoscope-based confocal endomicroscopy (eCLE) the objective is built into the distal tip of the endoscope. (**b**) The distal tip of a probe-based confocal laser endomicroscopy (pCLE) miniprobe is threaded through any 2.8 mm or larger accessory port of a standard endoscope

adjustable depth of penetration along the *z*-axis into the mucosa from 0 to 250 μm. Images can be obtained at a rate of 0.8–1.4 frames per second [2].

Probe-based CLE (Cellvizio™; Mauna Kea Technologies, Inc., Paris, France) is a standalone confocal system that is mediated by a series of interchangeable application-specific "miniprobes" designed to be passed via a 2.8 mm or larger accessory channel of virtually any endoscope (Fig. 6.2). Miniprobes are comprised of fiberoptic imaging bundles containing tens of thousands of fibers interfaced with a common freestanding confocal laser scanning unit and terminated by a fixed working-distance fluorescence microscope objective at the distal tip. In the laser scanning unit, a 488 nm laser source is focused into a scanning module which uses a series of lenses and two perpendicular mirrors to focus the beam into each fiber of the imaging bundle. Laser light travels through the fibers to excite the tissue. Fluorescent light is then emitted back into the imaging bundle and collected in a detector, one fiber at a time. This information is sent to a computer system, which then reconstructs the image. For luminal gastrointestinal endoscopy, placement of the probe tip is guided in real time by the endoscopic view. As such, unlike eCLE, pCLE is observed simultaneously with endoscopic views permitting dynamic microscopy within the context of macroscopic surroundings. Miniprobes are considered a consumable item in that they can be reprocessed up to 20 times before they must be replaced.

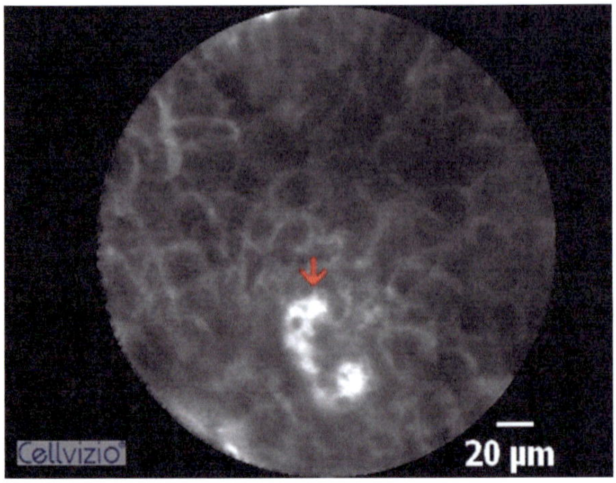

Fig. 6.2 Normal squamous cells in the esophagus are flat and scale-like, without any apparent crypts or villi. Bright blood vessels, or intrapapillary capillary loops, may be seen in the papillae (*red arrow*). By definition, squamous epithelium does not contain any columnar cells, glands, or goblet cells

Unlike the eCLE platform, pCLE probes have a fixed imaging depth of 40–70 μm depending on the miniprobe selected. Field of view ranges from 240 × 240 μm to 600 × 600 μm with lateral resolutions of 1 μm to 3.5 μm, respectively, based on the miniprobe selected. Images are captured at 12 frames per second and presented to the operator as near-video rate microscopic images in real time.

The advantages of eCLE are a high resolution, wider field of view and adjustable imaging depth: eCLE is also fully reprocessable and thus does not incur costs for consumables beyond the initial capital investment. Advantages of pCLE are the ability to observe simultaneous microscopic and endoscopic views in real time, compatibility with virtually any endoscope, and a frame-rate that enables real-time videos of novel in vivo dynamic processes such as microvascular blood flow. Because it is a standalone system, pCLE can be used ad hoc in conjunction with any state-of-the-art endoscope or probe-based technology to affect true multimodal imaging. The disadvantages of both systems compared to standard endoscopy include a restricted field of view due to the point-source nature of endomicroscopy, additional costs for the technology, the need for an exogenous contrast agent, added time for targeting and image interpretation, intra-observer variability, and the not-insignificant technical and interpretation learning curves involved [3].

Groundbreaking work with eCLE proved the concept that fluorescence microscopy could be incorporated into an endoscope and used clinically in the upper and lower GI tract [4]. During endoscopy, eCLE enabled "virtual biopsies" by visualizing the tissue architecture and blood flow in real time [4, 5]. With such capabilities, supplementing standard endoscopic procedures with CLE has the potential to change current diagnostic paradigms for a variety of diseases of the luminal gastrointestinal tract. The ability to perform "real-time histology," in theory, improves the diagnostic yield of a procedure by enabling the endoscopist to find and biopsy regions that are more likely to harbor abnormal tissue. Additionally, with training, endoscopists can make real-time decisions regarding management, potentially eliminating delays in care and repeat endoscopies which are de rigueur when tissue is sent for ex vivo histopathology.

Key Clinical Indications

Barrett's Esophagus and Esophageal Adenocarcinoma

Dysplasia Surveillance in Barrett's Esophagus

At present, endoscopic surveillance of patients with Barrett's metaplasia is the best option available to detect and treat dysplasia or intra-epithelial cancer in its early stages, prior to progression to invasive adenocarcinoma. Practically speaking, the current standard for monitoring patients with Barrett's metaplasia, as outlined by the Seattle Protocol [6], is cumbersome and ripe for improvement. The Seattle Protocol entails evaluation every 3–5 years under white light endoscopy to obtain targeted and random four-quadrant biopsies every 1–2 cm within the Barrett's segment [6]. For biopsy findings of dysplasia, intensive surveillance every 3–12 months or definitive treatment plus continued surveillance is required [6]. Needless to say, the time-intensive and biopsy-intensive nature of the Seattle Protocol is associated with low rates of adherence to guidelines [7, 8]. Moreover, the mistargeting of endoscopically inapparent dysplasia on random biopsies likely reduces the effectiveness of preventive surveillance [7, 8]. Frequent biopsies can also lead to reparative fibrosis that can render subsequent endoscopic therapy problematic. As such, there is a need to improve the diagnostic efficiency of surveillance in Barrett's metaplasia.

To this end, advanced imaging with targeting can improve sensitivity and reduce the number of biopsies necessary for the detection of Barrett's dysplasia. A randomized controlled prospective double-blind study showed that targeting biopsies with eCLE doubled the diagnostic yield of dysplasia compared to high definition white light endoscopy with random Seattle Protocol biopsies [9]. Subsequent larger controlled studies with both eCLE and pCLE have extended this observation. In a multicenter, randomized controlled trial of 101 consecutive patients with Barrett's Esophagus, adding pCLE to high definition white light endoscopy with narrow band imaging increased the sensitivity for dysplasia from 45.0 to 75.8 %, with a minor reduction in specificity from 88.2 to 84.2 % [10]. Moreover, a subsequent prospective, single-blinded multicenter randomized controlled trial of 192 patients comparing high definition white light endoscopy with random biopsies to high definition white light endoscopy plus eCLE with targeted biopsies showed that eCLE increased the yield of neoplasia from 7 to 34 % and would have obviated biopsies in 65 % of patients without underdiagnosing any dysplasia [11]. Thus, high confidence CLE readings that exclude dysplasia in a region of interest identified on widefield views may be able to obviate biopsies [12, 13].

The decision to forgo biopsy based on pCLE requires a very high level of confidence. Given the risk of leaving potentially dysplastic or neoplastic tissues behind without taking a biopsy, an approach must achieve a high sensitivity and high negative predictive value. Performance thresholds have been suggested by the American Society of Gastrointestinal Endoscopy's Preservation and Incorporation of Valuable Endoscopic Innovations (PIVI) on Barrett's surveillance where image-guided biopsies should have a per-patient sensitivity of >90 %, a negative predictive value of >98 % for detecting high-grade dysplasia or early adenocarcinoma, and a specificity of 80 % to enable a reduction in the number of biopsies over the Seattle Protocol [14]. CLE approaches these performance metrics and may permit it to replace random biopsies for the surveillance of Barrett's esophagus.

Guiding Endoscopic Eradication Therapy

CLE may also have a role in guiding treatment when dysplasia is found. Given the increasing number of well-tolerated endoscopic treatment options that prevent progression to Barrett's adenocarcinoma, detected dysplasia warrants consideration for endoscopic mucosal resection, radio frequency ablation, cryoablation, and/or photodynamic therapy as appropriate [6]. Preliminary indications are that CLE may also be useful for assessing the completeness of eradication and/or resection of Barrett's mucosa during treatment: in a small case series, pCLE revealed lesions not otherwise recognized and was used to assess for residual dysplasia at resection margins, thus enabling decisions to perform and/or extend endoscopic mucosal resection in real-time [15]. It should be noted, however, that assessing post-resection margins may be difficult due to dye extravasation and cautery artifact.

In addition to the potential utility of pCLE *during* endoscopic treatment for Barrett's esophagus, a related area of investigation involves the use of pCLE in identifying residual dysplasia *following* endoscopic eradication therapy. In a randomized controlled trial comparing high definition white light endoscopy to high definition white light endoscopy plus pCLE, there was no significant difference in the detection of residual BE or neoplasia following radio frequency ablation treatments [16]. However, this may have been due to an unexpectedly high rate of residual lesions resulting in an insufficient sample size to power this study adequately [2, 16]. In addition, an imaging depth of 40–70 μm may not be optimal for neoplasia detection in post-radio frequency ablation patients, as potentially dysplastic glands can occur beneath the neosquamous epithelium [17].

Gastric Adenocarcinoma

Chronic gastric injury, inflammation, infection with Helicobacter pylori, and atrophy are associated with the development of gastric intestinal metaplasia (GIM), which can degenerate into dysplasia and ultimately adenocarcinoma [18].

The presence of GIM is associated with a ten-fold higher relative risk of developing gastric cancer [19] and, as such, chronic atrophic gastritis, GIM, and dysplasia are considered precancerous lesions [20].

As a result, in countries with a high prevalence of gastric cancer such as Japan and South Korea, regular screening for gastric cancer typically commences at age 40 [21] with endoscopy being preferred over radiological imaging for high-risk individuals [19]. There is a crucial, largely unmet need to identify mucosa with the potential to become dysplastic or cancerous. White light endoscopy alone is neither sensitive nor specific for this purpose, and the large surface area of the stomach cannot be surveyed adequately using a random biopsy protocol. Therefore, it is desirable to be able to identify and biopsy regions that are likeliest to harbor premalignant lesions. Widefield imaging modalities used to help identify metaplastic or dysplastic tissue include narrow band imaging [22] and dye spray chromoendoscopy [23]. Unlike CLE, however, these modalities do not permit examination of tissue in vivo at the microscopic level.

CLE has shown promise for identifying microscopic changes in the epithelium associated with GIM and dysplasia. In a prospective study of 132 patients, eCLE identified specific gastric pit patterns that correlated to gastric cancer on index pathology with a sensitivity and specificity of 90.0 % and 99.4 %, respectively [24]. In a prospective study of 53 patients, eCLE was able to detect the presence of GIM with a sensitivity and specificity of 98 % and 95 %, respectively, compared to conventional endoscopy which detected GIM with a sensitivity and specificity of 37 % and 92 %, respectively [25]. Furthermore, pCLE has shown promise for defining the borders of intramucosal gastric cancer as well. In a prospective study of 46 patients undergoing endoscopic submucosal dissection or endoscopic mucosal resection for known gastric neoplasia, pCLE was able to identify the extent of neoplastic tissue accurately in 91 % of the cases [26]. These studies demonstrate that CLE can play a role in the early detection, prevention, and endoscopic treatment of gastric adenocarcinoma in high-risk patients.

Augmenting Endoscopic Mucosal Resection in the Colon

Endoscopic mucosal resection (EMR) is a non-surgical treatment for removing large precancerous polyps and early-stage intramucosal cancers in the colon [27, 28]. There are two uses for CLE in EMR: the first is to define accurately the margins of large flat colonic polyps prior to resection, and the second for post-resection surveillance to obviate the need for repeated colonoscopies [13, 27].

Following EMR of advanced polyps, close follow-up is required, especially following piecemeal removal [29] where the recurrence rate can be as high as 55 % [29]. Thus, repeat colonoscopy is recommended in 2–6 months [30] in order to biopsy EMR scars for histopathological assessment. If residual neoplasia is found, the patient must undergo yet another colonoscopy for removal and/or ablation. A shortcoming of this management paradigm is the inadequate sensitivity of sampling methods during follow-up colonoscopy. Virtual chromoendoscopy (narrow band imaging and Fuji Intelligent Color Enhancement) can be used to enhance detection of residual neoplasia [27]. However, in a prospective study of 92 patients, virtual chromoendoscopy alone had a sensitivity, specificity, positive predictive value, and negative predictive value of only 72 %, 77 %, 49 %, and 91 %, respectively [27]. Supplementing virtual chromoendoscopy with pCLE improved these values to 97 %, 77 %, 55 %, and 99 %, respectively [27]. In addition, when both modalities were in agreement, the performance profile approached that of the gold standard of histopathology, with a sensitivity, specificity, positive predictive value, and negative predictive value of 100 %, 87 %, 67 %, and 100 %, respectively [27]. Thus, in expert hands, the extent of therapy for residual neoplasia post-EMR can be guided in real time by CLE together with virtual chromoendoscopy. Absence of residual neoplasia by both CLE and virtual chromoendoscopy obviates the need for repeat colonoscopy in this setting [13].

Inflammatory Bowel Disease

Confocal laser endomicroscopy shows increasing promise for the management of inflammatory bowel diseases. A major advantage of CLE over conventional biopsy with histopathology is the ability to detect inflammatory bowel disease activity during endoscopy, even in apparently normal mucosa. In addition to cellular architecture, CLE can visualize dynamic process in vivo that relate to inflammation, intestinal barrier function, and vascular permeability [13]. As a result, CLE can visualize disease activity related to the pathophysiology of inflammatory bowel disease, which cannot be appreciated on ex vivo histopathology.

Disease Activity in Inflammatory Bowel Disease

CLE has an emerging role in monitoring disease activity to guide therapy, especially in patients who do not have endoscopically apparent inflammation. Traditionally, the decision to step up or step down inflammatory bowel disease therapy was guided by symptoms and quality of life assessments. More recently, "mucosal healing," or the absence of inflammation, has become a primary therapeutic endpoint [31]. Since endoscopic appearance underestimates the presence of inflammation, assessment for mucosal healing requires an extensive random biopsy protocol. CLE has shown promise in replacing the need for random biopsies to assess for inflammation in endoscopically normal-appearing tissue. Indeed, preliminary reports have shown that CLE performed in real time could predict histological inflammation with a sensitivity, specificity, positive predictive value, and negative predictive value of 94 %, 81 %, 82 %, and 94 %, respectively [32].

It may be possible to tailor therapy based on the extent of mucosal inflammation seen by optical biopsy. To this end, mucosal changes on CLE have been quantified in a recently described Crohn's Disease Endomicroscopic Activity Score (CDEAS) [33]. The CDEAS takes into account microscopic changes in crypts, the presence of micro-erosions, lamina propria vascularity and cellular infiltrate, and the density of goblet cells to yield a score from 0 to 8 [33]. In a prospective validation study, patients with active Crohn's disease (median C-reactive protein of 24.5) were found to have a median CDEAS score of 5, while patients with inactive disease (median C-reactive protein of 2.8) had a CDEAS of 2 [33]. Thus, CLE may help to guide therapy at the time of endoscopy based on real-time microscopic evaluation of the mucosa [13].

Monitoring disease activity in ulcerative colitis is also possible with CLE. A study of 153 patients from the University of Mainz established criteria for grading the level of inflammation in active colitis [34]. A subsequent study of 73 patients used simplified criteria involving crypt architecture alone to quantify active inflammation [35]. In both studies, CLE scores correlated well with index histopathology and were more accurate than white light endoscopy for assessing endoscopically normal tissue [35]. This further supports the use of CLE for detecting subclinical inflammation and tailoring individual therapy [13].

Dysplasia in Inflammatory Bowel Disease

Augmenting red flag techniques with CLE is an effective way to detect colonic dysplasia in patients with ulcerative colitis and Crohn's disease. Unlike conventional screening for sporadic colorectal cancer where precursor lesions are largely identifiable as polyps, precancerous lesions in inflammatory bowel disease very often consist of regions of flat dysplasia which are not necessarily visible by white light endoscopy [36, 37]. Therefore, to detect obscure dysplasia, inflammatory bowel disease patients undergo an onerous random biopsy protocol: in addition to biopsying endoscopically visible lesions, random samples are taken circumferentially in 4 quadrants every 10 cm along the length of the colon [37]. A minimum of 32 biopsies [38] yield a sensitivity of 90 % and 64 biopsies achieve a sensitivity of 95 % [37]. Because the vast majority of these biopsies contain no dysplasia, clinical and cost benefits would be realized if biopsies could be better targeted to dysplastic regions.

Modalities such as CLE that increase the *per-biopsy* yield of dysplasia are highly attractive. Indeed, in a trial of 161 patients with chronic ulcerative colitis, the combination of chromoendoscopy and eCLE increased the detection rate of intraepithelial neoplasia by 4.75-fold, while reducing the total number of biopsies taken by 50 % over a conventional random biopsy protocol. Moreover, the average number of biopsies per patient could have been reduced from 50 to 3.9 without missing any neoplastic lesions if only dysplastic lesions identified by CLE were biopsied [34]. As such, CLE can be used to target biopsies for dysplasia surveillance in inflammatory bowel disease patients. While this is not yet a standard of care in the United States, it has been adopted in European guidelines for the appropriate use of CLE [13].

Future Uses of CLE within the Luminal GI Tract

Custom Fluorophores Used as Tumor Markers

While not yet available clinically, there is ongoing research involving fluorophore-tagged peptides and antibodies that bind selectively to neoplastic cells, enabling CLE to identify and target specific tissue. To date, markers for identifying gastric cancer using CLE have been demonstrated ex vivo in human tissue, as well as in vivo in human gastric cancer xenografts in live mice [39]. Showing even more promise, fluorescent peptides with selective affinity for cancer cells have been used successfully, in vivo, to identify colorectal cancer [40], as well as high-grade dysplasia and esophageal adenocarcinoma [41].

Given the association between dysplasia and angiogenesis, fluorescent antibodies have been used to target vascular endothelial growth factor (VEGF) as a tumor marker. In one study using a murine model of colon cancer, as well as human samples ex vivo, a custom VEGF antibody was shown to bind selectively to colon cancer cells [42]. In addition to identifying cancer, fluorescently labeled antibodies detectable by CLE are being explored to assess the effectiveness of anti-angiogenic chemotherapies for colorectal cancer [43]. Continued progress in the field of fluorophore-labeled molecular imaging will make CLE indispensable for in vivo study of the gastrointestinal tract.

Squamous Cell Cancer of the Esophagus

The current standard for identifying squamous cell cancer of the esophagus, which is often subtle by white light endoscopy, is endoscopy with targeted biopsies using Lugol's stain [44, 45]. Preliminary studies using CLE to identify early squamous cell cancer of the esophagus have shown promising results [46–48]. In a series of 21 patients, CLE was able to identify squamous cell cancer with a sensitivity of 100 % and a specificity of 87 % [48]. In a subsequent study, CLE images from 64 patients with known squamous cell cancer revealed a distinct pattern of more tortuous, wider diameter intrapapillary capillary loops than patients without squamous cell cancer [47, 48]. While this information is promising, physical biopsy remains the gold standard for diagnosis. With additional study, CLE may prove to be useful for identifying and targeting biopsies in squamous cell cancer.

Screening and Prevention of Colorectal Cancer

At present, the prevention of sporadic colorectal cancer dominates the procedure volumes of most gastroenterologists in the United States and Europe. It is currently recommended that all average-risk individuals undergo a screening colonoscopy starting at age 50 in order to detect and remove premalignant polyps and disrupt the adenoma-to-carcinoma sequence. Because it is difficult to distinguish polyp types by standard white light endoscopy, all polyps are sent for histopathological examination, but the fact remains that the vast majority of polyps have no malignant potential and/or are diminutive (≤5 mm) and thus very rarely harbor cancer (<0.08 %) [49]. In addition, universal polypectomy for histopathology is costly and introduces incremental risks of bleeding and perforation [50, 51]. Nonetheless, histopathology is still an important part of assessing colorectal cancer risk and, therefore, post-polypectomy surveillance interval recommendations.

Given that the costs and risks of removing all diminutive polyps may outweigh the benefit, the American Society of Gastroenterology's Preservation and Incorporation of Valuable Endoscopic Innovations (PIVI) initiative developed performance targets for the purely optical management of diminutive polyps. For a technology to be used toward a "diagnose-and-leave" strategy of diminutive rectosigmoid polyps and/or a resect-and-discard approach for any diminutive polyp, it must have a negative predictive value of 90 % and result in a 90 % agreement with recommended surveillance intervals based on histopathology [52].

Based on a recent meta-analysis of 19 studies, to date the only advanced imaging modality to consistently achieve a negative predictive value sufficient to leave diminutive polyps behind in situ is narrow band imaging with a pooled negative predictive value of 91 % [52]. That said, CLE has been shown to provide highly accurate, near-histopathology-grade diagnosis in several reports that examined polyps of all sizes [3, 4, 53, 54]. Unfortunately, in the case of diminutive polyps, issues of image quality and stability, probe mistargeting, and operator expertise have emerged [54], such that CLE on its own has yet to meet PIVI thresholds. In an effort to improve overall performance, the combination of CLE with other modalities has yielded mixed results. A small study in 64 patients showed that the addition of pCLE to narrow band imaging did not increase the accuracy of diminutive polyp classification [55], but in another report, a sub-analysis of diminutive polyps showed promise [56].

Even if CLE meets the PIVI standards as part of a multimodal approach, operator factors may be a practical barrier to adoption for high-volume screening and surveillance colonoscopies. In a prospective study of 130 patients, experts in pCLE were able to identify adenomas with a sensitivity, specificity, positive predictive value, and negative predictive value of 96 %, 90 %, 97 %, and 88 %, respectively, while non-experts achieved rates of 88, 85, 94, and 71 %, respectively [57]. The implication is that studies from major academic centers, in which CLE is interpreted by experts, may overestimate the performance profile of CLE such that, in general practice, it falls short of PIVI thresholds to a greater degree than it would appear at first glance. Future progress in computer-assisted diagnosis has the potential to eliminate such operator variables, but its implementation into clinical practice is at minimum several years away [58].

CLE for Assessing Prognosis in Inflammatory Bowel Disease

The capability for dynamic in vivo microscopy with CLE has revealed novel mucosal features heretofore not visible by histopathology. These features may have prognostic utility for progression, treatment response, and disease classification in inflammatory bowel disease.

Epithelial gaps are the result of shed epithelial cells that can be appreciated by CLE in vivo as areas of epithelial drop-out and fluorescein leakage on small intestinal villi. In a case control study of 14 patients who were assessed with CLE, epithelial gap density was significantly higher in patients with Crohn's disease than controls [59]. The difference in gap density was replicated in a larger study of CLE in the terminal ileum in 28 patients with Crohn's disease or ulcerative colitis compared to 30 controls. [60]. Overall, in the inflammatory bowel disease group, increases in epithelial gap density were positively correlated with rates of future hospitalization [61, 62] and surgery [61]. As such, quantitative assessment of epithelial gap density may be a novel prognosticator of disease progression and therapeutic requirements.

In addition, fluorescent antibodies to membrane bound TNF (mTNF) have been used in a novel way to predict the response to biologic TNF inhibitors in Crohn's disease. In a study of 25 patients, fluorescent antibodies to mTNF were administered endoscopically prior to imaging with CLE. On CLE images, patients with high numbers of fluorescent cells, suggestive of the presence of mTNF-positive lymphocytes in the mucosa, were subsequently found to have a 92 % response rate to TNF inhibitors, compared to a 15 % response rate in patients who did not have detectable mucosal mTNF-positive cells [63]. This novel prognostic approach represents a large step forward for the application of personalized medicine to inflammatory bowel disease, given the great cost and potential side effects of biologic TNF inhibitor therapy that include an increased risk of lymphoma and infection.

Finally, approximately 15 % of inflammatory bowel disease patients have a constellation of symptoms, biomarkers, and radiographic findings, which overlap between ulcerative colitis and Crohn's disease that defies clinical classification. As such, they are labeled with indeterminate colitis [64], which can be problematic for therapeutic monitoring and decision making. In vivo imaging with CLE has shown promise for helping to better classify indeterminate colitis. In a prospective study of 79 patients, CLE revealed consistent differences in crypt architecture among ulcerative colitis and Crohn's disease patients, although the presence of granulomas and submucosal features could not be assessed [65]. The ability to classify indeterminate colitis impacts treatment and surveillance plans and is of crucial importance to patients being considered for surgical resection. However, further studies are required before CLE can be recommended for this purpose.

Irritable Bowel Syndrome

Irritable Bowel Syndrome, part of the spectrum of functional gastrointestinal disorders, is a highly prevalent and morbid condition in the United States. At present, irritable bowel syndrome remains a largely clinical diagnosis because specific disease biomarkers are lacking. However, novel in vivo observations using CLE show promise for expanding our understanding of the pathophysiology of irritable bowel syndrome. CLE has demonstrated that patients with irritable bowel syndrome have increased epithelial gaps and intestinal permeability compared to healthy controls

[66]. Moreover, in a study of 36 irritable bowel syndrome patients with suspected food intolerance, epithelial gaps could be induced with exposures to common antigens. Individuals were exposed to dilute food antigens including cow's milk, wheat, yeast, and soy via endoscopic infusions. In 22 patients, changes in the normal small intestinal mucosa could be appreciated by pCLE within 5 min of exposure, including increases in epithelial gaps, appearance of intervillous spaces, and increases in apparent intraepithelial lymphocytes. Subsequently, all patients were placed on exclusion diets for 12 months. Based on a symptom survey, patients who had mucosal changes on CLE reported a 74 % improvement, while patients who had no changes had no response to the exclusion diet [67]. While preliminary in scope, this study opens the door for future investigations regarding the pathophysiology of irritable bowel syndrome and gut permeability. Findings using CLE may help to individualize treatments including highly specific recommendations for exclusion diets.

Celiac Disease

Celiac disease is an immune-mediated disease of the gastrointestinal tract associated with dietary intake of wheat proteins that leads to intestinal inflammation accompanied by nutritional deficiencies, bloating, cramping, and diarrhea [68]. The gold standard for diagnosis is biopsy of the duodenum with histopathological evaluation, although patchy inflammation has been described [68]. Probe-based CLE may help to reduce the number of false negative biopsies for Celiac disease by helping to target biopsies during endoscopy. In a preliminary study of 17 patients with celiac disease and 14 non-celiac controls, pCLE was able to detect those subjects with celiac disease with a sensitivity and specificity of 94 % and 92 %, respectively [69]. This was achieved by noting features of villous atrophy and crypt hypertrophy in vivo [69]. Other studies in pediatric populations have shown that CLE can help to increase diagnostic yield by targeting biopsies within the duodenum [70, 71]. In the future, it is likely that CLE will assume a greater role in the diagnosis and management of celiac disease.

Techniques for CLE

Set up of CLE Systems

The eCLE system (EC3870K; Pentax, Tokyo, Japan) looks and feels like a larger caliber standard white light video endoscope, with a laser scanning confocal microscope built into the distal tip (Fig. 6.1). The dedicated upper endoscope or colonoscope selected for use is mated to an illumination/image processing box and monitor identical to a standard video endoscope cart. In addition to incorporating a fluorescence microscope, the endoscope is equipped with a 2.8 mm working channel and air and water nozzles. A 488 nm argon laser beam is used to excite the tissue via the microscope objective incorporated in the tip of the scope. The handle of the endoscope has two additional buttons for adjusting depth of field in the z-axis from 0 to 250 μm [72]. Fast scan mode permits low resolution video-rate imaging to enable targeting of the microscope to areas of interest. High resolution images with a field of view of 475×475 μm and a lateral resolution of 0.7 μm can then be captured as still frames at 0.8–1.4 per second [2].

The pCLE system (Cellvizio™; Mauna Kea Technologies, Inc., Paris, France) consists of a series of application-specific flexible fiberoptic confocal miniprobes, which are mated to a dedicated laser scanning unit, a detector, and a computer processor with a display screen, keyboard, and optional foot pedal triggers. Miniprobes are intended to be passed via the 2.8 mm or larger accessory channel of virtually any endoscope (Fig. 6.2). Depending on the clinical application, miniprobes for luminal pCLE include the GastroFlex, GastroFlexUHD, ColoFlex, and ColoflexUHD (Cellvizio™; Mauna Kea Technology, Paris, France). GastroFlex probes are 3 m long, intended for esophagogastroduodenoscopy, while the ColoFlex probes are 4 m and thus suited to colonoscopy and enteroscopy. Both "UHD" probes have a higher lateral resolution (1 μm) albeit a narrower field of view (240 μm) compared to their companion standard-definition probes, which have a lateral resolution of 3.5 μm and field of view of 600 μm.

Technique

Administering Fluorescein

Once the endoscopic procedure is underway and a region of interest identified on widefield views, 2.5–5 mL of 10% sodium fluorescein is administered intravenously as a slow bolus [73]. Dosing studies indicate that intravenous fluorescein achieves peak mucosal concentrations within 5–8 min and provides contrast with a signal-to-noise-ratio adequate for CLE for up to 30 min [74, 75]. In general, CLE imaging can be initiated approximately 1 min following the IV fluorescein bolus. If image quality and contrast are poor, a supplemental bolus up to the total maximum of 5 mL may be administered at any time within the 30 min imaging window. It is expected that image quality will deteriorate over time as dye equilibrates across aqueous compartments and is excreted in urine. That said, there is no additional benefit to image quality with additional fluorescein in excess of 5 mL [76]. While fluorescein persists at a low level in tissues which are sent for histopathological analysis, it does not interfere with ex vivo staining techniques, including immunohistochemistry and immunofluorescence microscopy [77]. Moreover, when the tissue sample is examined under fluorescence microscopy, it may aid in the assessment of vascular permeability by allowing the microscopist to assess for fluorescein in the extravascular space [77].

Interrogating a Tissue Sample

Endoscopic CLE

Since the eCLE probe is built into dedicated upper and lower endoscopes, the confocal microscope objective must be brought into contact with the desired tissue by manipulating and steering the scope into position such that the terminal face is fully apposed to the region of interest. The microscope objective is located at approximately 7 o'clock relative to the widefield forward endoscopic view. Thus, a region of interest should be positioned toward the bottom left hand corner of the video display. A blue laser beam can be seen to be projected onto the mucosa which can be used to guide the microscope objective beyond the tip of the endoscope. The microscope objective is placed in direct, gentle contact with the mucosa at which point the widefield endoscopic view is obscured. Gentle suction is then applied to hold the mucosa in place as the depth of the focal plane in the *z*-axis is adjusted using controls on the endoscope handle and as *x*- and *y*-axis image scans are obtained at a rate of approximately one per second. All image frames contain a scale marker to assist morphometric analysis. Of note, excessive suction force or pressure can alter blood flow, which can create artifacts for image classification and interpretation. For surveillance of endoscopically inapparent disease over a large area, the objective can be put in contact with the mucosa in a repetitive systematic geometric pattern to obtain image frames that can serve as optical or virtual biopsies. Physical biopsies of microscopically identified targets are obtained in relation to a faint residual suction ring left behind from scope stabilization that is adjacent to the imaged area.

Probe-Based CLE

When a region of interest is identified during endoscopy, the pCLE probe is advanced through the 2.8 mm or larger accessory channel of any standard endoscope. The probe will be visible once it protrudes beyond the tip of the endoscope and can be manipulated under direct visualization. The probe is advanced and the endoscope steered to place the probe in gentle contact with the mucosa in question. Due to peristalsis and respiratory excursion, probe stability can be problematic especially in the distal esophagus and in structures near the diaphragm. For this reason, some endoscopists choose to place a transparent cap at the tip of the endoscope in order to apply gentle pressure and/or suction, thus stabilizing the probe and minimizing motion artifacts. Once stably positioned, videos can be acquired by actuating a foot pedal. Endomicroscopic images are streamed at 12 frames per second in real-time and recorded digitally for cine-review and static frame analysis using an included trackball. All imaging with pCLE can be observed on the high definition monitor on the equipment tower, or fed to compatible external displays in the procedure suite. All images and videos have a scale marker to permit quantitative analysis. Technically speaking, while pCLE probes have a fixed working distance, applying very gentle pressure to the mucosa may allow for slightly deeper imaging. However, excessive pressure may artificially alter microvascular blood flow and impact image interpretation. Use of a double channel endoscope can be helpful for procedure flow and co-registration of optical and physical biopsies, as it enables continuous pCLE imaging via one port simultaneous with biopsy and/or marking with ink or cautery via the second port. For surveillance of endoscopically inapparent disease over a large area, the probe can be swept systematically in a circular or helical pattern to obtain a continuous video survey and additional interrogation of regions of interest by optical biopsy.

Assessment

In order to distinguish between normal and diseased tissue, it is useful to keep several general principles in mind when interpreting CLE images obtained with intravenous fluorescein contrast. Since CLE is magnified up to 1000-fold, much of what is visualized, albeit monochromatically, corresponds to histopathological structures as they would appear on a benchtop microscope. As such, many of the characteristics used on histopathological analysis, such as changes in the number of goblet cells, presence or absence of villi, and changes in cellular or crypt architecture, can be used for interpretation of CLE. That said, there are some features seen on histopathology which cannot be seen by CLE using fluorescein, for example, nuclear detail. However, by its in vivo nature, CLE can visualize features not seen on biopsies such as capillary blood flow and leakage patterns important for identifying inflammation and/or neoplasia. By combining traditional features analogous to histopathological findings and dynamic pathophysiological processes uniquely visualized by CLE, it is possible to create classification systems to aid in diagnosis.

When interpreting CLE images of a cell from any region of the GI tract, it is useful to classify the tissue based on the cellular architecture and surrounding blood vessels. A general trend is that as cells progress from normal tissue to neoplasia, there is a decreasing level of architectural organization, increase in the range of image contrast, and brighter, more prominent blood vessels. Another trend is that as the severity of inflammation increases, there is an increase in the size and tortuosity of blood vessels, an increased disorder in crypt architecture, and an increase in non-epithelial cellular infiltration. Finally, normal tissues along the GI tract are often regenerating, and much as for histopathology, it can be challenging to distinguish normal regeneration from pathological inflammation and/or neoplasia. These trends and concepts are encompassed in several classification systems that have been used over time for the study, validation, and clinical use of CLE.

Esophagus and Esophageal Diseases

The normal esophagus is lined by stratified squamous epithelial cells, but can be lined by columnar epithelium, typically cardia mucosa and/or specialized intestinal metaplasia associated with Barrett's esophagus. Descriptions of CLE of these mucosal types, as well as the changes associated with the progression from metaplasia to dysplasia, are detailed in the Miami Classification for pCLE and the Mainz Classification for eCLE (see Tables 6.1 and 6.2.). Not surprisingly, the two

Table 6.1 Miami classification

Tissue type	Vessel architecture	Cellular architecture
Normal squamous epithelium	Bright vessels within papillae (intra-papillary capillary loops)	Flat cells without crypts or villi
Non-dysplastic Barrett's esophagus	NA	Columnar cells. Dark goblet cells
High-grade dysplasia	Dilated irregular vessels	Villiform structures. Dark, irregularly thickened epithelial borders
Adenocarcinoma	Dilated irregular vessels	Disorganized/loss of villiform structure and crypts. Dark columnar cells
Normal stomach	NA	Regular round crypts, cobblestone appearance of normal glands
Gastritis	NA	Increased fluorescence in stroma, cellular infiltrate between crypts
Gastric dysplasia	NA	Irregular crypt lumen. Dark, irregular, thickened epithelium
Gastric adenocarcinoma	NA	Dark and irregular epithelium which is completely disorganized. Fluorescein leakage
Normal duodenum	NA	Villiform architecture. Bright, uniform epithelium
Duodenal adenoma	NA	Villiform architecture. Dark, irregular epithelium
Duodenal celiac disease	NA	Blunting or loss of villi
Normal colon	Regular, narrow vessels	Round crypt structures, dark goblet cells
Hyperplastic polyp	Small vessels	Crypts with slit-like or stellate openings (pits). Bright, non-thickened and uniform epithelium. Dark goblet cells
Adenoma	Vessel architecture is not used by Miami criteria to identify adenomas	Irregular villiform structures (including tubular adenoma). Dark, irregularly thickened epithelium. Decreased goblet cells
Adenocarcinoma	Dilated vessels	Disorganized villiform or lack of structure. Dark, irregularly thickened epithelium
Colitis	Dilated, prominent, branching vessels	Crypt fusion and distortion. Bright epithelium

Adapted from [3]

Table 6.2 Mainz classification

Tissue type	Vessel architecture	Cellular architecture
Squamous cells	Capillaries leading to the luminal surface, such that they appear in cross-section	Individual cells with clear borders
Gastric type epithelium	Regular-shaped capillaries visible only in the deeper mucosal layers	Regular columnar-lined epithelium with round glandular openings
Barrett's epithelium	Regular-shaped capillaries beneath columnar-lined epithelium visible in superficial and deep mucosa	Columnar-lined epithelium with goblet cells containing dark mucin in superficial mucosa. In deeper mucosa, villous pattern of epithelial cells
Esophageal neoplasia	Irregular capillaries visible in superficial and deep mucosa. Fluorescein leakage causes a heterogeneous, brighter signal intensity within the lamina propria	Dark cells with irregular borders and high contrast compared to surrounding tissue
Normal colon	Pericryptal vessels in a regular hexagonal, honeycomb pattern in the stroma	Round and regularly shaped colonic crypts with goblet cells containing dark mucin. No cellular infiltrate
Regenerating colon	Minimal increase in the number of pericryptal vessels in a regular hexagonal, honeycomb pattern	Stellate luminal crypt openings or focal aggregates of regular-shaped crypts. Normal or decreased goblet cell numbers
Colon neoplasia	Dilated and distorted vessels with increased leakage; irregular architecture with little or no orientation to adjacent tissue	Ridged-lined irregular epithelial layer with loss of crypts and goblet cells. Irregular cell architecture with little or no mucin
Mild to moderate colitis	Dilated, distorted microvessels that are moderately increased in number	Differences in shape, size, and distribution of crypts; increased distance between crypts, focal crypt destruction. Cellular infiltration involving <50 % of crypts
Severe colitis	Marked increase in dilation and distortion of microvasculature. Leakage of fluorescein	Unequivocal crypt destruction. Cellular infiltration present in >50 % of crypts

Adapted from [4, 34, 78]

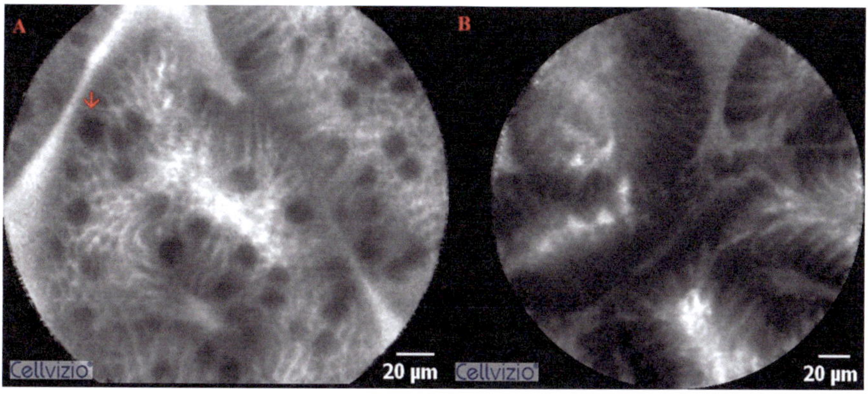

Fig. 6.3 (**a**) Non-dysplastic Barrett's esophagus is characterized by dark goblet cells (*red arrow*), well-organized villiform architecture, and columnar cells. Image Courtesy of Mauna Kea Technologies with permission. (**b**) As tissue progresses from non-dysplastic Barrett's to dysplasia, multilayered columnar epithelium, dark regions, dye leakage into the lamina propria, and paucity of goblet cells are observed

classification schemes overlap substantially with certain common general patterns. By CLE, normal stratified squamous epithelium, as seen in Fig. 6.2, is readily identified as flat, scale-like cells without visible crypts or villous projections. Bright, tightly-coiled blood vessels, or intrapapillary capillary loops (IPCLs), project up from the *lamina propria* into papillae [3]. Blood flow in IPCLs can be appreciated as moving circular shadows, representing red blood corpuscles displacing intravascular fluorescein [78]. By definition, squamous epithelium does not possess columnar cells, villous projections, or glandular structures, so when they are observed by CLE, the area being examined is most likely region of Barrett's esophagus and/or cardia mucosa.

In addition to columnar epithelium, villi, and/or glands, the diagnosis of specialized intestinal metaplasia in the esophagus requires the identification of goblet cells. Goblet cells can be seen readily by pCLE as large, round dark regions within the epithelial monolayer due to the exclusion of fluorescein by their high mucin content (Fig. 6.3). Another feature that distinguishes Barrett's esophagus from gastric mucosa is that Barrett's has regular appearing capillaries which can be seen beneath the epithelium in the lamina propria as well as deeper in the mucosa [78].

As tissue progresses from Barrett's metaplasia to dysplasia, there is a loss of regularity in both cellular architecture and vessel patterns. In high-grade dysplasia, as seen in Fig. 6.3, villiform structures and crypts still occur, but are characterized by multilayered columnar epithelium. Crypt glands are no longer uniformly sized or spaced and there are enlarged and irregularly shaped microvessels in the superficial and deeper layers of the mucosa [3]. Esophageal adenocarcinoma exhibits further disorganization, with the loss of villiform structures and crypts as seen in Fig. 6.4. Cells appear much darker compared to surrounding tissue, and goblet cells are no longer clearly identifiable. The microvasculature remains dilated and tortuous [3].

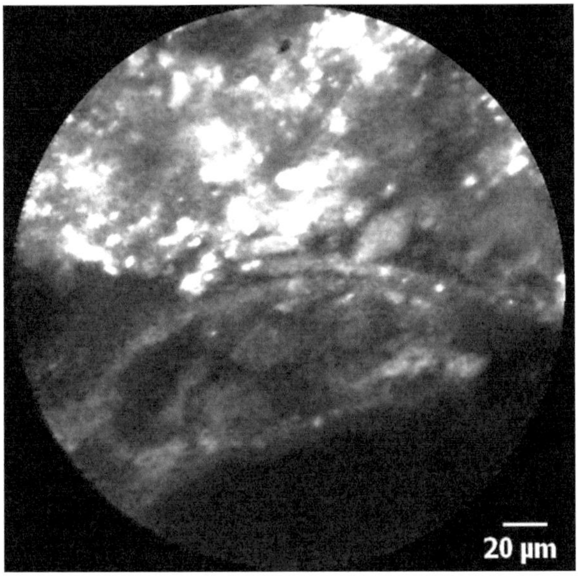

Fig. 6.4 In adenocarcinoma, there is disorganization and loss of villiform architecture. Other features of adenocarcinoma include dark columnar cells and irregular vessels with fluorescein leakage

Table 6.3 Kansas city criteria (requires at least 2 of 6 features) [79]

Criteria
Irregular, saw-toothed appearance of epithelium
Enlarged, irregular cells
Paucity of goblet cells
Variable glandular shape (budding, branching, crowding)
Variable thickness of glandular epithelium
Variable size and uneven spacing of glands

It should be noted that the Mainz Classification groups all esophageal neoplasia into one category, whereas the Miami classification has separate descriptions for high-grade dysplasia and esophageal adenocarcinoma. Another distinct, validated classification system with a specific focus on grading dysplasia using pCLE is known as the Kansas City Criteria. It describes six features, of which ≥2 must be present in order to label tissues as dysplasia (see Table 6.3). Relevant classification features of the Kansas City Criteria were identified by a panel of experts who reviewed pCLE videos with known pathology, which were then tested prospectively in cohorts of experts and non-experts who were given 1 h of training [79]. It has garnered favor over the Miami Classification due to its ease of use and validated accuracy.

Stomach and Diseases of the Gastric Mucosa

In the distal esophagus, there is typically a well-demarcated transition from squamous epithelium to the columnar epithelium of the cardia and the proximal stomach. Normal gastric mucosa is characterized by regular columnar-lined epithelium with

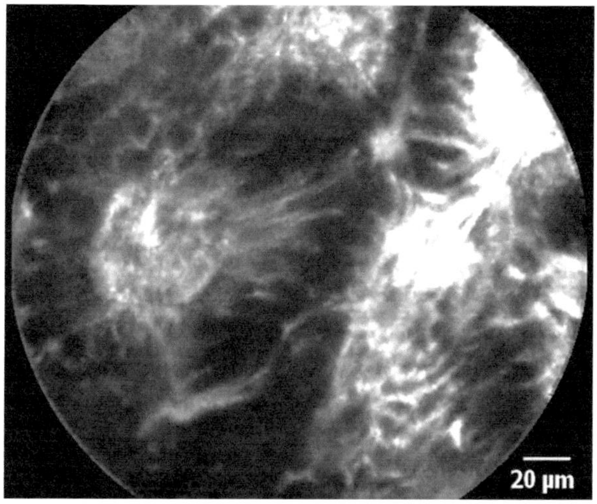

Fig. 6.5 Gastric adenocarcinoma is characterized by disorganized epithelium, with dark cells, and leakage of fluorescein. Image courtesy of Mauna Kea Technologies with permission

round gland openings, also referred to as "pits," in a cobblestone pattern. Unlike squamous epithelium, observed blood vessels are only present in the deeper mucosal layers.

Deviations from this pattern are seen in gastritis, gastric dysplasia, and gastric adenocarcinoma (Fig. 6.5). While tissue classification in the stomach based on CLE is a work in progress [3], the Miami Classification (as summarized in Table 6.1) notes several patterns for identifying different gastric pathologies [3].

Duodenum and Duodenal Diseases

Much like what is seen by histopathology, CLE of normal duodenal mucosa reveals individual intestinal villi with a vascular core lined with a bright, uniform epithelium with numerous interspersed goblet cells. Blunting of villi and expansion of the lamina propria are seen in celiac disease and can be used to target duodenal biopsies to increase the diagnostic yield compared to random biopsies. CLE may play a role in assessing adenomatous tissue within the duodenum especially involving the ampulla of Vater, where biopsies are associated with increased morbidity. While it has not been established that CLE can obviate the need for duodenal biopsies, it can help to target biopsies to abnormal regions. While still an area of study, known features of duodenal pathology by CLE are described by the Miami Classification, as outlined in Table 6.1 [3].

Colon

Inflammatory Bowel Disease

When using CLE in the assessment of patients with IBD, it is useful to look at cellular and vessel architecture, as well as dynamic processes such as epithelial leakage and gaps. The Mainz Criteria can be used to qualitatively describe active colitis, differentiating mild to moderate from severe colitis, while The Miami Classification describes the presence or absence of colitis. Additionally, there are more specific classification systems for assessing disease activity in inflammatory bowel disease or dysplasia in flat lesions.

Normal colon tissue has rounded crypt structures, dark goblet cells that exclude fluorescein, and regular peri-cryptal blood vessels, as seen in Fig. 6.6 [80]. Cellular architecture consists of regular luminal openings and distribution of crypts covered by a homogeneous layer of epithelial cells. In the absence of inflammation, there is no cellular infiltrate [34].

Mild to moderate colitis is characterized by a cellular infiltrate involving < 50 % of observed crypts. There is notable heterogeneity in the size, shape, and distribution of crypts, as well as sporadic crypt destruction. In the setting of inflammation, blood vessels, which are easily visible with fluorescein, become dilated and tortuous, as seen in Fig. 6.7 [34]. These changes in tissue and vessel architecture become more prominent in severe colitis where there is marked crypt destruction and cellular infiltrate that involves > 50 % of crypts, with further enlargement of microvessels and increased fluorescein leakage [34].

In clinical practice, there are additional scoring systems which may be used to grade the activity of IBD. For ulcerative colitis, there is a simplified scoring system based solely on crypt architecture to grade disease activity, described in Table 6.4 [35]. To quantify disease activity in Crohn's disease, images from either eCLE or pCLE can

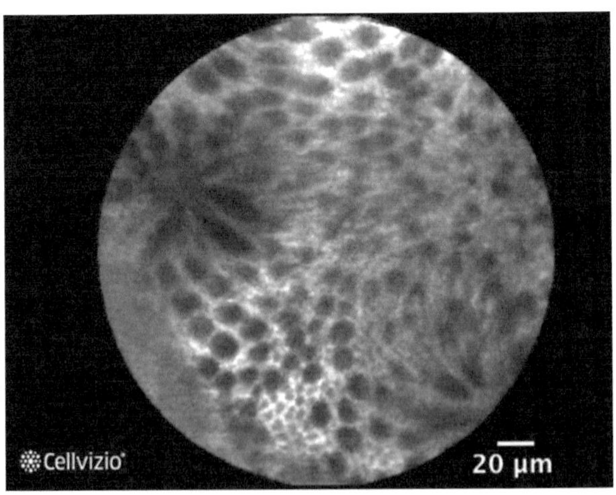

Fig. 6.6 Normal Colon is characterized by round crypts, dark goblet cells, and regular narrow vessels. Image. Courtesy of Mauna Kea Technologies with permission

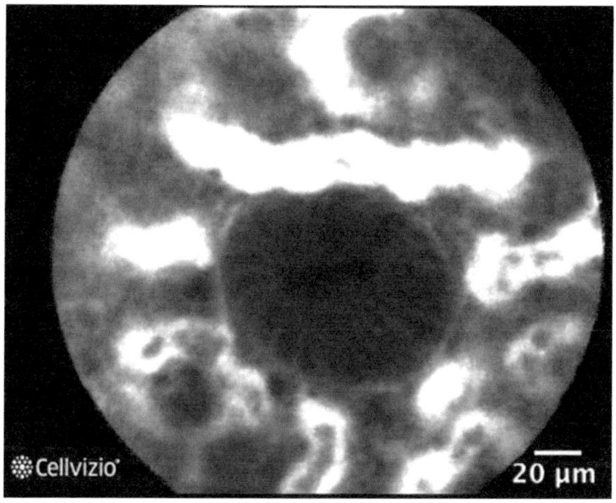

Fig. 6.7 Active colitis is characterized by distorted crypts, bright epithelium, and dilated, prominent branching vessels. In this image, crypts become widely spaced such that only one is visible in the pCLE viewing field. Image courtesy of Mauna Kea Technologies with permission

Table 6.4 UC: Endoscopic CLE for the assessment of mucosal changes in ulcerative colitis

Category	Crypt architecture description
A	Regular arrangement and size of crypts
B	Irregular arrangement of crypts, enlarged spaces between crypts
C	Dilation of crypt openings, more irregular arrangement of crypts, and enlarged spaces between crypts as compared to type B
D	Crypt destruction and/or crypt abscess

Adapted from [35]

Table 6.5 Crohn's Disease Endomicroscopic Activity Score (CDEAS)

Assign 1 point for any of the features below
Crypt number increased
Crypt number decreased
Crypt distortion present
Microerosions present
Cellular infiltrate increased
Vascularity increased
Goblet cells increased
Goblet cells decreased

Adapted from [33]

be used to determine a Crohn's Disease Endomicroscopic Activity Score (CDEAS), described in Table 6.5 [33].

In addition to using CLE to assess IBD activity, CLE can be used to target biopsies during surveillance for flat dysplasia. Even in the absence of a clearly demarcated polyp, there are changes in cellular and vessel architecture associated with dysplasia in patients with chronic ulcerative colitis. Dysplasia may be classified in ulcerative colitis by using the Mainz classification with eCLE to augment diagnosis with chromoendoscopy (see Table 6.2).

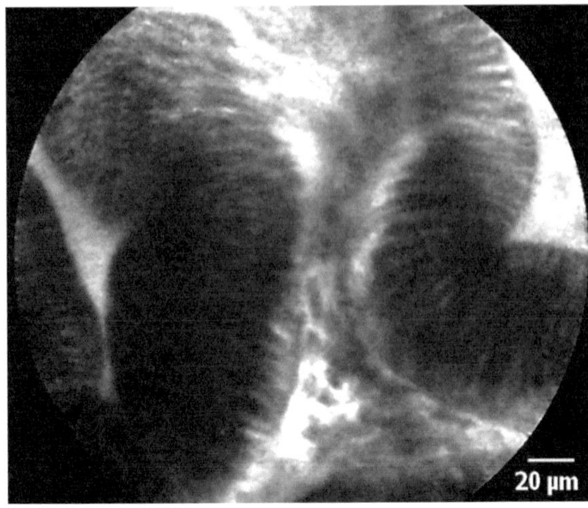

Fig. 6.8 Tubular adenomas are characterized by irregular or villiform structures, dark, multilayered columnar epithelium, and decreased goblet cells

As cells progress to neoplasia, blood vessels dilate with increased leakage and distortion, cellular architecture becomes irregular, and the number of goblet cells per field decreases presumably due to being crowded out by less differentiated, rapidly proliferating epithelial cells [34].

Polyps and Colorectal Cancer

As mentioned, colonic mucosa by CLE is described using crypt and vessel architecture, the details of which are outlined in Table 6.1 for pCLE and Table 6.2 for eCLE.

Neoplastic tissue in the colon is much less organized than normal or hyperplastic tissue. Features of adenomas, seen in Fig. 6.8, include irregular or villiform structures, a darkened and irregularly thickened epithelial layer, and a decrease in the number of goblet cells compared to normal or hyperplastic tissue [3]. Adenocarcinoma is characterized by further loss of tissue organization, as well as dilated capillaries with fluorescein extravasation. In addition to the dark, irregularly thickened epithelium which is present in adenoma, adenocarcinoma can feature disorganized villiform structures as well (Fig. 6.9) [3].

It is important to distinguish between neoplasia and cells which are either hyperplastic or regenerating as part of natural intestinal turnover and/or repair. Hyperplastic polyps are characterized by crypts with slit-like or stellate openings, uniform epithelium of normal width, and often increased numbers of dark goblet cells (Fig. 6.10) [3]. Regenerating cells are characterized by a mild increase in capillary density and flow, albeit without the distortion and vessel leakage seen in neoplasia. Likewise, the crypt architecture in regenerating mucosa is characterized by stellate crypt openings or focal aggregates of regular-shaped crypts in a more regular pattern compared to neoplasia [4]. Finally, neoplastic tissue is associated with a loss of goblet cells compared to normal or regenerating tissue [4].

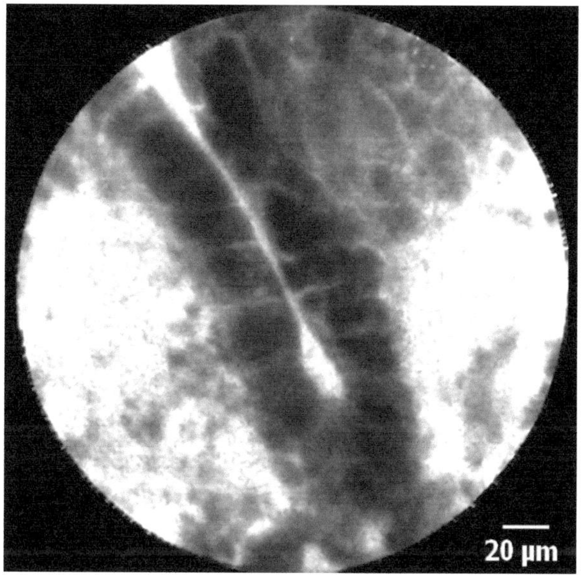

Fig. 6.9 Colorectal adenocarcinoma is typified by dark/light dye leaky and disorganized structures with marked heterogeneity in the layering of the epithelium. Image courtesy of Mauna Kea Technologies with permission

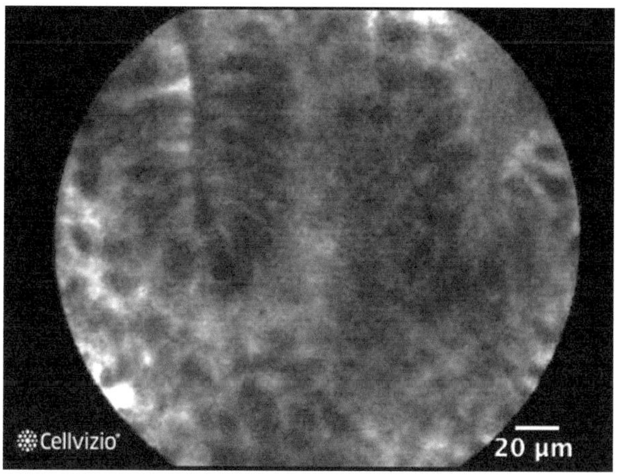

Fig. 6.10 Hyperplastic polyps are characterized by crypts with slit or stellate openings, and bright, non-thickened uniform epithelium. They have dark goblet cells and small blood vessels. Compared to neoplasia, hyperplastic polyps have smaller-caliber blood vessels and more organized tissue architecture. Image Courtesy of Mauna Kea Technologies with permission

Safety and Cost Considerations

Safety Profile of Commonly Used Fluorophores

The main risks associated with CLE are associated with administration of intravenous fluorescein. Depending on institutional policies, it is advisable to discuss the administration of intravenous fluorescein during the consent process, as CLE requires an "off label" use of the drug. Two expected effects are temporary yellowing of the skin [4, 73] and urine [2]. Mild side effects which occur in <2 % of patients include nausea, transient hypotension without shock, injection site erythema, diffuse rash, and mild epigastric pain [73]. While a large multicenter study of intravenous fluorescein for imaging of the gastrointentestinal tract showed no major adverse reactions [73], a broader review of over 12,000 patients in whom fluorescein was used for any purpose revealed that anaphylaxis occurred in slightly less than 0.10 % of subjects [81]. Other rare but serious side effects that have been documented in non-gastrointestinal uses include arterial ischemia, shock, thrombophlebitis, and seizure [73]. While these reactions are extremely rare, some endoscopists favor the use of diphenhydramine as part of sedation in order to, in theory, blunt any potential histamine reaction.

Cost

While a capital equipment investment is required for CLE, the additional costs can be justified if improved patient care and a reduction in the overall costs of endoscopic procedures are realized. Optical biopsies with CLE may prove to be cost effective by eliminating the need for tissue histopathology in certain circumstances, by enabling real-time interventions that can reduce the number of follow-up procedures required, and/or by avoiding hospitalizations and surgeries. In the case of Barrett's surveillance, CLE can reduce the number of histopathological specimens required by increasing the biopsy yield for dysplasia. In addition, there may be savings associated with better-tailored therapy and reduced numbers of biopsies for dysplasia surveillance in the care of patients with IBD. Real-time decision making with CLE during endoscopic therapy for Barrett's esophagus and large colonic polyps can reduce the number of procedures required, thus lowering expenses related to facility utilization, staffing, equipment, and histopathology [14]. At this time, however, no large cost benefit analysis has been performed to assess the impact of CLE on Barrett's esophagus, inflammatory bowel disease, or colonic endoscopic mucosal resection, and thus, projections on cost savings remain theoretical.

While using CLE in colorectal cancer screening is not yet a standard of care, there has been extensive analysis on how "optical biopsies" may provide cost savings. If CLE can obviate the need for polypectomy in the future, cost saving may be achieved by one of two strategies: a "diagnose and leave strategy," in which diminutive polyps may be left in situ, or a "resect and discard" strategy, in which diminutive polyps are resected but not sent to a pathologist. A "diagnose and leave" strategy, it could save up to $1 billion dollars annually in the United States, based on a polypectomy cost of $179 [52], while computer simulations predict that a "resect and discard" strategy could save $33 million annually [82].

Conclusion and Future Directions

The future of CLE depends on its ability to reduce the need for conventional tissue sampling and histopathological analysis. This is achieved through assessment of cellular architecture, as well as the ability to see novel features which are not available on conventional microscopy, such as capillary blood flow and endothelial leakage. In order for this to become a reality, it is necessary to adhere to pre-defined standards, such as those outlined by the Preservation and Incorporation of Valuable Endoscopic Innovations (PIVI) guidelines. This may be feasible for monitoring patients with BE, augmenting endoscopic mucosal resections, and possibly screening for colorectal cancer. Other areas which show promise include monitoring cancer and precancerous lesions in the stomach, as well as disease activity and flat dysplasia in patients with inflammatory bowel disease.

In addition to refining the application of CLE technology to meet the test parameters required for widespread clinical use, it is also necessary to train endoscopists in in vivo microscopy. Training specific to CLE must focus on both technical and cognitive aspects of performance [13]. Technical aspects include proper use of contrast to achieve adequate image quality, as well as optimal probe position and pressure, while cognitive aspects include the recognition and use of standardized features and nomenclature to describe CLE findings. Other potential barriers to wide adoption of CLE include the medico-legal consequences of forgoing biopsies and the costs associated with CLE systems and consumables. Thus, in the future, it will be necessary to utilize prospectively verified classification systems that can be readily adopted with a short learning curve, with performance characteristics that can augment endoscopic clinical decision making and/or histopathological analysis.

Helpful Hints

- Hold miniprobes with three fingers and an opposed thumb while feeding them into the biopsy channel in order to prevent tight bending and buckling that can break glass fibers
- To maximize stability when interrogating tissue by pCLE, have the miniprobe protrude only minimally from the end of the endoscope
- Use a dual lumen scope to ensure accurate targeting and co-registration of biopsies to areas visualized by pCLE
- You may fit a clear 4 mm cap to the distal tip of the endoscope during pCLE, with or without gentle suction to stabilize the miniprobe
- You may apply gentle suction to tissue during eCLE interrogation to ensure stability, however excessive suctioning may alter capillary flow dynamics
- Apply CLE objectives gently to tissue, as excessive pressure will alter microvascular flow dynamics
- Fluorescein may be injected incrementally but not in excess of 5 mL to prolong imaging time and/or further enhance contrast as needed

References

1. Goetz M, Memadathil B, Biesterfeld S, Schneider C, Gregor S, Galle PR, et al. In vivo subsurface morphological and functional cellular and subcellular imaging of the gastrointestinal tract with confocal mini-microscopy. World J Gastroenterol. 2007;13(15):2160–5.
2. Nakai Y, Isayama H, Shinoura S, Iwashita T, Samarasena JB, Chang KJ, et al. Confocal laser endomicroscopy in gastrointestinal and pancreatobiliary diseases. Dig Endosc. 2014;26 Suppl 1:86–94.
3. Wallace M, Lauwers GY, Chen Y, Dekker E, Fockens P, Sharma P, Meining A. Miami classification for probe-based confocal laser endomicroscopy. Endoscopy. 2011;43(10):882–91.
4. Kiesslich R, Burg J, Vieth M, Gnaendiger J, Enders M, Delaney P, et al. Confocal laser endoscopy for diagnosing intraepithelial neoplasias and colorectal cancer in vivo. Gastroenterology. 2004;127(3):706–13.
5. Polglase AL, McLaren WJ, Delaney PM. Pentax confocal endomicroscope: a novel imaging device for in vivo histology of the upper and lower gastrointestinal tract. Expert Rev Med Devices. 2006;3(5):549–56.
6. Spechler SJ, Sharma P, Souza RF, Inadomi JM, Shaheen NJ. American Gastroenterological Association medical position statement on the management of Barrett's esophagus. Gastroenterology. 2011;140(3):1084–91.
7. Peters FP, Curvers WL, Rosmolen WD, de Vries CE, Ten Kate FJ, Krishnadath KK, et al. Surveillance history of endoscopically treated patients with early Barrett's neoplasia: nonadherence to the Seattle biopsy protocol leads to sampling error. Dis Esophagus. 2008;21(6):475–9.
8. Abrams JA, Kapel RC, Lindberg GM, Saboorian MH, Genta RM, Neugut AI, et al. Adherence to biopsy guidelines for Barrett's esophagus surveillance in the community setting in the United States. Clin Gastroenterol Hepatol. 2009;7(7):736–42.
9. Dunbar KB, Okolo 3rd P, Montgomery E, Canto MI. Confocal laser endomicroscopy in Barrett's esophagus and endoscopically inapparent Barrett's neoplasia: a prospective, randomized, double-blind, controlled, crossover trial. Gastrointest Endosc. 2009;70(4):645–54.
10. Sharma P, Meining AR, Coron E, Lightdale CJ, Wolfsen HC, Bansal A, et al. Real-time increased detection of neoplastic tissue in Barrett's esophagus with probe-based confocal laser endomicroscopy: final results of an international multicenter, prospective, randomized, controlled trial. Gastrointest Endosc. 2011;74(3):465–72.
11. Canto MI, Anandasabapathy S, Brugge W, Falk GW, Dunbar KB, Zhang Z, et al. In vivo endomicroscopy improves detection of Barrett's esophagus-related neoplasia: a multicenter international randomized controlled trial (with video). Gastrointest Endosc. 2014;79(2):211–21.
12. Berzosa M, Wallace MB. Surveillance of Barrett's esophagus: why biopsy if you can endomicroscopy. Gastrointest Endosc. 2014;79(2):222–3.
13. Wang KK, Carr-Locke DL, Singh SK, Neumann H, Bertani H, Galmiche J-P, et al. Use of probe-based confocal laser endomicroscopy (pCLE) in gastrointestinal applications. A consensus report based on clinical evidence. United Eur Gastroenterol J. 2015;3(3):230–54.
14. Sharma P, Savides TJ, Canto MI, Corley DA, Falk GW, Goldblum JR, et al. The American Society for Gastrointestinal Endoscopy PIVI (Preservation and incorporation of valuable endoscopic innovations) on imaging in Barrett's esophagus. Gastrointest Endosc. 2012;76(2):252–4.
15. Johnson EA, De Lee R, Agni R, Pfau P, Reichelderfer M, Gopal DV. Probe-based confocal laser endomicroscopy to guide real-time endoscopic therapy in Barrett's esophagus with dysplasia. Case Rep Gastroenterol. 2012;6(2):285–92.
16. Wallace MB, Crook JE, Saunders M, Lovat L, Coron E, Waxman I, et al. Multicenter, randomized, controlled trial of confocal laser endomicroscopy assessment of residual metaplasia after mucosal ablation or resection of GI neoplasia in Barrett's esophagus. Gastrointest Endosc. 2012;76(3):539–47. e1.
17. Gray NA, Odze RD, Spechler SJ. Buried metaplasia after endoscopic ablation of Barrett's esophagus: a systematic review. Am J Gastroenterol. 2011;106(11):1899–908. quiz 909.

18. Kapadia CR. Gastric atrophy, metaplasia, and dysplasia: a clinical perspective. J Clin Gastroenterol. 2003;36(5 Suppl):S29–36. discussion S61-2.
19. Yoon H, Kim N. Diagnosis and management of high risk group for gastric cancer. Gut Liver. 2015;9:5–17.
20. Dinis-Ribeiro M, Areia M, de Vries AC, Marcos-Pinto R, Monteiro-Soares M, O'Connor A, et al. Management of precancerous conditions and lesions in the stomach (MAPS): guideline from the European Society of Gastrointestinal Endoscopy (ESGE), European Helicobacter Study Group (EHSG), European Society of Pathology (ESP), and the Sociedade Portuguesa de Endoscopia Digestiva (SPED). Endoscopy. 2012;44(1):74–94.
21. Lee KS, Oh DK, Han MA, Lee HY, Jun JK, Choi KS, et al. Gastric cancer screening in Korea: report on the national cancer screening program in 2008. Cancer Res Treat. 2011;43(2):83–8.
22. Ezoe Y, Muto M, Horimatsu T, Minashi K, Yano T, Sano Y, et al. Magnifying narrow-band imaging versus magnifying white-light imaging for the differential diagnosis of gastric small depressive lesions: a prospective study. Gastrointest Endosc. 2010;71(3):477–84.
23. Areia M, Amaro P, Dinis-Ribeiro M, Cipriano MA, Marinho C, Costa-Pereira A, et al. External validation of a classification for methylene blue magnification chromoendoscopy in premalignant gastric lesions. Gastrointest Endosc. 2008;67(7):1011–8.
24. Zhang JN, Li YQ, Zhao YA, Yu T, Zhang JP, Guo YT, et al. Classification of gastric pit patterns by confocal endomicroscopy. Gastrointest Endosc. 2008;67:843–53.
25. Guo YT, Li YQ, Yu T, Zhang TG, Zhang JN, Liu H, et al. Diagnosis of gastric intestinal metaplasia with confocal laser endomicroscopy in vivo: a prospective study. Endoscopy. 2008; 40(7):547–53.
26. Bok GH, Jeon SR, Cho JY, Cho JH, Lee WC, Jin SY, et al. The accuracy of probe-based confocal endomicroscopy versus conventional endoscopic biopsies for the diagnosis of superficial gastric neoplasia (with videos). Gastrointest Endosc. 2013;77(6):899–908.
27. Shahid MW, Buchner AM, Coron E, Woodward TA, Raimondo M, Dekker E, et al. Diagnostic accuracy of probe-based confocal laser endomicroscopy in detecting residual colorectal neoplasia after EMR: a prospective study. Gastrointest Endosc. 2012;75:525–33.
28. Larghi A, Waxman I. Endoscopic mucosal resection: treatment of neoplasia. Gastrointest Endosc Clin N Am. 2005;15:431–54. viii.
29. Khashab M, Eid E, Rusche M, Rex DK. Incidence and predictors of "late" recurrences after endoscopic piecemeal resection of large sessile adenomas. Gastrointest Endosc. 2009; 70:344–9.
30. Winawer SJ, Zauber AG, Fletcher RH, Stillman JS, O'Brien MJ, Levin B, et al. Guidelines for colonoscopy surveillance after polypectomy: a consensus update by the US Multi-Society Task Force on Colorectal Cancer and the American Cancer Society. CA Cancer J Clin. 2006;56:143–59. quiz 84–5.
31. Vaughn BP, Shah S, Cheifetz AS. The role of mucosal healing in the treatment of patients with inflammatory bowel disease. Curr Treat Options Gastroenterol. 2014;12(1):103–17.
32. Neumann H, Coron E, Mönkemüller K, Neurath MF, Vieth M. 702 Development of a new classification for confocal LASER endomicroscopy in IBD. Gastrointest Endosc. 2013;77(5):AB163.
33. Neumann H, Vieth M, Atreya R, Grauer M, Siebler J, Bernatik T, et al. Assessment of Crohn's disease activity by confocal laser endomicroscopy. Inflamm Bowel Dis. 2012;18(12):2261–9.
34. Kiesslich R, Goetz M, Lammersdorf K, Schneider C, Burg J, Stolte M, et al. Chromoscopy-guided endomicroscopy increases the diagnostic yield of intraepithelial neoplasia in ulcerative colitis. Gastroenterology. 2007;132:874–82.
35. Li CQ, Xie XJ, Yu T, Gu XM, Zuo XL, Zhou CJ, et al. Classification of inflammation activity in ulcerative colitis by confocal laser endomicroscopy. Am J Gastroenterol. 2010;105:1391–6.
36. Tytgat GN, Dhir V, Gopinath N. Endoscopic appearance of dysplasia and cancer in inflammatory bowel disease. Eur J Cancer. 1995;31A(7–8):1174–7.
37. Itzkowitz SH, Harpaz N. Diagnosis and management of dysplasia in patients with inflammatory bowel diseases. Gastroenterology. 2004;126:1634–48.

38. Leighton JA, Shen B, Baron TH, Adler DG, Davila R, Egan JV, et al. ASGE guideline: endoscopy in the diagnosis and treatment of inflammatory bowel disease. Gastrointest Endosc. 2006;63:558–65.
39. Li Z, Zuo XL, Li CQ, Zhou CJ, Liu J, Goetz M, et al. In vivo molecular imaging of gastric cancer by targeting MG7 antigen with confocal laser endomicroscopy. Endoscopy. 2013;45(2):79–85.
40. Hsiung PL, Hardy J, Friedland S, Soetikno R, Du CB, Wu AP, et al. Detection of colonic dysplasia in vivo using a targeted heptapeptide and confocal microendoscopy. Nat Med. 2008;14(4):454–8.
41. Sturm MB, Joshi BP, Lu S, Piraka C, Khondee S, Elmunzer BJ, et al. Targeted imaging of esophageal neoplasia with a fluorescently labeled peptide: first-in-human results. Sci Transl Med. 2013;5(184). 184ra61.
42. Foersch S, Kiesslich R, Waldner MJ, Delaney P, Galle PR, Neurath MF, et al. Molecular imaging of VEGF in gastrointestinal cancer in vivo using confocal laser endomicroscopy. Gut. 2010;59(8):1046–55.
43. Cartana T, Saftoiu A, Gruionu LG, Gheonea DI, Pirici D, Georgescu CV, et al. Confocal laser endomicroscopy for the morphometric evaluation of microvessels in human colorectal cancer using targeted anti-CD31 antibodies. PLoS One. 2012;7, e52815.
44. Lightdale CJ. Esophageal cancer. American College of Gastroenterology. Am J Gastroenterol. 1999;94:20–9.
45. Mori M, Adachi Y, Matsushima T, Matsuda H, Kuwano H, Sugimachi K. Lugol staining pattern and histology of esophageal lesions. Am J Gastroenterol. 1993;88(5):701–5.
46. Deinert K, Kiesslich R, Vieth M, Neurath MF, Neuhaus H. In-vivo microvascular imaging of early squamous-cell cancer of the esophagus by confocal laser endomicroscopy. Endoscopy. 2007;39(4):366–8.
47. Liu H, Li YQ, Yu T, Zhao YA, Zhang JP, Zuo XL, et al. Confocal laser endomicroscopy for superficial esophageal squamous cell carcinoma. Endoscopy. 2009;41(2):99–106.
48. Pech O, Rabenstein T, Manner H, Petrone MC, Pohl J, Vieth M, et al. Confocal laser endomicroscopy for in vivo diagnosis of early squamous cell carcinoma in the esophagus. Clin Gastroenterol Hepatol. 2008;6:89–94.
49. Rex DK, Kahi C, O'Brien M, Levin TR, Pohl H, Rastogi A, et al. The American Society for Gastrointestinal Endoscopy PIVI (Preservation and incorporation of valuable endoscopic innovations) on real-time endoscopic assessment of the histology of diminutive colorectal polyps. Gastrointest Endosc. 2011;73:419–22.
50. Levin TR, Zhao W, Conell C, Seeff LC, Manninen DL, Shapiro JA, et al. Complications of colonoscopy in an integrated health care delivery system. Ann Intern Med. 2006;145(12):880–6.
51. Rex DK, Johnson DA, Anderson JC, Schoenfeld PS, Burke CA, Inadomi JM. American College of Gastroenterology guidelines for colorectal cancer screening 2009 [corrected]. Am J Gastroenterol. 2009;104:739–50.
52. Abu Dayyeh BK, Thosani N, Konda V, Wallace MB, Rex DK, Chauhan SS, et al. ASGE Technology Committee systematic review and meta-analysis assessing the ASGE PIVI thresholds for adopting real-time endoscopic assessment of the histology of diminutive colorectal polyps. Gastrointest Endosc. 2015;81(3):502. e1–e16.
53. Buchner AM, Shahid MW, Heckman MG, Krishna M, Ghabril M, Hasan M, et al. Comparison of probe-based confocal laser endomicroscopy with virtual chromoendoscopy for classification of colon polyps. Gastroenterology. 2010;138(3):834–42.
54. Shahid MW, Buchner AM, Raimondo M, Woodward TA, Krishna M, Wallace MB. Accuracy of real-time vs. blinded offline diagnosis of neoplastic colorectal polyps using probe-based confocal laser endomicroscopy: a pilot study. Endoscopy. 2012;44(4):343–8.
55. Kuiper T, van den Broek FJ, van Eeden S, Fockens P, Dekker E. Feasibility and accuracy of confocal endomicroscopy in comparison with narrow-band imaging and chromoendoscopy for the differentiation of colorectal lesions. Am J Gastroenterol. 2012;107(4):543–50.

56. Shahid MW, Buchner AM, Heckman MG, Krishna M, Raimondo M, Woodward T, et al. Diagnostic accuracy of probe-based confocal laser endomicroscopy and narrow band imaging for small colorectal polyps: a feasibility study. Am J Gastroenterol. 2012;107:231–9.
57. Ignjatovic A, East JE, Suzuki N, Vance M, Guenther T, Saunders BP. Optical diagnosis of small colorectal polyps at routine colonoscopy (Detect InSpect ChAracterise Resect and Discard; DISCARD trial): a prospective cohort study. Lancet Oncol. 2009;10:1171–8.
58. Andre B, Vercauteren T, Buchner AM, Krishna M, Ayache N, Wallace MB. Software for automated classification of probe-based confocal laser endomicroscopy videos of colorectal polyps. World J Gastroenterol. 2012;18(39):5560–9.
59. Liu JJ, Madsen KL, Boulanger P, Dieleman LA, Meddings J, Fedorak RN. Mind the gaps: confocal endomicroscopy showed increased density of small bowel epithelial gaps in inflammatory bowel disease. J Clin Gastroenterol. 2011;45(3):240–5.
60. Liu JJ, Wong K, Thiesen AL, Mah SJ, Dieleman LA, Claggett B, et al. Increased epithelial gaps in the small intestines of patients with inflammatory bowel disease: density matters. Gastrointest Endosc. 2011;73(6):1174–80.
61. Turcotte JF, Wong K, Mah SJ, Dieleman LA, Kao D, Kroeker K, et al. Increased epithelial gaps in the small intestine are predictive of hospitalization and surgery in patients with inflammatory bowel disease. Clin Transl Gastroenterol. 2012;3, e19.
62. Kiesslich R, Duckworth CA, Moussata D, Gloeckner A, Lim LG, Goetz M, et al. Local barrier dysfunction identified by confocal laser endomicroscopy predicts relapse in inflammatory bowel disease. Gut. 2012;61:1146–53.
63. Atreya R, Neumann H, Neufert C, Waldner MJ, Billmeier U, Zopf Y, et al. In vivo imaging using fluorescent antibodies to tumor necrosis factor predicts therapeutic response in Crohn's disease. Nat Med. 2014;20(3):313–8.
64. Chutkan RK, Scherl E, Waye JD. Colonoscopy in inflammatory bowel disease. Gastrointest Endosc Clin N Am. 2002;12(3):463–83. viii.
65. Tontini GE, Mudter J, Vieth M, Atreya R, Gunther C, Zopf Y, et al. Confocal laser endomicroscopy for the differential diagnosis of ulcerative colitis and Crohn's disease: a pilot study. Endoscopy. 2015;47(5):437–43.
66. Turcotte JF, Kao D, Mah SJ, Claggett B, Saltzman JR, Fedorak RN, et al. Breaks in the wall: increased gaps in the intestinal epithelium of irritable bowel syndrome patients identified by confocal laser endomicroscopy (with videos). Gastrointest Endosc. 2013;77(4):624–30.
67. Fritscher-Ravens A, Schuppan D, Ellrichmann M, Schoch S, Rocken C, Brasch J, et al. Confocal endomicroscopy shows food-associated changes in the intestinal mucosa of patients with irritable bowel syndrome. Gastroenterology. 2014;147(5):1012–20. e4.
68. National Institutes of Health Consensus development conference statement on celiac disease, June 28–30, 2004. Gastroenterology. 2005;128:S1–9.
69. Leong RW, Nguyen NQ, Meredith CG, Al-Sohaily S, Kukic D, Delaney PM, et al. In vivo confocal endomicroscopy in the diagnosis and evaluation of celiac disease. Gastroenterology. 2008;135:1870–6.
70. Venkatesh K, Cohen M, Evans C, Delaney P, Thomas S, Taylor C, et al. Feasibility of confocal endomicroscopy in the diagnosis of pediatric gastrointestinal disorders. World J Gastroenterol. 2009;15(18):2214–9.
71. Venkatesh K, Abou-Taleb A, Cohen M, Evans C, Thomas S, Oliver P, et al. Role of confocal endomicroscopy in the diagnosis of celiac disease. J Pediatr Gastroenterol Nutr. 2010;51(3):274–9.
72. Hoffman A, Goetz M, Vieth M, Galle PR, Neurath MF, Kiesslich R. Confocal laser endomicroscopy: technical status and current indications. Endoscopy. 2006;38(12):1275–83.
73. Wallace MB, Meining A, Canto MI, Fockens P, Miehlke S, Roesch T, et al. The safety of intravenous fluorescein for confocal laser endomicroscopy in the gastrointestinal tract. Aliment Pharmacol Ther. 2010;31:548–52.
74. Sharman MJ, Mansfield CS, Whittem T. The exogenous fluorophore, fluorescein, enables in vivo assessment of the gastrointestinal mucosa via confocal endomicroscopy: optimization of intravenous dosing in the dog model. J Vet Pharmacol Ther. 2013;36(5):450–5.

75. Becker V, von Delius S, Bajbouj M, Karagianni A, Schmid RM, Meining A. Intravenous application of fluorescein for confocal laser scanning microscopy: evaluation of contrast dynamics and image quality with increasing injection-to-imaging time. Gastrointest Endosc. 2008;68:319–23.
76. Shahid MW, Crook JE, Meining A, Perchant A, Buchner A, Gomez V, et al. Exploring the optimal fluorescein dose in probe-based confocal laser endomicroscopy for colonic imaging. J Interv Gastroenterol. 2011;1(4):166–71.
77. Coron E, Mosnier JF, Ahluwalia A, Le Rhun M, Galmiche JP, Tarnawski AS, et al. Colonic mucosal biopsies obtained during confocal endomicroscopy are pre-stained with fluorescein in vivo and are suitable for histologic evaluation. Endoscopy. 2012;44(2):148–53.
78. Kiesslich R, Gossner L, Goetz M, Dahlmann A, Vieth M, Stolte M, et al. In vivo histology of Barrett's esophagus and associated neoplasia by confocal laser endomicroscopy. Clin Gastroenterol Hepatol. 2006;4:979–87.
79. Gaddam S, Mathur SC, Singh M, Arora J, Wani SB, Gupta N, et al. Novel probe-based confocal laser endomicroscopy criteria and interobserver agreement for the detection of dysplasia in Barrett's esophagus. Am J Gastroenterol. 2011;106(11):1961–9.
80. Wallace M. et al. Miami classification for probe-based confocal laser endomicroscopy. 2011;43(10):882–91.
81. Ha SO, Kim DY, Sohn CH, Lim KS. Anaphylaxis caused by intravenous fluorescein: clinical characteristics and review of literature. Intern Emerg Med. 2014;9(3):325–30.
82. Hassan C, Pickhardt PJ, Rex DK. A resect and discard strategy would improve cost-effectiveness of colorectal cancer screening. Clin Gastroenterol Hepatol. 2010;8:865–9. 9 e1–3.

Chapter 7
Optical Coherence Tomography: Clinical Applications in Gastrointestinal Endoscopy

Cadman L. Leggett, Daniel K. Chan, and Kenneth K. Wang

Principles of Optical Coherence Tomography

Optical coherence tomography (OCT) is analogous in many ways to B-mode endoscopic ultrasonography. An ultrasound probe contains multiple acoustic transducers that emit high frequency (5–15 MHz) sound pulses capable of propagating through tissue at a speed determined by its physical properties. Sounds waves that encounter denser tissue structures are reflected back to the transducer and are said to be hyperechoic, producing a stronger acoustic signal compared to the surrounding tissue. OCT uses infrared light (λ 750–1300 nm) rather than sound waves. Propagation of coherent monochromatic light through biological tissue is dependent on the absorptive and scattering properties of the tissue. The relatively longer wave length of infrared light decreases absorption by tissue and allows detection of reflected or backscattered light. The high velocity of light (299,792,458 m/s) compared to sound (343.2 m/s), however, does not allow direct electronic measurement of reflected light. To do so, an interferometer (Fig. 7.1) is employed to compare the phase difference of two light paths or "arms": a sample arm (tissue) and a reference arm (mirror). Light reflected from the tissue specimen is combined with light that has

C.L. Leggett, M.D. • D.K. Chan, M.D.
Division of Gastroenterology and Hepatology, Mayo Clinic, Rochester, MN, USA

K.K. Wang, M.D. (✉)
Barrett's Esophagus Unit, Division of Gastroenterology and Hepatology, Mayo Clinic, 200 First St. SW, Rochester, MN 55905, USA
e-mail: wang.kenneth@mayo.edu

V.J.A. Konda, I. Waxman (eds.), *Endoscopic Imaging Techniques and Tools*,
DOI 10.1007/978-3-319-30053-5_7

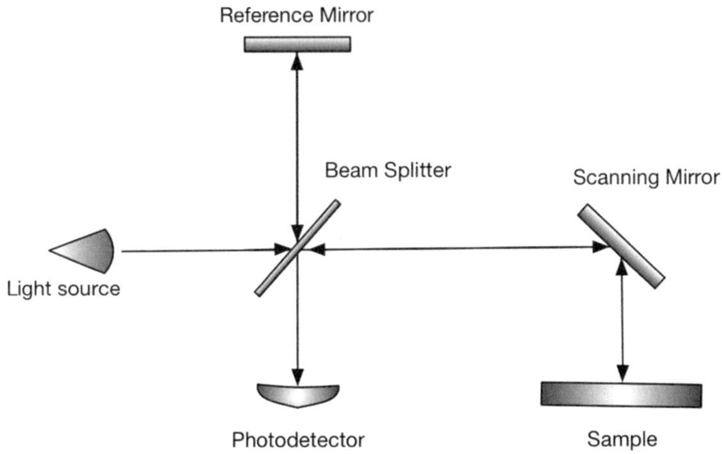

Fig. 7.1 Schematic diagram showing basic optical principles of optical coherence tomography. Infrared light (λ 750–1300 nm) reflected from a scanning mirror (sample) is combined with light reflected from a reference mirror and known to have traveled a set distance. The combined light waves are captured by a photodetector and generate an interference intensity profile

traveled a known distance through the reference arm and focused onto a photodetector. The interference profile generated by the combined light waves is said to be "constructive" if the two light waves are in phase with one another (even multiple of $\lambda/2$) and "destructive" if they are out of phase (odd multiple of $\lambda/2$). Constructive interference generates a strong OCT signal, while destructive interference generates a weak OCT signal.

In time-domain OCT, the reference mirror is scanned across a range of positions that match different depths in the sample tissue. Image acquisition speed is therefore dependent on the scanning speed of the reference mirror. The image is constructed through a rasterized image of these points that represent depth and longitudinal surface. Fourier domain OCT refers to second-generation OCT imaging systems that measure the interference signal as a function of a slight frequency shift and therefore does not require a scanning reference mirror. This approach results in imaging speeds that are 10–200 times faster and a detection sensitivity that is 10–100 greater than time-domain OCT. [1] Fourier domain OCT includes two types of techniques, spectral domain OCT and optical Fourier domain imaging; also known as swept source OCT or more recently termed volumetric laser endomicroscopy (VLE).

Commercially Available OCT Systems

OCT-based microscopes were first developed for imaging the retina which was an ideal application given the optically clear focused pathways to the layered structure and the fovea. These devices now can visualize the cell bodies, receptors, and

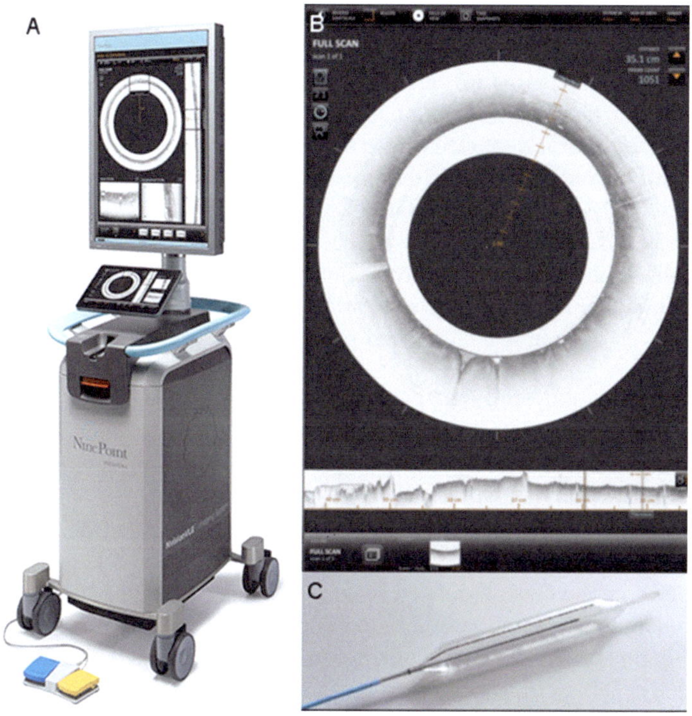

Fig. 7.2 (**a**) Nvision volumetric laser endomicroscopy imaging console (Nine Point Medical, MA), (**b**) User interface showing cross-sectional transverse and longitudinal views as well as magnified region of interest, (**c**) VLE imaging balloon probe. *Axial resolution*; *Transverse resolution*: 30 μm; *Imaging depth*: >3 mm; *Dynamic range*: >45 dB; *Balloon diameters*: 14, 17, 20 mm; *Balloon length*: 6 cm; *Endoscope channel compatibility*: ≥2.8 mm

vascular structures in the retina and are invaluable for the treatment of retinopathies. OCT probes were originally designed for use in the fields of cardiology and were subsequently applied to gastrointestinal imaging [2, 3]. Coronary OCT allows the visualization of unstable coronary plaques that are responsible for the majority of sudden death events. OCT systems differ from each other in their scanning depth, resolution, speed of image acquisition, and scanning method (radial vs. linear). The image acquisition speed and high signal to noise ratio of VLE make this type of OCT system well-suited for imaging of the gastrointestinal tract. The most recent commercially available OCT system is the Nvision VLE Imaging System (Nine Point Medical, MA), which consists of a console, monitor, and optical probe (Fig. 7.2). The Nvision VLE system was designed for imaging of the esophagus. Its optical probe is centered by a balloon (diameter: 14, 17, 20 mm; length: 6 cm) that is deployed through a gastroscope's instrument channel (2.8 mm or larger). The balloon is used to keep tissue at the optimal imaging distance for the focal length of the probe. Imaging is performed by automatic helical pullback of the probe from the distal to the proximal end of the balloon over 90 s. VLE images have an axial resolution of 7 μm and a transverse resolution of ~30 μm and can reach an imaging depth of up to 2–5 mm. A total of 1200 cross-sectional images are acquired over a 6 cm VLE scan. VLE scans are viewed using a software interface that allows simultaneous examination of cross-sectional transverse and longitudinal views.

The VLE catheter is deployed across the gastroesophageal junction with the distal 1–2 cm of the probe located in the stomach. The balloon catheter is then inflated at low-pressure (5–15 psi) using an insufflation device and pressure gauge. A scout image can be obtained to determine adequate centering of the balloon prior to full scan imaging and to ensure proper positioning of the balloon across the esophagus. The scout imaging allows image acquisition in approximately 20 s. After imaging acquisition, the balloon is deflated and removed through the gastroscope's instrument channel.

The first-generation Nvision VLE imaging system was evaluated in a safety and feasibility trial that enrolled 100 patients with suspected or confirmed Barrett's esophagus (BE) across three academic centers. [4] VLE was successfully completed in 87 patients (87 %), defined as having at least one complete 6 cm full scan that showed the proximal stomach, gastroesophageal junction, and distal esophagus. VLE was not completed in nine patients due to optical probe-related issues and in three patients due to console-related issues. The Nvision company has produced a second-generation imaging system addressing the probe and console limitations observed in this study. There were no device-related serious adverse events reports in this study. However, two minor device-related adverse events were reported including a small esophageal mucosal tear in two patients that did not require specific intervention. The balloon used in this was 25 mm in diameter, which has subsequently resulted in the creation of the smaller sizes to ensure appropriate size balloon for the esophageal diameter. The device was deemed safe for patients with suspected or confirmed BE.

Gastrointestinal Applications of Optical Coherence Tomography

Esophagus

OCT has a wide range of applications in benign and neoplastic esophageal imaging. The normal esophagus demonstrates a five-layered architecture under OCT: low scattering epithelium, high scattering lamina propria, low scattering muscularis mucosa, high scattering submucosa, and low scattering muscularis propria (Fig. 7.3a, b) [5]. In contrast, Barrett's esophagus lacks a layered architecture and often shows heterogenous scattering and epithelial glands (Fig. 7.3c) [6, 7]. Studies have shown that OCT can distinguish between Barrett's esophagus, gastric cardia, and squamous epithelium at the gastroesophageal junction with 85 % sensitivity, 95 % specificity, and high interobserver agreement [8].

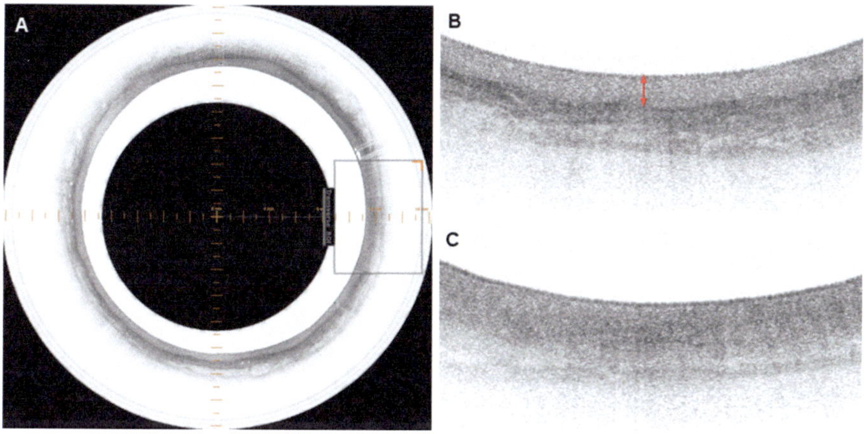

Fig. 7.3 (**a**) In-vivo volumetric laser endomicroscopy showing (**b**) squamous epithelium and an island of (**c**) Barrett's esophagus (*region of interest box*). Squamous epithelium shows a layered architecture with low scattering epithelium (*double head arrow*) and high scattering submucosa. Barrett's esophagus lacks a layered architecture and shows heterogenous scattering

The use of OCT to detect dysplasia associated with Barrett's esophagus is an emergent field. OCT can be used to assess epithelial surface maturation and glandular architecture. These features have been applied to a four point scoring index for differentiating intramucosal adenocarcinoma/high-grade dysplasia from low-grade dysplasia/non-dysplastic Barrett's esophagus [9]. A score of greater than or equal to two has been associated with 83 % sensitivity and 75 % specificity in the detection of Barrett's associated neoplasia with OCT (Fig. 7.4) [9]. The use of these criteria with VLE showed decreased diagnostic performance at the same dysplasia score threshold [10]. The optimal diagnostic performance was found to be a score of ≥3, which was associated with 70 % sensitivity, 60 % specificity, and 67 % diagnostic accuracy compared to other scores. The increased dysplasia score threshold required for VLE was attributed to the fact that the diagnostic criteria were developed using a first-generation form of OCT that is different from VLE, which uses second-generation OCT technology and a balloon catheter. Furthermore, compared with OCT used in prior studies in which single, ~5 mm wide images were used for diagnosis, image interpretation using VLE is performed over a much wider field of view (6 cm, 1200 frames) that may have frame-to-frame variation in surface signal intensity. A recent study has introduced modified criteria for use with VLE that take into account wide field imaging capabilities of second generation OCT optics (Fig. 7.5) [10]. These criteria contain specific VLE features associated with neoplasia, including lack of mucosal layering, increased surface signal intensity, and quantification of atypical glandular structures. Ex-Vivo validation of these criteria showed a sensitivity of 86 %, specificity of 88 %, and diagnostic accuracy of 87 % in the diagnosis of BE-associated dysplasia.

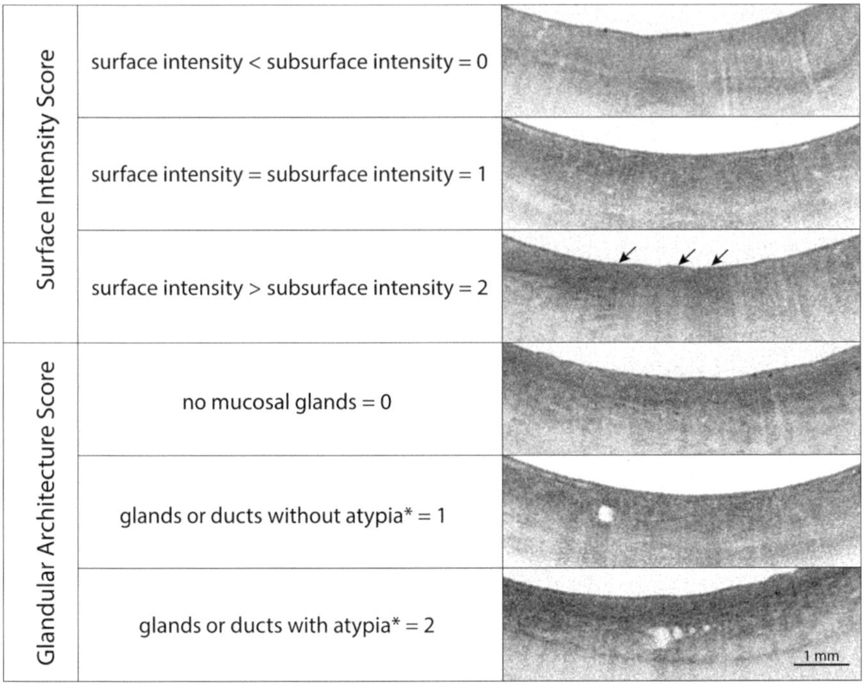

Fig. 7.4 Optical coherence tomography scoring index for detection of Barrett's esophagus (BE)-associated dysplasia. The scoring index consists of two independent criteria (surface to subsurface signal intensity and glandular architecture) that are added to calculate a dysplasia score. A dysplasia score of ≥2 is associated with a sensitivity of 83 % and a specificity of 75 % for the diagnosis of neoplasia in BE. *Black arrows* show areas of increased surface intensity. Adapted with permission from Leggett CL, Gorospe EC, Chan DK, et al. Comparative Diagnostic Performance of Volumetric Laser Endomicroscopy and Confocal Laser Endomicroscopy in the Detection of Dysplasia Associated with Barrett's Esophagus. Gastrointestinal endoscopy 2015; Ahead of print. © Elsevier [10]. *Asterisk* Glandular atypia is defined by the presence of irregular and/or dilated glands

Endoscopic mucosal ablation is a commonly employed treatment modality for dysplastic Barrett's esophagus. Measurement of Barrett's esophagus epithelium thickness using OCT has shown to predict response to radiofrequency ablation. A threshold thickness of 333 μm derived from receiver operating characteristic curves corresponded to a 92 % sensitivity, 85 % specificity, and 88 % accuracy in predicting the presence of Barrett's epithelium on follow-up endoscopy [11].

Reports of subsquamous esophageal adenocarcinoma that arises after mucosal ablation have given rise to concern for the neoplastic potential of buried intestinal metaplasia [12, 13]. The cross-sectional imaging capability of OCT allows closer examination of the esophageal submucosa and several studies have used OCT to detect buried glands under neosquamous epithelium following radiofrequency ablation. A study that used a three-dimensional OCT probe to evaluate for buried glands at the esophagogastric junction in patients undergoing radiofrequency ablation

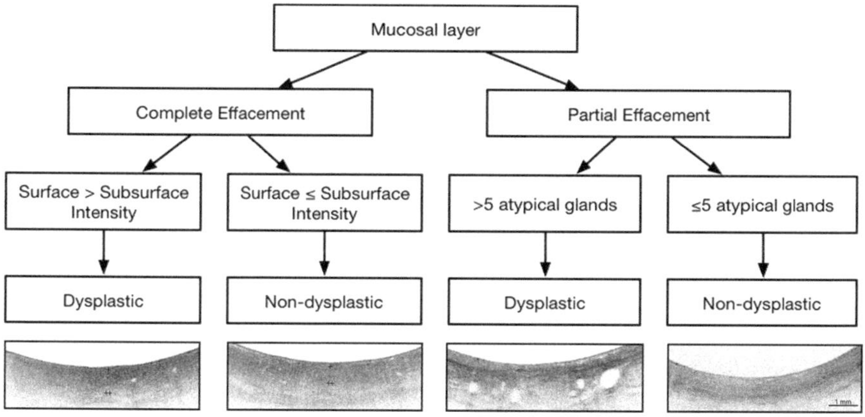

Fig. 7.5 Volumetric laser endomicroscopy diagnostic algorithm for detection of Barrett's esophagus (BE)-associated dysplasia. Interpretation of the diagnostic algorithm is performed over a longitudinal distance of 1 cm of Barrett's esophagus (BE). Partial effacement of the mucosal layer is defined by a mucosal layer present in ≥50 % of the scan. Complete effacement of the mucosal layer is defined by a mucosal layer over <50 % of the scan. A rating of image surface to subsurface intensity corresponds to the most prevalent ratio (surface > subsurface intensity vs. surface ≤ subsurface intensity) present in ≥50 % of the scan. The single asterisk represents the VLE surface signal intensity and the double asterisk the subsurface intensity. Adapted with permission from Leggett CL, Gorospe EC, Chan DK, et al. Comparative Diagnostic Performance of Volumetric Laser Endomicroscopy and Confocal Laser Endomicroscopy in the Detection of Dysplasia Associated with Barrett's Esophagus. Gastrointestinal endoscopy 2015; Ahead of print. © Elsevier [10]

showed the presence of glands in 72 % of patients before achieving complete eradication of intestinal metaplasia and in 63 % of patients after complete response [14]. A limitation of this study was the lack of histological confirmation of the submucosal structures observed. A more recent study using VLE detected submucosal glandular structures in 76 % of post-radiofrequency ablation patients that reached complete eradication of intestinal metaplasia [15]. These structures were targeted with endoscopic mucosal resection and found to correspond to normal histological structures (dilated glands and blood vessels) in 92 % of cases. Only a single endoscopic mucosal resection specimen contained evidence of buried glands. A case report showed subsquamous adenocarcinoma imaged with VLE in a freshly excised endoscopic mucosal resection specimen (Fig. 7.6) [16].

OCT has also been shown to have high accuracy in the preoperative staging of superficial esophageal squamous cell carcinoma. A single-center study that compared OCT imaging to histological staging of submucosal dissection specimens showed an overall imaging staging accuracy of 92.7 % [17]. The developed criteria were based on the visualization of squamous epithelial layers grouped into three categories (epithelium/lamina propria, muscularis mucosa, submucosa). A subsequent study showed that the accuracy of OCT in staging tumors limited to the epithelium/lamina propria was significantly higher than high-frequency probe-based endoscopic ultrasound (95 % vs. 81 %, $p < 0.01$) [17]. The authors of this study note

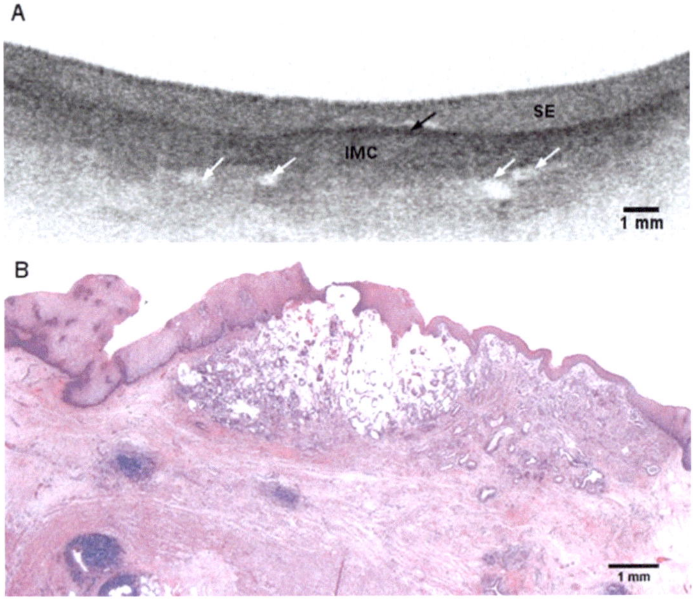

Fig. 7.6 (**a**) Volumetric laser endomicroscopy of endoscopic mucosal resection with features suggestive of intramucosal adenocarcinoma including increased signal intensity (*black arrow*) and atypical appearing glands and dilated ducts (*white arrow*) underneath a layer of squamous epithelium. (**b**) Endoscopic mucosal resection showing subsquamous moderate to poorly differentiated adenocarcionoma invading into the lamina propria and muscularis mucosa. Adapted with permission from Leggett CL, Gorospe E, Owens VL, et al. Volumetric laser endomicroscopy detects subsquamous Barrett's adenocarcinoma. American Journal of Gastroenterology 2014;109:298–9. © Nature Publishing Group [16]

that the diagnostic performance of OCT is limited by depth of penetration, the sample area of OCT, and the inability of OCT to distinguish between cancer invasion and inflammatory cell infiltration. There are currently no published reports on the use of VLE in staging esophageal squamous cell carcinoma.

Finally, few reports describe the use of OCT in differentiating heterotropic gastric mucosa (cervical inlet patch) in the upper esophagus from squamous epithelium [18].

Stomach

The application of OCT to the stomach is largely limited by the high reflectivity of glandular epithelium that restricts imaging of deeper layers. OCT images of the stomach are characterized by lack of contrast, a high reflective surface, vertical crypt and pit architecture, and a broad, regular gland architecture. Gastritis is described as having more surface reflectivity and more pronounced crypt and pit architecture compared to the normal stomach [19].

Small Bowel and Colon

There are limited applications of OCT to imaging of the small bowel. Although OCT can clearly distinguish normal villous architecture from villous atrophy found in celiac disease, it is unable to tell apart normal villous architecture with and without increased intraepithelial lymphocytes, an important histological hallmark of this condition (Fig. 7.7) [20].

Colonic mucosa imaged with OCT is characterized by a regular, uniform mucosal crypt pattern, a highly scattering submucosa, a weakly scattering muscularis propria, and a highly scattering serosal stripe (Fig. 7.8a) [21]. OCT can distinguish between normal colon and inflammatory conditions such as ulcerative colitis and Crohn's disease (Fig. 7.8b, c). A study that evaluated OCT patterns of colonic mucosa in patients with ulcerative colitis found that OCT can correctly identify several disease features endoscopically [22]. An OCT scoring index that included mucosal backscattering alterations (0–3°) delimited darker areas (absent/present)

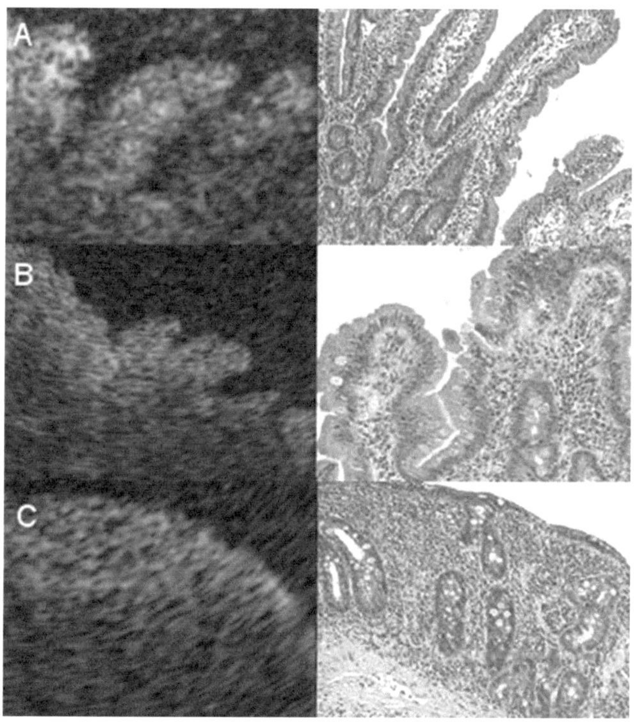

Fig. 7.7 Optical coherence tomography of (**a**) normal villous morphology with corresponding histology, (**b**) celiac disease with mild villous atrophy, and (**c**) celiac disease with marked villous atrophy. Adapted with permission from Masci E, Mangiavillano B, Albarello L, et al. Pilot study on the correlation of optical coherence tomography with histology in celiac disease and normal subjects. Journal of gastroenterology and hepatology 2007;22:2256–60. © John Wiley and Sons [20]

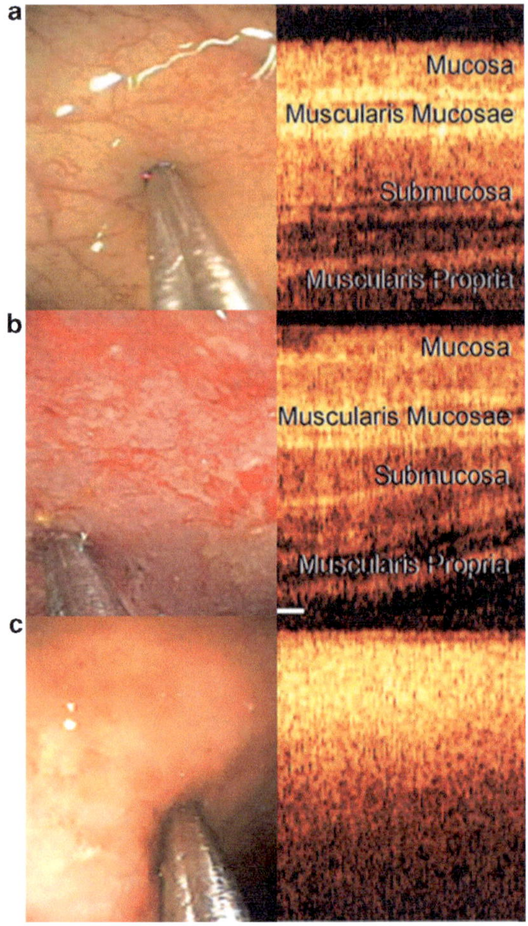

Fig. 7.8 Endoscopic and optical coherence view of (**a**) normal colonic mucosa showing a layered architecture, (**b**) ulcerative colitis showing preserved layered architecture, and (**c**) Crohn's disease showing disrupted layered architecture. Adapted with permission from Shen B, Zuccaro G, Jr., Gramlich TL, et al. In vivo colonoscopic optical coherence tomography for transmural inflammation in inflammatory bowel disease. Clinical gastroenterology and hepatology: the official clinical practice journal of the American Gastroenterological Association 2004;2:1080–7. © Elsevier [24]

and alterations in the layered structure of the colonic wall (evident/present/absent) correlated with histological features of mucosal inflammation (0–3°), lymphoid aggregate (present/absent), granuloma (present/absent), and crypt abscess (present/absent). The authors of this study report that OCT can reliably distinguish between mild–moderate ulcerative colitis and severe disease.

OCT has also been used to assess the degree of disruption of the colon's layered architecture, a feature associated with transmural inflammation often found in Crohn's disease. A study that performed OCT on colectomy specimens of patients with ulcerative colitis and Crohn's disease found that the sensitivity and specificity for OCT to detect transmural disease was 86 % and 91 %, respectively [23]. Eight patients with a preoperative diagnosis of ulcerative colitis and features of transmural inflammation on OCT were found to have Crohn's disease based on histological evidence of transmural disease found in the colectomy specimens. A follow-up study by the same investigators validated the use of OCT to distinguish between Crohn's disease and ulcerative colitis in-vivo [24]. Using the clinical diagnosis as the gold standard, a disrupted layered architecture on OCT had a diagnostic sensitivity and specificity of 90 % and 83 %, respectively, for the diagnosis of Crohn's disease. The use of OCT to distinguish between types of inflammatory bowel disease in practice is challenged by image interpretation of various colonic regions ranging from normal mucosa/slight inflammation in Crohn's disease that can produce images with normal layered mucosa and severe inflammation in ulcerative colitis that can produce images with a disrupted layered architecture.

The use of OCT has also been studied in the assessment of colonic adenomatous and hyperplastic polyps. Hyperplastic polyps are described as having an organized crypt pattern and scattering intensity similar to normal colonic mucosa [25]. In contrast, adenomatous polyps demonstrate an absence of an organized crypt pattern and a decrease in scattering intensity compared to normal colonic mucosa. This observation was later confirmed in a study that measured the scattering coefficient of adenomatous polyps and found it to be between the values obtained for normal and malignant tissues [26]. The use of OCT as a real-time diagnostic tool for colorectal polyps requires further evaluation and in-vivo validation.

Pancreatobiliary

OCT probes designed for use during endoscopic retrograde cholangiopancreatography allow in-vivo imaging of the pancreatobiliary ductal system [27]. The normal common bile duct and pancreatic duct are described as having three distinct layers: a low scattering inner layer that represents the epithelium (mean thickness 0.05 mm), a highly scattering intermediate layer that represents the submucosa (mean thickness 0.41 mm), and an outer low scattering layer that represents the serosa. All three layers have a homogenous scattering signal with greater distinction between the inner and intermediate layers compared to the outer and intermediate layers [28].

Fibrotic changes in the pancreatobiliary ductal system demonstrate an increased thickness of the intermediate layer and preserved three-layer architecture. Inflammatory changes, on the other hand, demonstrate an increased thickness of the inner epithelial layer with higher scattering of the intermediate layer [29]. These features, however, may be subtle and not specific enough to distinguish acute from chronic inflammatory changes in the main pancreatic duct.

Dysplastic and neoplastic changes of the pancreatobiliary ductal system can be observed with OCT. The presence of dysplasia in the main pancreatic duct epithelium is characterized by a thickened inner layer with a heterogenous scattering profile with the interphase between the inner and intermediate layer appearing irregular [30, 31]. Neoplastic changes often show a disorganized layer architecture and heterogenous light scattering. The diagnostic performance of OCT for malignant pancreatobiliary strictures is reported in few in-vivo studies. A study that evaluated 16 patients with benign biliary strictures and 19 patients with malignant strictures (confirmed by brush cytology and/or biopsy) showed a sensitivity of 84 % for detecting malignancy when combining OCT criteria and brushing/biopsy results [32].

A study of 12 patients with main pancreatic duct strictures showed that the accuracy of OCT for detecting neoplastic tissue was 100 % compared to 66.7 % for brush cytology alone [31].

OCT has also been used to describe specific morphological features of pancreatic cysts. Freshly excised pancreatic specimens containing mucinous (mucinous cystic neoplasms and intraductal papillary mucinous neoplasms) and serous (serous cyst adenomas) cysts demonstrated differences in cystic wall morphology and the scattering profile of cystic fluid [33]. The application of these diagnostic features to endoscopic retrograde cholangiopancreatography, however, is limited by the depth of imaging of OCT and the location of pancreatic cysts in relation to the main pancreatic duct.

Conclusion and Further Directions

OCT is capable of high-resolution real-time imaging of the gastrointestinal tract. Its role in gastrointestinal endoscopy, however, is yet to be defined. An evolving clinical application of OCT is the detection of dysplasia associated with BE. The commercially available Nvision VLE system can provide comprehensive views of the human esophagus and may allow detection of dysplasia that is missed on surveillance biopsies. The use of VLE to guide biopsies is not feasible with the current Nvision system that uses a balloon catheter for imaging acquisition. A laser cautery marking device has been developed in which the operator can select a target region. A pilot study of 22 patients showed that this device had 93 % accuracy between the intent to biopsy site identified with VLE and the histopathology diagnosis [34]. A tethered capsule endomicroscopy device has also been developed as a minimally invasive form of VLE (Fig. 7.9) [35]. This device was tested in 26 patients, of whom

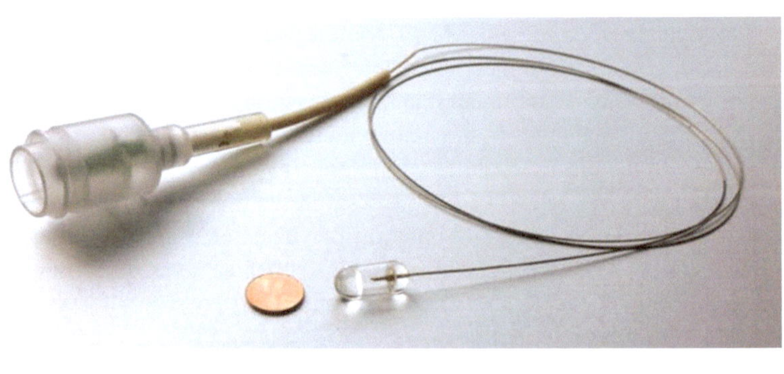

Fig. 7.9 The tethered capsule endomicroscopy catheter photographed with the capsule adjacent to a penny for scale. Adapted from Gora MJ, Sauk JS, Carruth RW, et al. Tethered capsule endomicroscopy enables less invasive imaging of gastrointestinal tract microstructure. Nature medicine 2013;19:238–40. © Nature Publishing Group [35]

2 were unable to swallow the capsule. Images were acquired through four passes over an average of 6 min. Most participants reported preferring this imaging approach to conventional endoscopy.

The addition of Doppler measurement to OCT has allowed detection of subtle changes in mucosal and submucosal microcirculation [36]. Endoscopic OCT angiography has been recently described using an ultrafast OCT device that allows visualization of microvasculature by detecting the intensity decorrelation of erythrocytes [37]. This device has promising applications for identification of subtle microvascular changes associated with BE dysplasia.

References

1. Tsai T-H, Fujimoto J, Mashimo H. Endoscopic optical coherence tomography for clinical gastroenterology. Diagn. 2014;4:57.
2. Tearney GJ, Brezinski ME, Boppart SA, et al. Images in cardiovascular medicine. Catheter-based optical imaging of a human coronary artery. Circulation. 1996;94:3013.
3. Drexler W, Morgner U, Ghanta RK, et al. Ultrahigh-resolution ophthalmic optical coherence tomography. Nat Med. 2001;7:502–7.
4. Wolfsen HC, Sharma P, Wallace MB, et al. Safety and feasibility of volumetric laser endomicroscopy in patients with Barrett's esophagus (with videos). Gastrointest Endosc. 2015;82(4):631–40.
5. Zuccaro G, Gladkova N, Vargo J, et al. Optical coherence tomography of the esophagus and proximal stomach in health and disease. Am J Gastroenterol. 2001;96:2633–9.
6. Suter MJ, Vakoc BJ, Yachimski PS, et al. Comprehensive microscopy of the esophagus in human patients with optical frequency domain imaging. Gastrointest Endosc. 2008;68:745–53.
7. Vakoc BJ, Shishko M, Yun SH, et al. Comprehensive esophageal microscopy by using optical frequency-domain imaging (with video). Gastrointest Endosc. 2007;65:898–905.
8. Evans JA, Bouma BE, Bressner J, et al. Identifying intestinal metaplasia at the squamocolumnar junction by using optical coherence tomography. Gastrointest Endosc. 2007;65:50–6.
9. Evans JA, Poneros JM, Bouma BE, et al. Optical coherence tomography to identify intramucosal carcinoma and high-grade dysplasia in Barrett's esophagus. Clin Gastroenterol Hepatol. 2006;4:38–43.
10. Leggett CL, Gorospe EC, Chan DK, et al. Comparative diagnostic performance of volumetric laser endomicroscopy and confocal laser endomicroscopy in the detection of dysplasia associated with Barrett's esophagus. Gastrointest Endosc. 2015; Ahead of print.
11. Tsai TH, Zhou C, Tao YK, et al. Structural markers observed with endoscopic 3-dimensional optical coherence tomography correlating with Barrett's esophagus radiofrequency ablation treatment response (with videos). Gastrointest Endosc. 2012;76:1104–12.
12. Gray NA, Odze RD, Spechler SJ. Buried metaplasia after endoscopic ablation of Barrett's esophagus: a systematic review. Am J Gastroenterol. 2011;106:1899–908. quiz 1909.
13. Titi M, Overhiser A, Ulusarac O, et al. Development of subsquamous high-grade dysplasia and adenocarcinoma after successful radiofrequency ablation of Barrett's esophagus. Gastroenterology. 2012;143:564–6. e1.
14. Zhou C, Tsai TH, Lee HC, et al. Characterization of buried glands before and after radiofrequency ablation by using 3-dimensional optical coherence tomography (with videos). Gastrointest Endosc. 2012;76:32–40.
15. Swager AF, Boerwinkel DF, de Bruin DM, et al. Detection of buried Barrett's glands after radiofrequency ablation with volumetric laser endomicroscopy. Gastrointest Endosc. 2016;83(1):80–8.

16. Leggett CL, Gorospe E, Owens VL, et al. Volumetric laser endomicroscopy detects subsquamous Barrett's adenocarcinoma. Am J Gastroenterol. 2014;109:298–9.
17. Hatta W, Uno K, Koike T, et al. A prospective comparative study of optical coherence tomography and EUS for tumor staging of superficial esophageal squamous cell carcinoma. Gastrointest Endosc. 2012;76:548–55.
18. Zhou C, Kirtane T, Tsai TH, et al. Three-dimensional endoscopic optical coherence tomography imaging of cervical inlet patch. Gastrointest Endosc. 2012;75:675–7. discussion 677.
19. Brand S, Poneros JM, Bouma BE, et al. Optical coherence tomography in the gastrointestinal tract. Endoscopy. 2000;32:796–803.
20. Masci E, Mangiavillano B, Albarello L, et al. Pilot study on the correlation of optical coherence tomography with histology in celiac disease and normal subjects. J Gastroenterol Hepatol. 2007;22:2256–60.
21. Adler DC, Zhou C, Tsai TH, et al. Three-dimensional endomicroscopy of the human colon using optical coherence tomography. Opt Express. 2009;17:784–96.
22. Familiari L, Strangio G, Consolo P, et al. Optical coherence tomography evaluation of ulcerative colitis: the patterns and the comparison with histology. Am J Gastroenterol. 2006;101:2833–40.
23. Shen B, Zuccaro G, Gramlich TL, et al. Ex vivo histology-correlated optical coherence tomography in the detection of transmural inflammation in Crohn's disease. Clin Gastroenterol Hepatol. 2004;2:754–60.
24. Shen B, Zuccaro Jr G, Gramlich TL, et al. In vivo colonoscopic optical coherence tomography for transmural inflammation in inflammatory bowel disease. Clin Gastroenterol Hepatol. 2004;2:1080–7.
25. Pfau PR, Sivak Jr MV, Chak A, et al. Criteria for the diagnosis of dysplasia by endoscopic optical coherence tomography. Gastrointest Endosc. 2003;58:196–202.
26. Wang C, Zhang Q, Wu X, et al. Quantitative diagnosis of colorectal polyps by spectral domain optical coherence tomography. BioMed Res Int. 2014;2014:570629.
27. Poneros JM, Tearney GJ, Shiskov M, et al. Optical coherence tomography of the biliary tree during ERCP. Gastrointest Endosc. 2002;55:84–8.
28. Testoni PA, Mangiavillano B. Optical coherence tomography for bile and pancreatic duct imaging. Gastrointest Endosc Clin N Am. 2009;19:637–53.
29. Seitz U, Freund J, Jaeckle S, et al. First in vivo optical coherence tomography in the human bile duct. Endoscopy. 2001;33:1018–21.
30. Testoni PA, Mangiavillano B, Albarello L, et al. Optical coherence tomography to detect epithelial lesions of the main pancreatic duct: an Ex Vivo study. Am J Gastroenterol. 2005;100:2777–83.
31. Testoni PA, Mariani A, Mangiavillano B, et al. Intraductal optical coherence tomography for investigating main pancreatic duct strictures. Am J Gastroenterol. 2007;102:269–74.
32. Arvanitakis M, Hookey L, Tessier G, et al. Intraductal optical coherence tomography during endoscopic retrograde cholangiopancreatography for investigation of biliary strictures. Endoscopy. 2009;41:696–701.
33. Iftimia N, Cizginer S, Deshpande V, et al. Differentiation of pancreatic cysts with optical coherence tomography (OCT) imaging: an ex vivo pilot study. Biomed Opt Express. 2011;2:2372–82.
34. Suter MJ, Gora MJ, Lauwers GY, et al. Esophageal-guided biopsy with volumetric laser endomicroscopy and laser cautery marking: a pilot clinical study. Gastrointest Endosc. 2014;79:886–96.
35. Gora MJ, Sauk JS, Carruth RW, et al. Tethered capsule endomicroscopy enables less invasive imaging of gastrointestinal tract microstructure. Nat Med. 2013;19:238–40.
36. Yang VX, Tang SJ, Gordon ML, et al. Endoscopic Doppler optical coherence tomography in the human GI tract: initial experience. Gastrointest Endosc. 2005;61:879–90.
37. Tsai TH, Ahsen OO, Lee HC, et al. Endoscopic optical coherence angiography enables 3-dimensional visualization of subsurface microvasculature. Gastroenterology. 2014;147:1219–21.

Chapter 8
Endocytoscopy: Endoscopic Imaging Techniques and Tools

Valerio Balassone and Haruhiro Inoue

Abbreviations

BE	Barrett's esophagus
ECA	Endocytoscopic atypia classification
ECT	Endocytoscopy
ESSC	Esophageal squamous cell cancer
IOA	Inter-observer agreement
NBI	Narrow band imaging
NPV	Negative predictive value
PPV	Positive predictive value

Technology Overview

> *The ability to establish an immediate endoscopic diagnosis that is virtually consistent with the histopathology has been the ultimate objective of Endoscopy since the very earliest phases of its development.*
>
> S.E. Kudo

Prediction of histology has been a goal of endoscopic imaging since it first began [1]. For this purpose, the use of magnifying observation of the gastrointestinal tract was first reported in 1985 [2]. The ordinary magnifying power of the endoscope was

V. Balassone, M.D. • H. Inoue, M.D., Ph.D., F.A.S.G.E. (✉)
Digestive Diseases Center, Showa University Koto Toyosu Hospital,
Toyosu 5-1-38, Koto-Ku, Tokyo 135-8577, Japan
e-mail: valerio.balassone@gmail.com; haruinoue777@yahoo.co.jp

V.J.A. Konda, I. Waxman (eds.), *Endoscopic Imaging Techniques and Tools*,
DOI 10.1007/978-3-319-30053-5_8

of ×45. A clinical application of a prototype for ultra-high magnification endoscopy with a magnifying capacity of up to ×150 was described in 1996 [3]. Endocytoscopy (ECT) is the subsequent evolutional step based on the same light-microscopy principle [4, 5]. The light-focusing depth of this contact-microscopy technology ranges between 0 and 50 μm. Thus, the observation is limited to the very superficial mucosal layer. The appeal of ECT lies in the real-time integration of *structural* and *cellular* atypia information obtained from the "in vivo" observation of very superficial epithelium. ECT not only enables the prediction of histology, but also allows a real-time observation of living cells.

The differentiation of metaplastic/neoplastic from non-neoplastic mucosa has been the primary application of ECT in gastrointestinal endoscopy [6]. In the benignancy field, the use of ECT has been purposed as an additional tool in the work up of several digestive diseases like celiac sprue, ulcerative colitis, and *Helicobacter pylori*-related gastritis [7–9].

The structures susceptible of ECT observation are selected under a normal white light or narrow band imaging (NBI) endoscopy. Subsequently, a contact light endocytoscopy is carried out. To better visualize specific irregularities in mucosal glands structure and cell nuclei, different staining spray solutions have been employed.

Technique

Two optical systems, using probe-based or endoscope-based technology, have been used for ECT. A technical comparison is provided in Table 8.1. The probe-based endocytoscopes can provide a magnified image of ×450 or ×1390 on a separate monitor and the probe diameter is 3.2 mm. Thus, a therapeutic gastroscope or a colonoscope with a 3.7 mm working channel is required. The endocytoscopy

Table 8.1 Endocytoscopes technical overview

	Probe-based		Endoscope-based			
	XEC 300	XEC 120	XGIF-Q260EC1	XCF-Q260EC1	GIF-Y0001	CF-Y0020-I
Diameter (mm)	3.2		11.6	13.6	10.7	
Total length (cm)	380		103	133	103	
Standard magnification	N/A		×85	×110	×80–100	
Endocytoscopy magnification (digital)	×450–570	×1100–1390	×580		×450	×380
Field of view (μm)	300×300	120×120	400×400		400×400	700×600
Horizontal resolution	4.2	1.7	4.0		3.7	
Imaging light depth (μm)	30		5		50	

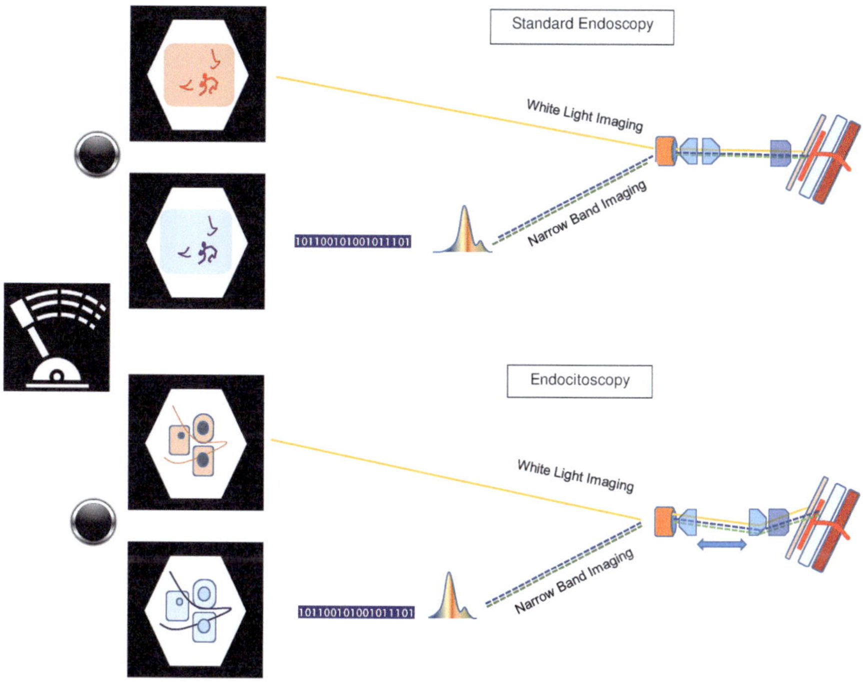

Fig. 8.1 Scheme of last-generation endoscope-based endocytoscope technology

facilities have been progressively integrated into a standard endoscope-based endocytoscope. This technical evolution has substantially improved the feasibility of the in vivo observation [10]. Since a continuous magnification from a standard overview to ×1400 fold is provided, the last generation of ECT scope-based models represents the "all-in-one" prototype [11]. In these endocytoscopes, optical and digital imaging technologies are combined (Fig. 8.1).

Mucosal Preparation

Because of the ECT contact microscopy principle, an optimal preparation of the mucosa is essential. Mucolysis with *N*-acetyl-cysteine and a pre-staining with an adsorptive agent are required for esophageal and gastric mucosa observation. The presence of mucus can substantially impair the quality of endocytoscopy images by preventing epithelium staining and by making a correct focus of the entire observation field impossible (Fig. 8.2).

For the study of head/neck mucosa, the subsequent administration of an 8 % lidocaine spray can improve the patient tolerance to the examination [12]. In addition, a bowel prep is necessary for colon ECT [13]: it consists of the administration of 2–3 L of polyethylene glycol solution in the morning before the procedure.

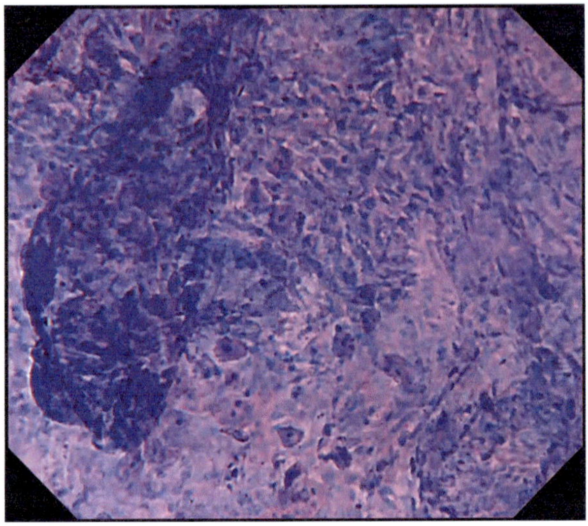

Fig. 8.2 Quality of images before and after mucolysis, adenocarcinoma in a Barrett's esophagus. In the lower part of the endocytoscopic image, the presence of mucus prevents a complete epithelium staining and a clear focusing. The post-processing virtual chromo-endoscopy enhances the *bluish* components (nuclei cells)

Epithelium Staining

The mucosa eligible to ECT observation is identified with conventional endoscopy. Subsequently, a staining solution is usually delivered onto the mucosal surface using standard spraying catheters. Better conditions for ECT mucosal imaging were reported after staining a mixed solution of 0.05 % crystal violet and 0.5 % methylene blue. Crystal violet alone effectively dyes the cytoplasm, whereas methylene blue reveals details of cell structure, including nuclei and cytoplasm [14]. The use of toluidine blue or methylene blue as a single staining is also reported [13]. After the appropriate time of exposure (from 5 to 60 s) to the dye, repeated washes of the mucosa are necessary to remove the excess contrast dye. For extended observation, staining of the mucosa may be repeated [13]. The black pigment of tattoo used for suspicious lesions can decrease the ECT image quality by interfering with the staining of crypts [15].

Image Acquisition

A stable position of the endoscope is essential and the patient is generally under intravenous sedation/anesthesia. Once an adequate position is obtained, a hand-operated lever is used to allow gradual magnification at the center of the monitor, ensuring that the area of interest is accurately located [16]. High-resolution images are taken and videos are recorded.

Assessment Criteria

ECT can distinguish between normal and pathological mucosa based on the assessment of both architectural (cellular density, size/arrangement of cells, vascular structures) and cytological features (size and shape of nuclei, nucleus-to-cytoplasm ratio, staining pattern) [11]. Specific criteria will be discussed for any ECT application. An overview of reported ECT criteria validated by an in-vivo experience and compared with histopathology as a gold standard is reported in Table 8.2.

Limitations of the Technique

ECT is not a feasible tool for wide screening of mucosa. It must be considered as an adjunctive technique for targeted assessment of lesions identified by conventional or other imaging. Therefore, its application is subject to the diagnostic performance of previous white light/NBI endoscopy. In inexpert hands, the procedure can be time-consuming and labor-intensive because it involves a multistep process of mucosal washing, staining, and imaging, compounded by limitations of visual interference by the presence of mucus or blood, inconsistent image quality, and image degradation from motion artifacts [13]. Furthermore, because of its surface microscopy principle, ECT is not a useful technique to directly assess the invasion depth of early neoplastic lesions. Nevertheless, a number of endocytoscopy atypia criteria have been demonstrated to be able to predict the level of submucosal invasion in colonic lesions [4].

Key Clinical Indications

Esophageal Squamous Cell Cancer and Atypia

Observation of esophageal squamous cell cancer (ESSC) and atypia is one of the most important applications of ECT. The staining features of superficial esophageal cancer were first assessed in a prospective study enrolling 72 patients and reporting a diagnostic accuracy of 76 % [17]. An ECT feasibility of 94.5 % was reported in another preliminary experience conducted on 87 patients using a probe-based endocytoscope [18]. With the ×450 probe, it was possible to assess cells' nuclei and nucleolus in esophageal mucosa. Blood cell circulation was observed with the ×1100 probe. Several cytological and architectural atypia characteristics of esophageal mucosa were subsequently integrated among the ECT diagnostic criteria of esophageal squamous cell cancer.

In a preliminary experience including 12 patients, nuclei/cytoplasm ratio and cells density were successfully assessed using a probe-based endocytoscope [19].

Table 8.2 Overview of reported diagnostic criteria for endocytoscopy, sorted by purposed disease and year. Ex vivo studies and descriptive experiences excluded IOA= inter-observer agreement, PPV=positive predictive value, NPV=negative predictive value

Disease	Author (year) / Study design (patient no.)	Purposed ECT criteria	Reported diagnostic performance
Esophageal squamous cell carcinoma	Inoue et al. (2006) [10]	*Classification of atypia: ECA (endocytoscopy atypia classification)*	Sensitivity 83.3 %; specificity 93.7 %; accuracy 82 %
	Prospective (28)	– *ECA 1*. Large, cytoplasm-rich cells with a rhomboid shape in a regular arrangement. Small nuclei are located at their center (healthy squamous epithelium)	
		– *ECA 2*. The cell margin becomes round. Different-sized, smaller nuclei are observed (inflammation/reactive)	
		– *ECA 3*. The cell becomes smaller in size, but the nuclei are still compact (borderline)	
		– *ECA 4*. Cell density and nucleus/cytoplasm ratio increase (suggestive for malignant lesion)	
		– *ECA 5*. Cells of various sizes are arranged irregularly, with a high nucleus/cytoplasm ratio (definitively recognized endoscopically as a malignant lesion)	
	Minami (2012) [14]	*ECA classification after double staining*	Sensitivity 91.7 %; specificity 91.0 %; accuracy 91.3 %; PPV 90.6 %; NPV 92.0 %
	Prospective (14)		
Barrett's esophagus	Pohl (2009) [8]	*Neoplasia vs. non-neoplasia: cyto-architecture criteria*	×450: feasibility 51 %; PPV 29 %; NPV 44 %
	Prospective (8)	Polarity of cells and nuclei (spacing, orientation); Abnormalities in size, shape, and uniformity of nuclei; chromatin; nucleoli; nucleus/cytoplasm ratio	×1125: feasibility 22 %; PPV 44 %; NPV 82 %; IOA kappa 0.45
H. Pylori related gastritis	Sato et al. (2015) [9]	*Normal vs. inflammation or atrophic mucosa*: staining features, architectural or cytological abnormalities	n-Pit: sensitivity 78.9 %; specificity 60.8 %; PPV 88.6; NPV 42.9; kappa 0.857
	Prospective (9)	– *n-Pit* (normal pit predominant pattern mucosa)	n-Pap: sensitivity 52.9 %; specificity 89.5 %, PPV 93.1; NPV 41.5; kappa 0.769
		– *n-Pap* (normal pap predominant pattern mucosa)	
Gastric cancer	Kaise et al. (2015) [26]	*Atypia cyto-architectural classification criteria*	Feasibility 88 %; sensitivity 86 %; specificity 100, accuracy 96 %; PPV 100 %; NPV 94 %
	Prospective (26)	*High-grade atypia*: Any of: lumen absence or fusion, disappearance of gland structure, irregular nuclei showing three typical features (swelling, disarrangement, and heterogeneity of shape)	
		Low-grade atypia: mild irregularities in gland structure, lumen shortening and narrowing, absence or fusion of part of the lumen	

Colorectal lesions	Cipolletta (2009) [31]	Observation of *aberrant crypt* foci for the diagnosis of colon dysplasia	Sensitivity 91 %; specificity 100 %; IOA kappa 0.68
	Prospective (31)		
	Kudo et al. (2011) [1]	*Endocytoscopy classification* (EC) for colorectal lesions:	Sensitivity 100 %; specificity 100 %; accuracy 100 %; PPV: 98 %
	Prospective (1)	– *EC 1a* = Roundish lumens, Fusiform nuclei (normal)	
		– *EC 1b* = Narrow serrated lumens, Small roundish nuclei (hyperplastic)	
		– *EC 2* = Slit-like smooth lumens Uniform fusiform or roundish nuclei (dysplasia)	
		– *EC 3a* = Irregular and rough lumens. Large number of roundish nuclei (HGD, SMs cancer)	
		– *EC 3b* = Unclear gland formation Agglomeration of distorted nuclei (SMm cancer)	
	Mori et. al. (2013) [32]	*Endocytoscopy criteria* compared with modified Vienna Classification	Sensitivity 97.6 %; specificity 100 %; accuracy 94.1 %; IOA kappa 0.841
	Randomized controlled Trial (32)	Normal mucosa = Roundish lumens Fusiform nuclei = VCC1-2	
		Hyperplastic polyp = Narrow serrated lumens, Small roundish granules = VCC1-2	
		Low grade adenoma. = Slit-like lumens, Slightly swollen fusiform nuclei = VCC3	
		High grade adenoma = Slit-like or irregular lumens Swollen roundish nuclei = VCC4	
		Invasive cancer = Unclear gland formation Agglomeration of distorted nuclei = VCC5	
	Kudo et al. (2014) [4]	*PIT pattern + endocytoscopy*	Sensitivity 97.4 %; specificity 89.4 %; accuracy 96.5 %; PPV 94.9 %; NPV 96.6 %; IOA kappa 0.62
	Retrospective (4)	Pit pattern I-II = EC 1a-1B	
		Pit pattern IIIL-IIIS and IV-Vi (LG) = EC 2-3a	
		Pit pattern Vi (HG) and Vn = EC 3b	
	Kudo et al. (2015) [33]	*Endocytoscopy vascular (ECV) pattern for colorectal lesions:*	Sensitivity; specificity; accuracy
			95.5 %; 99.4 %; 99.0 %
			97.5 %; 61.3 %; 75.8 %
	Retrospective (33)	– *EC-V1* = fine and obscure microvessels (non-neoplastic)	74.6 %; 97.2 %; 88.6 %
		– *EC-V2* = regular network (neoplastic)	IOA kappa 0.88
		– *EC-V3* = irregular microvessels (invasive cancer)	

Finally, a 5-scale comprehensive classification—namely Endocytoscopic Atypia Classification (ECA)—was validated by two prospective studies, enrolling 28 and 110 patients, respectively [10, 14]. By using an endoscope-based endocytoscope with a ×380 magnifying power and a double-staining solution, it was possible to evaluate the following ECA criteria: nuclei size, nuclei/cytoplasm ratio, cellular shape, and arrangement (Fig. 8.3). A strong correlation with histology was demonstrated (Fig. 8.4).

Another comprehensive classification, integrating the iodine staining features observed during standard endoscopy (Fig. 8.5) and cyto-architectural endocytoscopic atypia characteristics of esophageal squamous epithelium, was reported by Kumagai in 2009. The in-vivo and ex-vivo ECT's findings were compared with the histopathology of the resected specimen. Because of the high level of diagnostic

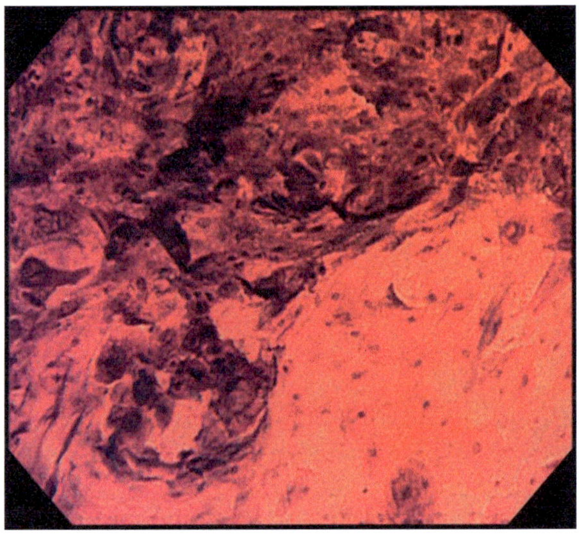

Fig. 8.3 Endocytoscopy of an esophageal squamous cell carcinoma. The transition between squamous cell epithelium (*bottom right*) and squamous cancer (*top left*) is centered in the observation field. In the squamous cancer area, the nuclei density and nuclei/cytoplasm ratio is higher and cells with heterogeneous size are arranged (ECA 5)

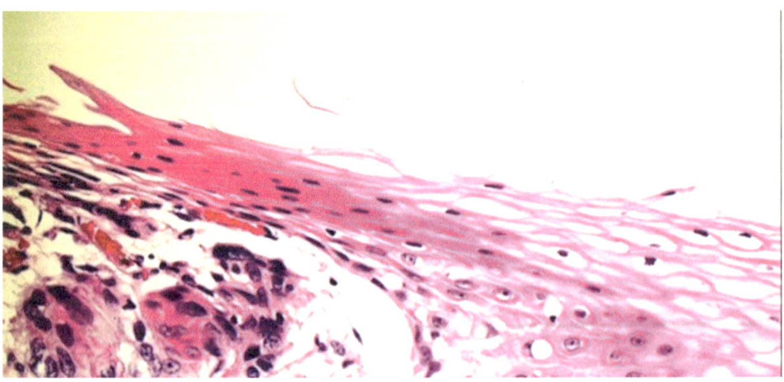

Fig. 8.4 The standard Hematoxylin-Eosin staining histopathology of the resected lesion confirmed a squamous cell carcinoma of the esophagus

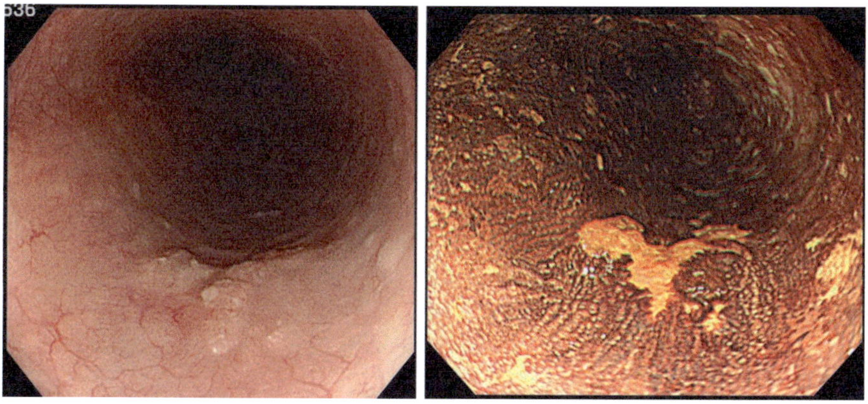

Fig. 8.5 White light endoscopy of an early squamous esophageal cancer carcinoma (0-IIA). *Left*: Standard endoscopy. *Right*: After Iodine staining, the lesion is recognized as an unstained area

accuracy reported, the potential of ECT to reduce the need for standard biopsies in low-graded ECT atypia esophageal mucosa was suggested [20–22].

Since the histopathological knowledge may vary among endoscopists, an ex-vivo study on 10 resected esophagi for cancer aimed to assess the accuracy of computer-aided endocytoscopy diagnosis [23]. ECS pictures from pathological and non-pathological mucosa were assessed with a dedicated software in order to calculate density and shape of stained nuclei. A good correlation with computed findings and histopathology was confirmed.

Barrett's Epithelium and Esophageal Adenocarcinoma

In the first study assessing the diagnostic performance of ECT in Barrett's esophagus (BE), a probe-based endocytoscope was employed [24]. Endocytoscopy images were recorded from pre-marked areas in the Barrett's segment using a magnification of ×1125 or ×450. Biopsies were taken from the same area. In order to allow a precise comparison with histology, they were independently assessed. In this study, the ECT diagnostic performance and feasibility were reported as unsatisfactory especially because of the inadequate image quality. These limitations were imputed to the major difficulty of ECT of assessing a normal targeted area rather than just comparing larger areas of grossly normal mucosa with obvious neoplastic lesions. The ECT feasibility may have been further impaired by the use of old-generation, probe-based endocytoscopes.

A pilot ex-vivo assessment of ECT performance in the diagnosis of BE has been reported in 2013 [25]. A simple diagnostic classification system was purposed and an acceptable accuracy in the diagnosis of squamous epithelium, non-dysplastic BE, dysplastic BE, and esophageal adenocarcinoma was reported. The Inter-observer agreement to classify each category was excellent, even among inexperi-

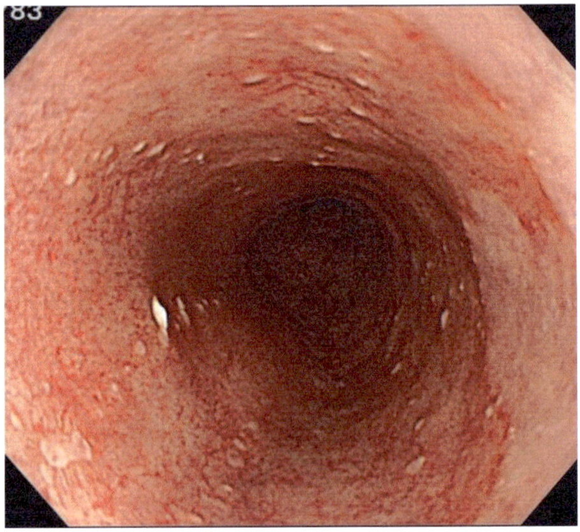

Fig. 8.6 White light endoscopy of Barrett's esophagus

enced observers. At the present time, no in vivo studies have confirmed the reliability of purposed criteria.

The first in-vivo use of an endoscope-based ECT in the diagnosis of BE has been recently reported [16]. The metaplastic mucosa was identified during standard magnification endoscopy (Fig. 8.6). With a ×380 magnifying power endocytoscopy (Fig. 8.7), the esophageal papillary squamous cell islands surrounded by glandular Barrett's epithelium were observed and a complete correspondence with targeted biopsies was confirmed.

Early Gastric Cancer

The initially reported limited feasibility of endocytoscopy for the diagnosis of gastric cancer was probably a consequence of using probe-based endocytoscopes [11]. A prospective study enrolling 82 patients with gastric lesions susceptible of histopathological assessment after endoscopic resection has demonstrated a highly satisfactory feasibility of endoscope-based ECT in early gastric cancer [26]. The accuracy of endocytoscopy for gastric cancer diagnosis was compared with the subsequent histopathological findings as gold standard. Specific irregularities in gland structure and cell nuclei were assessed to establish the diagnosis of atypia. In non-neoplastic gastric mucosa, the gland lumen was well-preserved and cells lining the mucosa were regularly arranged. Low-grade ECT atypia was defined by mild irregularities in gland structure, lumen shortening, and narrowing or absence or fusion of part of the

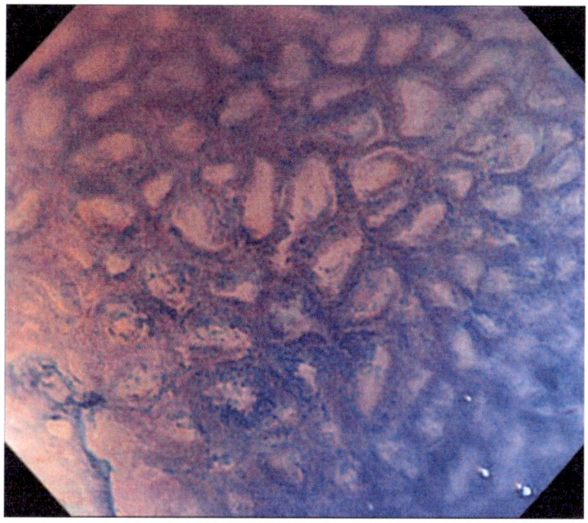

Fig. 8.7 Endocytoscopy observation of Barrett's esophagus glandular structure

lumen. High-grade ECT atypia diagnosis was defined by the presence of any of the following criteria: lumen absence or fusion, disappearance of gland structure, and irregular nuclei showing three typical features (swelling, disarrangement, and heterogeneity of shape). The use of ECT in signet cell gastric cancer was first reported as an ex-vivo observation of a surgically resected stomach [27]. During normal white light endoscopy, the gastric lesion can be observed as an ulcerated area surrounded by normal mucosa (Fig. 8.8). The subsequent endocytoscopy observation can confirm the presence of cytoplasmic halo and peripheral nuclei (Fig. 8.9).

Gastric H. pylori-*Related Inflammation and Intestinal Metaplasia*

The diagnosis of gastrointestinal infections has been one of the first adjunctive ECT applications [28]. In 2006, upon ex-vivo ECT observation of gastric mucus supernatant from a patient with gastric ulcer, the visualization of alive, moving *H. pylori* was achieved. Direct observation of bacteria can be difficult and time-consuming. Therefore, a prospective study has employed the ECT to demonstrate the normality of gastric mucosa and to indirectly exclude an *H. pylori*-related inflammation [9]. Seventy patients were enrolled in the study and a comparison with histological specimen and serum pepsinogen test was employed to validate the endocytoscopic criteria that were employed to distinguish between normal and pathological mucosa.

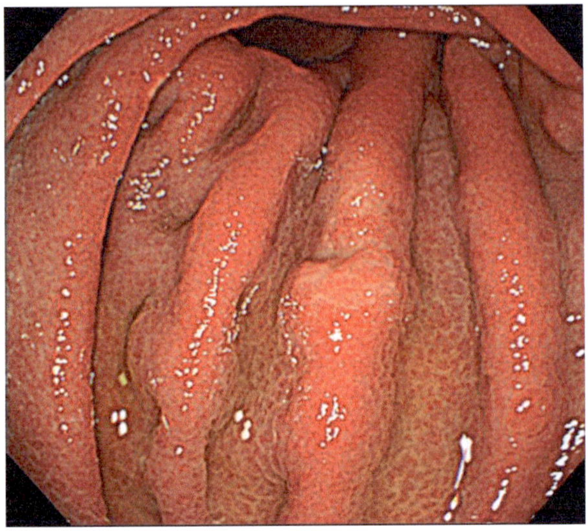

Fig. 8.8 White light endoscopy of an ulcerated lesion of the gastric antrum

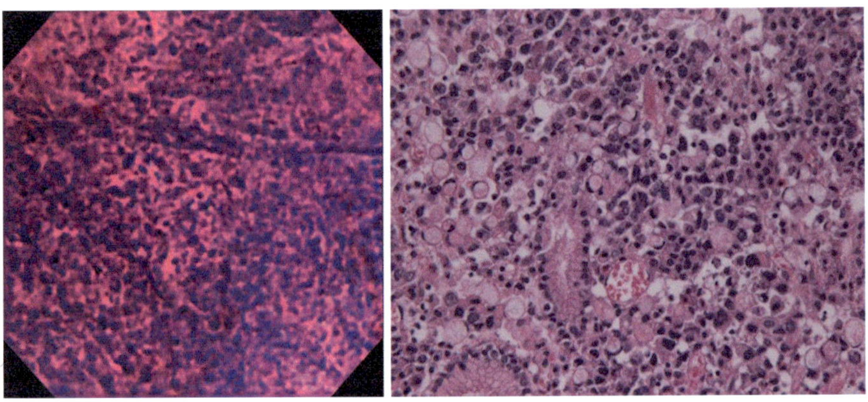

Fig. 8.9 Endocytoscopy observation strongly suggestive for a Signet ring cell stomach carcinoma. *Left*: The cytoplasmic halo and peripheral nuclei are visible in the highlighted box. *Right*: The histology with Hematoxylin-Eosin staining confirmed the diagnosis of signet ring cell carcinoma

Celiac Disease

A prospective study enrolling 16 patients, 8 with clinically active and 8 with non-clinically active celiac disease has reported a sensibility of 88 % and a specificity of 100 % for the ECT diagnosis compared with histopathology as gold standard. Dynamic and morphologic parameters were employed to establish the ECT diagnosis. The use of in-vivo ECT observation of duodenal mucosa was purposed as a future less invasive technique to assess the activity of celiac disease [29].

On the other hand, another study enrolling 40 patients with diagnosis of celiac disease assessed the diagnostic accuracy of probe-based ×450 and ×1100 magnification Endocytoscopy in comparison with histopathology [8]. In the assessment of microstructural changes in celiac disease, four criteria were significant predictors of advanced disease (Marsh III pathology): a number <3 of villi per visual field, confluence of villi, irregular epithelial lining, and inability to delineate loop capillaries. Nevertheless, none of the mentioned criteria could predict an early stage disease (Marsh I pathology) and no additional information was provided by the ×1100 magnification probe observation. To date, no studies have assessed the accuracy of ECT using the new endoscope-based system for the first-time diagnosis of celiac disease.

Colorectal Lesions

The first prospective application of ECT in the observation of colon atypia has been reported by Sasajima in 2006 [30]. In a blinded study enrolling 60 patients, the following aspects were assessed: (1) pattern of the cellular arrangement; (2) size, shape, and arrangements of colonic glands (pits); (3) size and shape of the cells; (4) size and shape of the nuclei; and (5) nuclear-cytoplasmic ratio. When compared with histopathology as a gold standard, the overall diagnostic accuracy was 93.3 %.

In another study enrolling 48 consecutive patients, the presence of aberrant crypt foci was observed using a probe-based endocytoscope. All the 48 lesions were resected endoscopically and the histopathology confirmed a sensitivity of 91 % and a specificity of 100 % [31].

A prospective randomized controlled trial enrolling 203 patients with colonic polyps evaluated the diagnostic accuracy of endocytoscopy versus standard biopsy. The histopathology of resected lesions was employed as gold standard comparison [32]. The definitive histological examination confirmed the expected non-inferior diagnostic accuracy of endocytoscopy (94.1 % vs. 96 % of standard biopsy). A retrospective analysis on 455 patients has compared the diagnostic accuracy of pit pattern classification obtained from standard high-magnification endoscopy and pit pattern with the addition of endocytoscopy criteria. Pit pattern classification confirmed a high diagnostic accuracy and no significant differences were found with the addition of endocytoscopy criteria for the recognition of neoplastic changes. Nevertheless, endocytoscopy improved the diagnostic accuracy for predicting submucosal invasion from 93.6 to 96.8 %. The same diagnostic improvement was confirmed in a retrospective analysis of 198 colorectal lesions subsequently reported by the same group and employing a ×450 all-in-one NBI endocytoscope without mucosal staining [33]. A simplified and time-saving endocytoscopic classification based on the microvascular pattern was purposed. The diagnostic accuracy of ECT was comparable with the data obtained from high-magnification endoscopy and not affected by the lesion size or the macroscopic type. A very high inter-observer agreement of 0.88 is reported. On the other hand, in the differentiation between adenoma and invasive cancer, the diagnostic accuracy of microvascular pattern was limited

(88 %). Because the endoscopic resection is the standard treatment for both intramucosal cancer and adenoma, the clinical impact of this limitation was considered irrelevant [33].

Safety and Cost Considerations

Safety of endocytoscopy is comparable to a standard flexible diagnostic endoscopy. No relevant complications related to ECT observation have been reported. A 9.2 % incidence of minor and self-stopping bleeding caused by endocytoscope contact has been reported in a preliminary experience with probe-based endocytoscope [34].

Endocytoscopy technology is not yet widely available. Most reported clinical experiences were carried out using prototypes. For these reasons, the room for cost/effectiveness consideration is actually limited. The endocytoscopy potential to reduce the necessity of histopathology for low-graded atypia has been suggested by several authors. Furthermore, the possible clinical impact of smart biopsies, together with the possibility of real-time decision-making, must be taken into account when economical information is available.

Conclusion and Future Directions

Endocytoscopy provides a safe and reliable in-vivo observation of intestinal mucosa. This optical microscopy technology has been employed to assess cyto-architectural and microvascular modification with the main intent of predicting mucosal histological abnormalities. The recent integration of endocytoscopy facilities into an all-in-one endoscope has substantially improved the feasibility of the in vivo observation. Nevertheless, endocytoscopy generally requires mucosal preparation and staining, which can be time-consuming. Thus, the observation with endocytoscopy is indicated for selected clinical situations where the use standard or high-magnification endoscopy cannot clarify or predict the presence of mucosal abnormalities.

The future directions for endocytoscopy are two: technical improvement and extended applications. The expected technological improvement is represented by the computer-aided diagnosis. The use of dedicated softwares can facilitate the gathering of high-quality images in a faster and more "user-friendly" fashion for the observer. Some relevant endocytoscopy criteria like nuclei density and nuclei/cytoplasm ratio could be automatically calculated. Another expected direction for ECT is to improve its diffusion as an integrational tool in the management of benign digestive diseases. According to the preliminary experiences on celiac sprue, gastritis, and ulcerative colitis, the utility of real-time observation of vascular and cyto-architectural characteristics is not limited to the classification of atypia: it can also provide some unique information in the diagnosis of several benignant diseases.

References

1. Kudo S-E, Wakamura K, Ikehara N, Mori Y, Inoue H, Hamatani S. Diagnosis of colorectal lesions with a novel endocytoscopic classification—a pilot study. Endoscopy. 2011;43:869–75. http://www.ncbi.nlm.nih.gov/pubmed/21837586.
2. Furuta Y, Kobori O, Shimazu H, Morioka Y, Okuyama Y. A new in vivo staining method, cresyl violet staining, for fiberoptic magnified observation of carcinoma of the gastric mucosa. Gastroenterol Jpn. 1985;20:120–4. http://www.ncbi.nlm.nih.gov/pubmed/2411618.
3. Inoue H, Honda T, Yoshida T, Nishikage T, Nagahama T, Yano K, et al. Ultra-high magnification endoscopy of the normal esophageal mucosa. Dig Endosc. 1996;8:134–8. http://doi.wiley.com/10.1111/j.1443-1661.1996.tb00429.x.
4. Kudo S, Mori Y, Wakamura K, Ikehara N, Ichimasa K, Wada Y, et al. Endocytoscopy can provide additional diagnostic ability to magnifying chromoendoscopy for colorectal neoplasms. J Gastroenterol Hepatol. 2014;29:83–90. http://www.ncbi.nlm.nih.gov/pubmed/23980563.
5. Kato M, Shimizu Y, Nakagawa S, Yamamoto J, Asaka M. Usefulness of magnifying endoscopy in upper gastrointestinal tract: history and recent studies. Dig Endosc. 2005;17:S5–10. http://doi.wiley.com/10.1111/j.1443-1661.2005.00515.x.
6. Goetz M, Malek NP, Kiesslich R. Microscopic imaging in endoscopy: endomicroscopy and endocytoscopy. Nat Rev Gastroenterol Hepatol. 2014;11:11–8. http://www.ncbi.nlm.nih.gov/pubmed/23897286.
7. Kiesslich R, Goetz M, Lammersdorf K, Schneider C, Burg J, Stolte M, et al. Chromoscopy-guided endomicroscopy increases the diagnostic yield of intraepithelial neoplasia in ulcerative colitis. Gastroenterology. 2007;132:874–82. http://linkinghub.elsevier.com/retrieve/pii/S0016508507001874.
8. Pohl H, Rösch T, Tanczos BT, Rudolph B, Schlüns K, Baumgart DC. Endocytoscopy for the detection of microstructural features in adult patients with celiac sprue: a prospective, blinded endocytoscopy-conventional histology correlation study. Gastrointest Endosc. 2009;70:933–41.
9. Sato H, Inoue H, Ikeda H, Sato C, Phlanusittepha C, Hayee B, Santi EGR, Yasutoshi Kobayashi SK. In vivo gastric mucosal histopathology using endocytoscopy. World J Gastroenterol. 2015;21:5002. http://www.wjgnet.com/1007-9327/full/v21/i16/5002.htm.
10. Inoue H, Sasajima K, Kaga M, Sugaya S, Sato Y, Wada Y, et al. Endoscopic in vivo evaluation of tissue atypia in the esophagus using a newly designed integrated endocytoscope: a pilot trial. Endoscopy. 2006;38:891–5. http://www.thieme-connect.de/DOI/DOI?10.1055/s-2006-944667.
11. Neumann H, Fuchs FS, Vieth M, Atreya R, Siebler J, Kiesslich R, et al. Review article: in vivo imaging by endocytoscopy. Aliment Pharmacol Ther. 2011;33:1183–93. http://doi.wiley.com/10.1111/j.1365-2036.2011.04647.x.
12. Shimizu Y, Takahashi M, Yoshida T, Ono S, Mabe K, Kato M, et al. Endoscopic in vivo cellular imaging of superficial squamous cell carcinoma of the head and neck by using an integrated endocytoscopy system (with video). Gastrointest Endosc. 2013;78:351–8. http://dx.doi.org/10.1016/j.gie.2013.03.1336.
13. Kwon RS, Wong Kee Song L-M, Adler DG, Conway JD, Diehl DL, Farraye FA, et al. Endocytoscopy. Gastrointest Endosc. 2009;70:610–3. http://linkinghub.elsevier.com/retrieve/pii/S0016510709021853
14. Minami H, Inoue H, Yokoyama A, Ikeda H, Satodate H, Hamatani S, et al. Recent advancement of observing living cells in the esophagus using CM double staining: endocytoscopic atypia classification. Dis Esophagus. 2012;25:235–41. http://doi.wiley.com/10.1111/j.1442-2050.2011.01241.x.
15. Fasoli A, Pugliese V, Gatteschi B, Truini M, Meroni E. Endocytoscopic imaging and tattooing: a caveat. Endoscopy. 2009;41:E41–2. http://www.thieme-connect.de/DOI/DOI?10.1055/s-0028-1119489.

16. Eleftheriadis N, Inoue H, Ikeda H, Onimaru M, Yoshida A, Hosoya T, et al. Endocytoscopic visualization of squamous cell islands within Barrett's epithelium. World J Gastrointest Endosc. 2013;5:174. http://www.wjgnet.com/1948-5190/full/v5/i4/174.htm.
17. Inoue H, Kumagai Y, Yoshida T, Kawano T. High-magnification endoscopic diagnosis of the superficial esophageal cancer. Dig Endosc. 2000;12:S32–5.
18. Inoue H, Kazawa T, Sato Y, Satodate H, Sasajima K, Kudo S, et al. In vivo observation of living cancer cells in the esophagus, stomach, and colon using catheter-type contact endoscope, "Endo-Cytoscopy system". Gastrointest Endosc Clin N Am. 2004;14. 589–94, x–xi. http://www.ncbi.nlm.nih.gov/pubmed/15261204.
19. Kumagai Y, Monma K, Kawada K. Magnifying chromoendoscopy of the esophagus: in-vivo pathological diagnosis using an endocytoscopy system. Endoscopy. 2004;36:590–4. http://www.thieme-connect.de/DOI/DOI?10.1055/s-2004-814533.
20. Kumagai Y, Kawada K, Yamazaki S, Iida M, Momma K, Odajima H, et al. Endocytoscopic observation for esophageal squamous cell carcinoma: can biopsy histology be omitted? Dis Esophagus. 2009;22:505–12. http://www.ncbi.nlm.nih.gov/pubmed/19302209.
21. Kumagai Y, Toi M, Kawada K, Kawano T. Angiogenesis in superficial esophageal squamous cell carcinoma: magnifying endoscopic observation and molecular analysis. Dig Endosc. 2010;22:259–67. http://doi.wiley.com/10.1111/j.1443-1661.2010.01010.x.
22. Banerjee R, Reddy DN, Rao GV, Shekharan A, Ramji C. Application of high-resolution narrow band imaging and endocytoscopy for early diagnosis of esophageal neoplasia. Indian J Gastroenterol. 2008;27:204–6. http://www.ncbi.nlm.nih.gov/pubmed/19112192.
23. Kodashima S, Fujishiro M, Takubo K, Kammori M, Nomura S, Kakushima N, et al. Ex vivo pilot study using computed analysis of endo-cytoscopic images to differentiate normal and malignant squamous cell epithelia in the oesophagus. Dig Liver Dis. 2007;39:762–6. http://www.ncbi.nlm.nih.gov/entrez/query.fcgi?cmd=Retrieve&db=PubMed&dopt=Citation&list_uids=17611178.
24. Pohl H, Koch M, Khalifa A, Papanikolaou I, Scheiner K, Wiedenmann B, et al. Evaluation of endocytoscopy in the surveillance of patients with Barrett's esophagus. Endoscopy. 2007;39:492–6. http://www.ncbi.nlm.nih.gov/pubmed/17554642.
25. Tomizawa Y, Iyer PG, Wongkeesong LM, Buttar NS, Lutzke LS, Tsung-Teh Wu KKWY. Assessment of the diagnostic performance and interobserver variability of endocytoscopy in Barrett's esophagus: a pilot ex-vivo study. World J Gastroenterol. 2013;19:8652. http://www.wjgnet.com/1007-9327/full/v19/i46/8652.htm.
26. Kaise M, Ohkura Y, Iizuka T, Kimura R, Nomura K, Kuribayashi Y, et al. Endocytoscopy is a promising modality with high diagnostic accuracy for gastric cancer. Endoscopy. 2015;47:19–25. http://www.thieme-connect.de/DOI/DOI?10.1055/s-0034-1377965.
27. Fasoli A, Pugliese V, Furnari M, Gatteschi B, Truini M, Meroni E. Signet ring cell carcinoma of the stomach: correlation between endocytoscopy and histology. Endoscopy. 2009;41:E65–6. http://www.ncbi.nlm.nih.gov/pubmed/19319785.
28. Kimura S, Inoue H, Sato Y, Aoyama Y, Shimojima M, Masuyama T, et al. Ex vivo visualization of Helicobacter pylori using an endocytoscopic probe. Biomed Res. 2006;27:255–7. http://www.ncbi.nlm.nih.gov/pubmed/17099290.
29. Matysiak-Budnik T, Coron E, Mosnier JF, Le Rhun M, Inoue H, Galmiche JP. In vivo real-time imaging of human duodenal mucosal structures in celiac disease using endocytoscopy. Endoscopy. 2010;42:191–6. http://www.ncbi.nlm.nih.gov/pubmed/20101565.
30. Sasajima K, Kudo SE, Inoue H, Takeuchi T, Kashida H, Hidaka E, et al. Real-time in vivo virtual histology of colorectal lesions when using the endocytoscopy system. Gastrointest Endosc. 2006;63:1010–7.
31. Cipolletta L, Bianco M, Rotondano G, Piscopo R, Meucci C, Prisco A, et al. Endocytoscopy can identify dysplasia in aberrant crypt foci of the colorectum: a prospective in vivo study. Endoscopy. 2009;41:129–32. http://www.thieme-connect.de/DOI/DOI?10.1055/s-0028-1103452.

32. Mori Y, Kudo S, Ikehara N, Wakamura K, Wada Y, Kutsukawa M, et al. Comprehensive diagnostic ability of endocytoscopy compared with biopsy for colorectal neoplasms: a prospective randomized noninferiority trial. Endoscopy. 2013;45:98–105. http://www.ncbi.nlm.nih.gov/pubmed/23307149.
33. Kudo S, Misawa M, Wada Y, Nakamura H, Kataoka S, Maeda Y, et al. Endocytoscopic microvasculature evaluation is a reliable new diagnostic method for colorectal lesions (with video). Gastrointest Endosc. 2015;1–12. http://linkinghub.elsevier.com/retrieve/pii/S0016510715023998.
34. Inoue H, Kudo SE, Shiokawa A. Observation of living cancer cells in the gastrointestinal tract. Clin Gastroenterol Hepatol. 2005;3:S61–3.

Chapter 9
In Vivo Agents and Markers for Endomicroscopy

Daniel P. Perl and Sharmila Anandasabapathy

Abbreviations

2-NBDG	2-[*N*-(7-nitrobenz-2-oxa-1,3-diaxol-4-yl) amino]-2-deoxyglucose
CLE	Confocal laser endomicroscopy
eCLE	Endoscopic-integrated CLE
ECS	Endocytoscopy
HRME	High-resolution microendoscopy
IBD	Inflammatory bowel disease
MCE	Magnification chromoendoscopy
MDM	Multispectral digital microscope
mTNF	Membrane-bound tumor necrosis factor
NIR	Near-infrared imaging
pCLE	Probe-based CLE
WLE	White-light endoscopy

D.P. Perl, M.D.
Internal Medicine, University of Michigan Health System,
Ann Arbor, MI, USA

S. Anandasabapathy, M.D. (✉)
Medicine and Gastroenterology, Baylor College of Medicine,
One Baylor Plaza, Houston, TX, USA
e-mail: Sharmila.Anandasabapathy@bcm.edu

V.J.A. Konda, I. Waxman (eds.), *Endoscopic Imaging Techniques and Tools*,
DOI 10.1007/978-3-319-30053-5_9

Types of In Vivo Agents

Vital-Dyes

Fluorescein

Fluorescein, a widely used, non-toxic, fluorescent agent can be applied intravenously and within a matter of seconds can be used for imaging for up to an hour. When given, this agent concentrates in the lamina propria, the intercellular spaces, and the capillaries thereby highlighting tissue architecture and deeper lesions. Overall, fluorescein is a safe agent that has been primarily studied with confocal laser endomicroscopy [1].

Acriflavine/Proflavine

In contrast to intravenous fluorescein, acriflavine and proflavine are vital-dye agents that are topically applied, absorbed by cells, and stain nuclei, providing cell-surface imaging thus aiding in diagnosing neoplasia in vivo. Because these agents are sprayed onto the epithelium, deeper structures cannot be resolved [2].

Methylene Blue, Toluidine Blue, and Crystal Violet

These topically applied agents accumulate in tissue depressions and are able to stain nuclei and cytoplasm. They are extensively used throughout the GI tract, many times in conjunction with ECS (endocytoscopy), with each dye having particular advantages. One ex vivo study that varied concentration and time of exposure of these agents found that in the esophagus, sixty seconds of 1 % methylene blue showed better contrast between the cytoplasm and nuclei, whereas in the stomach and colon 60 s of 0.25 % toluidine was better [3].

Unlike methylene blue and toluidine blue, crystal violet stains primarily the cytoplasm. While this agent alone was shown to be inferior to either methylene blue and toluidine blue [3], a more recent double-staining study in ECS found that the combination of crystal violet with methylene blue led to significantly faster identification of colonic glands [4]. As such, current imaging with ECS utilizes this double-staining technique [5].

Contrast Agents

Indigo Carmine

Unlike the vital-dyes that are absorbed, indigo carmine is a contrast agent that accumulates in crevices, crypts, and foveolae and thereby highlights the mucosal surface [6]. In combination with other topical agents, this agent has been studied in vivo throughout the gastrointestinal tract, showing clinical efficacy in detection of gastric and colon cancer. Additionally, it is recommended for use for colorectal cancer screening in inflammatory bowel disease (IBD) patients.

Targeted Agents

Peptides

A new field of study has emerged attempting to identify peptides that bind to cell-surface markers of organ-specific neoplasia. In general, *phage display* begins with biopanning the peptide library and removing those peptides that bind nonspecifically to normal mucosa. Then, the remaining peptides are biopanned against neoplastic mucosa and those that bind are selected and can be utilized as molecular probes [7].

Molecules

2-[*N*-(7-nitrobenz-2-oxa-1,3- diaxol-4-yl) amino]-2-deoxyglucose or 2-NBDG is a glucose analog that is transported into highly active cells, becomes fluorescent upon incorporation [8]. This agent has shown promise in ex vivo studies of Barrett's esophagus for differentiating inflammation from Barrett's metaplasia and Barrett's neoplasia (high grade or cancer) when combined with confocal microscopy.

Lectin

Surface glycan units have been shown to decrease during histological progression of normal esophageal tissue to adenocarcinoma. Thus, lectins, which are topically applied agents that can bind surface glycan units have shown utility ex vivo in discriminating benign esophageal mucosa from high-grade dysplasia and cancer with fluorescence endoscopes [9].

Antibodies

Fluorescently labelled antibodies targeting receptors and proteins have been used in animal models intravenously and in human tissue topically. Diseases including IBD and cancers of the colon and stomach have been studied. After application of the agent, confocal laser endomicroscopy with an excitation wavelength of 488 nm is typically employed for imaging.

Table 9.1 Features of imaging systems

	Imaging system		Resolution	Field of view	In vivo agents
Endomicroscopy devices	CLE	eCLE	0.7 μm	475 μm	IV fluorescein, topical acriflavine, peptides, molecular markers
		pCLE	1 μm	240–600 μm	
	ECS	×450	4.2 μm	300 μm	Topical methylene blue, indigo carmine, crystal violet
		×1100	1.7 μm	120 μm	
	HRME		4 μm	750 μm	Topical proflavine
Red flag imaging	MDM		50–100 μm	2.5 cm	Topical proflavine
	NIR		<10 μm	3.6 mm	Topical octapeptide

This table outlines the specific characteristics of each imaging system and organizes the contrast agents based on the systems they have been studied with

CLE confocal laser endomicroscopy, *eCLE* endoscopic-integrated CLE, *pCLE* probe-based CLE, *ECS* endocytoscopy, *HRME* high-resolution microendoscopy, *MDM* multispectral digital microscope, *NIR* near-infrared imaging

Mucolytics

Acetic Acid

In addition to being a mucolytic, this agent is absorbed by cells and, as a result, reversibly alters cellular protein structure thereby leading to whitening and opacification of normal mucosa. The amount and duration of whitening is greater in normal mucosa relative to neoplastic lesions [10]. Clinically, this agent has shown efficacy with chromoendoscopy in evaluating Barrett's esophagus and gastric lesions.

N-acetylcysteine and Simethicone

These topically applied mucolytic agents have shown clinical benefit in producing better visualization of the stomach and colon beyond simple saline solutions when applied to the mucosa prior to the administration of contrast agents (Table 9.1).

Esophagus

Barrett's Esophagus is the primary precursor to esophageal adenocarcinoma and patients with Barrett's have a 30–40 fold increased risk of developing this cancer when compared to patients without the condition [11]. Because of this increased risk, Barrett's patients undergo surveillance endoscopy at 1–3-year intervals based on pathologic grade. Despite these current guidelines, the current standard of white-light endoscopy with random four quadrant biopsies has been shown to miss up to

57 % of neoplasia [12]. Indeed, Barrett's associated neoplasia (high-grade dysplasia, intraepithelial cancer) can often be focal, flat, and indistinguishable from non-neoplastic mucosa on white-light endoscopy alone. In hopes of improving the early detection of neoplasia, several novel imaging technologies with nonspecific and more targeted contrast agents that highlight dysplastic features are being developed. Of them, fluorescein has seen the most clinical use in conjunction with confocal laser endomicroscopy (CLE).

Fluorescein and Confocal Laser Endomicroscopy

CLE provides in vivo microscopic assessments of the mucosa by using low-power laser light in conjunction with a fluorescent contrast agent to excite tissue. Emitted light from the tissue is refocused through a pinhole, thereby reducing background and out-of-focus light to create images that are 1–2 μm in spatial resolution and closely resemble standard histopathology. Confocal provides 1000-fold magnification of the tissue allowing endoscopists to view histological-grade images. This technology is available in both endoscope-integrated (eCLE) as well as probe-based (pCLE) platforms and has a 475-by-475 μm field of view with lateral resolutions of 0.7 μm in the eCLE and 1 μm in the pCLE [2, 13].

Kiesslich et al. were the first to demonstrate the power of eCLE clinically in the evaluation of Barrett's esophagus (see Fig. 9.1). Utilizing intravenous fluorescein, they showed in vivo that eCLE could accurately identify Barrett's metaplasia

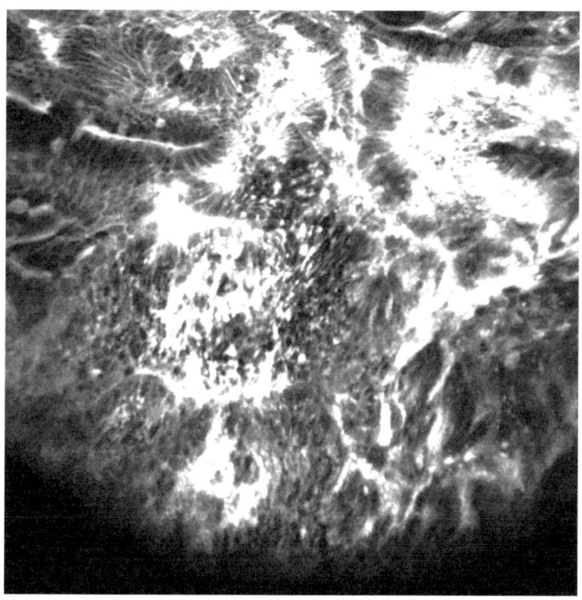

Fig. 9.1 This confocal laser endomicroscopy image with IV fluorescein depicts esophageal adenocarcinoma. The glandular architecture is completely effaced and the few glands that are visible are crowded

(96.8 %) and Barrett's-associated neoplasia (97.4 %). Moreover, the interobserver variability for histopathological diagnosis ($k = 0.843$) and intraobserver agreement ($l = 0.892$) was high [14]. The implications of these robust findings were demonstrated in a multicenter randomized controlled trial by Canto et al. that showed high-definition white-light endoscopy (WLE) with eCLE and targeted biopsy had a higher diagnostic yield compared to high-definition WLE and random biopsy alone (34 % vs. 7 %; $p < 0.0001$) and that eCLE increased the sensitivity for detecting cancer from 40 to 96 % with no significant drop in specificity [15]. In addition to adenocarcinoma, eCLE demonstrated some potential in diagnosing squamous cell carcinoma with accuracy, sensitivity, and specificity measures of 95 %, 100 %, and 87 %, respectively [16]. Studies evaluating the efficacy of fluorescein and pCLE also showed promising results. In a randomized controlled multicenter trial, high-definition WLE combined with pCLE significantly ($p = 0.002$) improved the sensitivity compared to high-definition WLE alone [17].

That said, in a meta-analysis conducted in 2014 on seven previous studies totaling 345 patients, Gupta et al. concluded that CLE should not replace random biopsy as of yet because of its low per-lesion sensitivity (68 %) and negative predictive ratio (0.24) [18]. Part of CLE's limitations, especially in terms of sensitivity, is related to its small field of view.

- CLE has been shown to improve the sensitivity of high-definition white-light endoscopy and significantly enhance diagnostic yield. If available, it should be used with IV flourescein to enhance Barrett's surveillance.

Acriflavine/Proflavine

Acriflavine and its principal component, proflavine, are topically applied vital-dyes that are absorbed by the epithelium and concentrate in cell nuclei. In the esophagus, these agents have been studied both as a wide-field, red-flagging tool as well as a high-resolution, diagnostic device. As a high-resolution device, an ex vivo study illustrated that high-resolution microendoscopy (HRME) could be applied to esophageal tissue and distinguish squamous epithelium, Barrett's metaplasia, and high-grade dysplasia (see Fig. 9.2) from one another [19]; separately, the same group developed an algorithm to objectively discriminate neoplastic versus benign sites that was 87 % sensitive and 85 % specific. Comparatively, the subjective analysis of two expert gastroenterologists and two expert pathologists showed much lower specificities (53 % and 68 %, respectively) though their sensitivity averaged 87 % [20]. Overall, HRME, like CLE, provides high-resolution images (lateral spatial resolution of 4 μm), yet the field of view of 750 μm remains impractical for screening.

The multispectral digital microscope (MDM), a device in prototype format undergoing testing in clinical trials and not commercially available, provides a field of view of 2.5 cm and spatial resolution of 50–100 μm. Using multiple filters, linear polarizers, and excitation wavelengths ranging from 365 to 450 nm, the

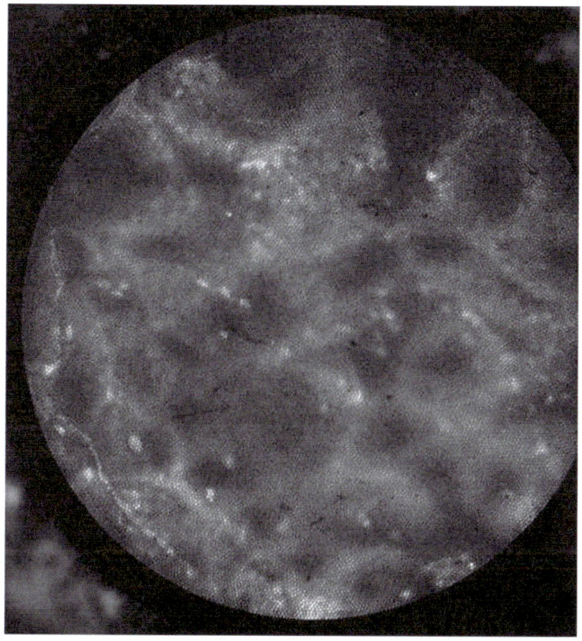

Fig. 9.2 This high-resolution microendoscopy image with topical proflavine depicts Barrett's esophagus with high-grade dysplasia. Cell nuclei appear crowded and the glandular architecture is heterogeneous throughout, with glands varying in size and shape

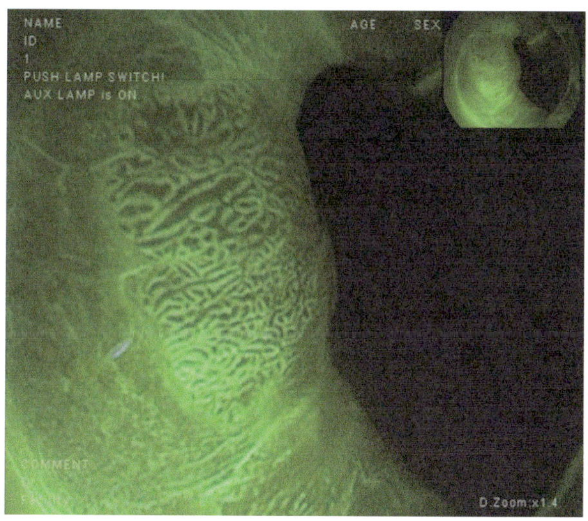

Fig. 9.3 This image taken with multispectral digital microscope and topical proflavine demonstrates normal tissue at the gastric–esophageal junction. Individual glands can be identified and the space in between the glands is homogenous throughout the tissue

MDM highlights the glandular architecture of the esophageal mucosa in vivo (see Fig. 9.3) and can distinguish benign Barrett's metaplasia from high-grade dysplasia and adenocarcinoma [21, 22]. And because the MDM, like the HRME, utilizes proflavine as its topical contrast agent, the two imaging modalities can be employed sequentially—the MDM as a red-flagging device and the HRME as a diagnostic tool; the efficacy of which is being tested in vivo.

Methylene Blue and Crystal Violet

ECS uses a topical agent to stain and highlight the surface of GI mucosa, as opposed to CLE that can also image the subsurface. With its two magnification settings, ECS can visualize the density of cells at its low magnification (×450, field of view 300 by 300 μm), and subcellular features at its high magnification (×1100, field of view 120 by 120 μm) [23]. Using methylene blue, Kumagai et al. demonstrated that ECS could resolve cellular changes in patients with esophageal squamous carcinoma. Taking into account cellular density to nucleus-to-cytoplasm ratios to heterogeneity in cellular shape and size, ECS was 95 % sensitive and 84 % specific for diagnosing squamous cell carcinoma in vivo [24]. Later, Minami et al. added topical crystal violet, which stains the cytoplasm in contrast to methylene blue that stains both the nucleus and cytoplasm [4]. With this double-staining technique, this group developed a new classification system for squamous atypia in the esophagus with an efficacy (91.3 %), comparable to that of hematoxylin and eosin staining [25].

Utility of ECS has also been shown in Barrett's esophagus. In 2013, Tomizawa et al. developed a classification system for differentiating Barrett's lesions using ECS that showed great efficacy (accuracy measures ranged from 83 to 100 %) and excellent ($k>0.897$) interobserver agreement [26]. Although ex vivo, this study supports the continued use of ECS in clinical practice.

Overall, ECS has been shown to be safe and efficacious in helping diagnose and target dysplastic lesions [23]; yet, more in vivo clinical trials are necessary before ECS can replace conventional histopathological biopsy.

Acetic Acid

Acetic acid is a topically applied agent that breaks down the mucus layer exposing epithelium to unbuffered acid. In turn, the mucosal pit pattern and villi become more pronounced as the tissue whitens, an effect that persists longer in non-dysplastic esophageal epithelium. When these features were tested, the interobserver ($k=0.571$) and intraobserver ($k=0.709$) agreement was moderate to substantial [27] and it led to significantly improved detection of neoplasia [12].

In 190 sites on 119 patients, Longcroft-Wheaton et al. found acetic acid chromoendoscopy to have a sensitivity and specificity of 95.5 % and 81 %, respectively, with zero missed cancers and four missed dysplasias (two high-grade, two low-grade) when compared to histology. Furthermore, when compared to WLE, acetic acid increased ($p=0.001$) the detection rate of neoplasia in vivo 2.5-fold [28]. In an even larger study ($n=263$), Bhandari et al. found acetic acid to double the rate of detection of Barrett's associated neoplasia to 96 % compared to the 48 % seen with WLE ($p=0.001$). Though acetic acid did have a 25 % false positive rate in this cohort, the authors estimated a 91–97 % cost reduction [29], all of which suggests that acetic acid chromoendoscopy is clinical and cost-effective.

Possible Future Agents

2-NBDG

2-NBDG has been shown to have high sensitivity and specificity for dysplastic Barrett's esophagus tissue. In two ex vivo studies, this topically applied agent had a higher mean fluorescent intensity in neoplastic biopsies compared to that of metaplastic biopsies with 96 % sensitivity and 90 % specificity [30]. While these results are encouraging, in vivo studies are necessary to determine 2-NBDG's future clinical applications.

Peptide Biomarkers

Using the technique of *phage display* (see section Targeted agents: Peptides), Lu et al. identified one target sequence, ASYNYDA that bound specifically to esophageal adenocarcinoma and linked it to a fluorescent marker; it was shown on confocal endomicroscopy to bind with a 3.8-fold greater intensity to dysplastic tissue in vivo, having a sensitivity of 75 % and specificity of 97 % [31]. And with more sequences being identified, the applications of this new imaging technology are promising.

Lectin

The expression of surface glycans has been shown to decrease throughout the progression of normal esophageal mucosa to dysplasia to adenocarcinoma. Bird-Lieberman et al. identified a group of lectins that bind surface glycan units and demonstrated decreased binding as the tissue progressed from normal mucosa to neoplasia ($p<0.05$). Of these lectins, WGA was selected both for its aforementioned property to distinguish benign from malignant tissue ($p<0.001$) and also for its presence in the human diet and thus decreased likelihood for toxicity.

In an ex vivo study on four specimens, fluorescently labelled WGA correlated strongly with the degree of histological assessment of dysplasia ($p=0.0002$). Importantly, there was no correlation between WGA fluorescence and acute ($p=0.68$) or chronic (0.82) inflammation. Additionally, because this agent does not rely on high-resolution endoscopy, it is not limited by a small field of view and could be effective as a red-flagging device. That said, the 10-min wait-time may be a concern clinically, and must be addressed in future in vivo trials [9].

Stomach

Part of the poor prognosis in gastric cancer is attributable to difficulty in distinguishing dysplastic lesions from benign gastritis as evidenced by the 77.8–84.0 % sensitivity of WLE alone [32]. To improve detection, a significant amount of research developing new imaging modalities has been done.

Fluorescein

The use of CLE with intravenous fluorescein has been extensively studied in the stomach. In 2008, two in vivo studies using intravenous fluorescein looked at the feasibility of CLE determining gastric histology. Guo et al. looked at the presence of goblet cells, columnar cells, and villiform foveolar epithelium to predict gastric intestinal metaplasia and found that CLE correlated with the histological findings ($k=0.94$), having a sensitivity and specificity of 98 % and 95 %, respectively. By comparison, the correlation between WLE and histopathology was 0.25, with WLE having a sensitivity and specificity of 36.9 % and 91.6 %, respectively. However, CLE had a much lower correlation (0.67) to histology when attempting to discriminate between complete and incomplete gastric intestinal metaplasia [33]. Alternatively, Zhang et al. classified based on gastric pit pattern alone and were able to differentiate moderate-to-severe activity, atrophy, and cancer with accuracies of 97.5 %, 95.8 %, and 97.1 %, respectively [34].

More than highlighting histopathology, CLE also accurately (92.8 %) identified *H. pylori* infection via white spots, microabscesses, or neutrophils with substantial ($k=0.78$) interobserver agreement [35]. In fact, Wang et al. showed that CLE could correctly diagnose *H. pylori* infection (sensitivity and specificity of 82.9 % and 90.9 %, respectively) while simultaneously categorizing the histological severity into normal mucosa, active inflammation, atrophy, and intestinal metaplasia all with sensitivity and specificity measures greater than 92.9 % [36].

In short, for the diagnosis of gastric intestinal metaplasia, real-time pCLE was more accurate than WLE ($p<0.001$) and autofluorescence imaging ($p<0.001$), and comparable to magnifying narrow-band imaging [37]. Moreover, in a randomized controlled trial comparing CLE with targeted biopsy to WLE with standard biopsy, the diagnostic yield of CLE was higher both in per-patient ($p=0.074$) and per-lesion ($p<0.001$) analysis with CLE decreasing ($p<0.001$) the mean number of biopsies by 68 % [38].

In moving on to gastric adenomas and superficial cancers, CLE also performed well clinically. With intravenous fluorescein and topical acriflavine, CLE was able to diagnose hyperplastic polyps and adenomas (accuracy = 90 %) and discriminate between them (accuracy = 97 %) in vivo with almost perfect intraobserver ($k=0.92$) and interobserver ($k=0.83$) agreement [39]. Later, Li et al. developed a two-tiered classification system setting low-grade intraepithelial neoplasia as the upper limit of "non-cancerous lesions" and high-grade intraepithelial neoplasia as the lower limit of "cancerous lesions." This system, when applied prospectively to 1572 patients, had a sensitivity and specificity of 88.9 % and 99.3 %, respectively, both of which were significantly ($p<0.05$) better than that of WLE [40].

CLE has also shown utility in pre- and post-endoscopic submucosal dissection (ESD) of gastric cancer. Prior to 31 patients undergoing ESD, CLE was performed and compared to endoscopic biopsy. Overall, CLE was significantly more accurate (94.2 %) than endoscopic biopsy (85.7 %) in diagnosing gastric adenomas and adenocarcinomas using post-ESD histopathology as the gold standard ($p=0.031$). On top of having a less accurate pre-procedural diagnosis, additional endoscopic biopsies can lead to fibrosis, which makes ESD technically more difficult, and can increase the risk of adverse events associated with ESD including bleeding and perforation [41].

Currently, no in vivo agent has replaced the gold standard of biopsy to diagnose neoplasia in the stomach. That said, CLE has been shown to be significantly better than WLE at identifying neoplasia.

- If a center possesses CLE, it can be used with IV fluorescein for assessing suspicious lesions, but is not ideal for screening because of its small field of view.

Indigocarmine and Acetic acid

Chromoendoscopy with indigo carmine, a topically applied contrast dye, is able to highlight mucosal changes that are not apparent with WLE. Rather than being absorbed, this dye accumulates in crevices, crypts, and foveolae and thereby normal tissue is stained blue and abnormal tissue is stained translucent pink [6]. Several studies have shown its clinical benefit, with the most recent 2008 study by Sakai et al. finding chromoendoscopy with indigo carmine accurately identifying 52.8 % of gastric lesions while conventional endoscopy accurately identifying just 17.0 % ($p<0.005$) [42]. Although a 3-fold improvement on WLE, the efficacy of indigo carmine alone was still lacking.

Acetic acid is absorbed by cells and, as a result, reversibly alters cellular protein structure thereby leading to whitening and opacification of normal mucosa. In applying this agent to abnormal gastric tissue, acetic acid was found to have shortened duration of whitening as the histological grade of the tissue became more severe [10]. Thus, in the aforementioned study by Sakai et al., gastric lesions were also assessed with acetic acid. Acetic acid alone performed similarly to indigo carmine alone (41.5 % vs. 52.8 %, $p<0.242$), but together the two agents achieved a significantly higher ($p<0.005$) diagnostic performance of 94.3 % [42].

A limitation of the above studies, however, is that most lesions analyzed were well-differentiated. Consequently, Lee et al. stratified the performance of the two in vivo agents in well-differentiated versus undifferentiated tissue. While chromoendoscopy with indigo carmine and acetic acid distinguished the cancerous border significantly more than conventional endoscopy in well-differentiated lesions (89.8 % vs. 68.5 %, $p<0.001$), the two imaging modalities did not differ ($p=0.494$) in efficacy for undifferentiated adenocarcinomas [43]. In summary, there have been many advancements in chromoendoscopy, namely the incorporation of both indigo carmine and acetic acid and the understanding that it is superior to conventional WLE only in differentiated lesions. As such, there is still need for a wide-field screening technique that can be applied to all types of gastric adenocarcinoma.

- Although superior to WLE in identifying gastric lesions, chromoendoscopy with acetic acid plus indigo carmine should not be used in undifferentiated cancers of the stomach.

Methylene Blue and Crystal Violet

In contrast to the research in the esophagus, ECS, which utilizes a topical stain and ultrahigh magnification, has seen more mixed results in the stomach. In 2007, Eberl et al. found that after the application of methylene blue, the sensitivity and specificity of ECS for predicting neoplasia in the stomach was 56 % and 89 % respectively. They attributed the low sensitivity in the stomach to the gastric secretions [44]. In hopes of minimizing this, Chiu et al. applied simethicone solution vigorously onto the gastric mucosa prior to staining with methylene blue. Despite this method, they reported unsatisfactorily that just 71 of 102 images were of good quality. That said, they were able to identify goblet cells significantly more in intestinal metaplasia compared to chronic gastritis ($p<0.0001$), and using the presence of goblet cells as the sole criterion for diagnosing gastric intestinal metaplasia, the study found a sensitivity of 89 % and specificity of 71 % [45]. Another study looking at the efficacy of ECS in diagnosing early gastric cancer assessed 82 lesions for glandular structural and cellular atypia. After performing similar in vivo prepping and staining techniques as the prior study, they were able to adequately image 88 % of lesions and, with their criteria, found a sensitivity and specificity of 86 % and 100 %, respectively, for discriminating cancer from benign tissue [46]. Taken together, these studies indicate the improving clinical capability of ECS, with perhaps its strongest limiting factor being obtaining adequate image quality. In addition to dimethicone, the second study added pronase to the mucus clearing solution, which significantly improved image quality ($p=0.00318$); yet, still 12 % of lesions were of poor quality. Thus, more research identifying a suitable agent to improve viewing is certainly warranted. Separately, while the efficacy of the prior studies are promising, larger patient populations validating the reproducibility of ECS is necessary as are studies looking at the intra- and interobserver variability amongst novel and experienced users.

Possible Future Agents

MG7

MG7 represents a molecular marker that is specific for gastric cancer. An in vivo study looking at transplanted human gastric cancers into mice, found that CLE could identify tumors with fluorescently labelled antibodies against MG7. Separately, this study stained ex vivo specimens of human gastric cancers and targeted MG7. They found fluorescence in 96 % of neoplastic lesions compared to 22 % of normal mucosa ($p<0.0001$) [47].

Colon: Adenocarcinoma

Colonoscopy has emerged as the gold standard for colorectal cancer screening and it has been shown to be efficacious, especially for large lesions. In one meta-analysis of adenomas and non-adenomatous polyps measuring greater than 10 mm, only 2.1 % and 0 % were missed, respectively. For smaller lesions, however, colonoscopy fails far more often. That is, adenomas and non-adenomatous polyps measuring less than 10 mm were missed 23 and 22 % of the time, respectively [48]. Currently, all lesions are excised and sent for pathology. This method not only increases the cost associated with the procedure, which in some countries is significant, but also if the specimen comes back malignant repeat colonoscopies may be necessary to determine resectability. As such, contrast agents that allow for better screening and in vivo diagnosis are being researched.

Methylene Blue, Indigo Carmine, and Crystal Violet

Magnification chromoendoscopy (MCE) with topically applied agents has been found to be useful in colonoscopy, specifically in lesions that are flat and depressed. In modifying Kudo's classification of colonic pit patterns into non-neoplastic (Type I and II) and neoplastic groups (Type III, IV and V), Tung et al. found in a prospective study that MCE had a sensitivity of 93.8 % and specificity of 64.6 % [49]. In another prospective study on 1850 patients, Hurlstone et al. similarly used the Kudo classification system and indigo carmine, and, unlike Tung et al., performed crystal violet staining for lesions that had central depressions, were indeterminate, or were type V. Using this method, this study found MCE to be 98 % sensitive and 92 % specific, the latter of which was a significant improvement relative to that found in Tung et al. Granted a clinical improvement for in vivo diagnosis, MCE cannot completely replace the need for histopathology [50].

Unlike MCE, which is able to magnify mucosa ×100 and visualize glandular architecture, ECS represents a more recent imaging device that offers ×450 magnification and thus is able to visualize cellular features in addition to pit patterns. By double-staining in ECS with crystal violet and methylene blue, one is able to identify cell nuclei better than with crystal violet alone. And with the addition of crystal violet, glands become apparent 47 s sooner ($p<0.001$) than with methylene blue alone [51]. In a prospective analysis on 206 patients, the accuracy of ECS was significantly better than conventional endoscopy (100 % vs. 96.7 %, $p=0.015$). And, in discriminating massively invasive submucosal cancers from other neoplastic tissue, ECS performed even better relative to conventional endoscopy reaching an overall accuracy of 95.9 % compared to that of 85.6 % ($p=0.001$). Notably, in this study, ten lesions from ten patients could not be analyzed with ECS because of poor image quality [52]. Despite this potential limitation, in another prospective randomized controlled trial on 203 lesions, ECS was shown to be non-inferior to standard biopsy for discriminating neoplastic lesions [53].

To compare MCE to ECS directly, in 2014, Kudo et al. performed MCE with crystal violet and then ECS with methylene blue and crystal violet. Diagnoses were recorded using only MCE imaging and compared to MCE plus ECS imaging. Overall accuracy for diagnosing neoplasia was comparable between the two modalities ($p=0.606$) with sensitivities and specificities ranging from 89.7 to 97.8 %. However, in predicting massively invasive submucosal cancer, MCE plus ECS was more specific ($p=0.041$) and accurate ($p=0.004$) than MCE alone [54].

Because both MCE and ECS are based on glandular and cellular patterns, Mori et al. developed and evaluated a computer program that translated ECS criteria into endoscopic diagnoses. They found that the computer software was similar in predicting neoplasia compared to expert endoscopists both in terms of sensitivity ($p=0.868$) and specificity ($p=0.256$) and was significantly better than novel endoscopists ($p<0.001$, $p<0.002$). Furthermore diagnosis was instant, occurring in less than a second. With its perfect reproducibility and 92.0 % sensitivity, the implementation of a computer-based ECS to general endoscopy practices seems to be within reach [55]. Currently though, the technology is limited to a few institutions [54] and it takes more than 5 m of additional time to image compared to conventional biopsy [53], thus obstacles remain before ECS becomes ingrained in standard practice.

Fluorescein and Acriflavine

As in previous sections, the use of CLE with intravenous fluorescein and acriflavine has found clinical applications in the colon. In the first in vivo study on CLE, Kiesslich et al. demonstrated that acriflavine staining was limited to the epithelium whereas intravenous fluorescein was also able to highlight deeper structures including the lamina propria and microvasculature. Consequently, in the prospective component of their study, only fluorescein was injected and sites were analyzed according to the study's classification system. Overall, they found CLE predicted neoplasia with a sensitivity of 97.4 %, specificity of 99.4 %, and an overall accuracy of 99.2 % [56]. This study, however, did not distinguish between low- and high-grade dysplastic lesions.

In 2010, Sanduleanu et al. attempted to make this distinction using both intravenous fluorescein and topical acriflavine, the latter of which allows improved visualization of cytonuclear changes. In combining these agents, the study created a CLE-based adenoma-dysplasia classification system that reliably discriminated between low- and high-grade dysplasia (accuracy = 96.7 %; $k=0.88$). Although promising, this study concluded that other nuclear features, such as hyperchromasia and nucleoli, could not be resolved and that other techniques would be helpful in this regard [57].

Whereas the prior studies examined screening colonoscopy, Shahid et al. looked at patients undergoing post-endoscopic mucosal resection surveillance and showed that real-time pCLE was more sensitive than virtual chromoendoscopy ($p=0.045$) in identifying residual neoplasia. And when used together, these imaging techniques approached sensitivity levels similar to histopathology (100 %). Altogether, the study concluded that by providing real-time diagnosis, CLE combined with other imaging could allow patients to forego repeat colonoscopies [58].

Instead of intravenous contrast, Wang et al. examined the efficacy of CLE with *topically* applied fluorescein. They found that after five seconds of application, imaging software could analyze objectively, the fluorescence intensity ratio between the lamina propria and crypt and accurately discriminates normal from neoplastic lesions (89 %, $p<0.001$), hyperplasia from adenoma (96 %, $p<0.001$), and tubular from villous adenoma (93 %, $p<0.001$). Moreover, procedural time lengthened by just 2–3 min per lesion [59].

Molecular Biomarkers

Cancer biomarkers can provide a multitude of prognostic information, from risk of progression to response to therapy, and simultaneously they can also improve diagnostic accuracy. In focusing on this last benefit, the number of potential molecular probes has steadily increased over the last few years. These probes can be divided into two groups, activatable, which are injected intravenously, absorbed by cells and become fluorescent upon enzymatic cleavage, and the more common peptide, which are applied topically. Generally, the peptide probes are non-toxic, non-immunogenic, and can be labelled easily and binds rapidly to tissues of interest. Yet activatable probes have their advantages, most notably providing fluorescence several centimeters below the surface mucosa as opposed to peptides, which in one study was able to provide images at a depth of 400 μm [60–62].

Using the technique of *phage display* (see section Targeted agents: Peptides), Hsiung et al. identified a heptapeptide sequence, conjugated it to fluorescein and demonstrated its in vivo accuracy (sensitivity = 81 %, specificity = 78 %) using a confocal microendoscope [63]. Since then, other peptides have been found and tested with other imaging devices, including near-infrared imaging (NIR). This system, which does not use visible light wavelengths, is less affected by scattering due to hemoglobin, autofluorescence, and background tissue artifact and can still provide subcellular imaging. Moreover, whereas the field of view for confocal imaging is ~100 μm, NIR has a field of view of 3.6 mm (resolution <10 μm), which is more optimal for large-surface screening. And in testing an octapeptide target with newly enhanced NIR system, Liu et al. was able to visualize several cellular features of dysplasia within mice colons and ex vivo in 6 of 8 human specimens [61].

- Although promising, NIR with biomarkers needs more clinical research before becoming part of routine practice.

Antibodies

VEGF represents another promising antibody-mediated imaging target. Foersch et al. showed that intravenously applied VEGF antibodies were detected in 13 of 15 tumor-positive mice and 9 of 10 human xenograft tumors. In comparison, healthy tissue showed almost no mucosa signal. And after incubating human specimens in VEGR antibody solution, 12 of 13 tumor-positive specimens showed fluorescence patterns similar to that of mice while 10 of 11 normal controls showed minimal signal [64]. A similar study on EGF-R also found that neoplastic tissue demonstrated significantly ($p = 0.0035$) more fluorescent than normal mucosa [65]. While significant, the injected antibodies took 24 h to reach optimal imaging results, which, in translating to clinical practice, may be problematic. Moreover, some tumors may be VEGF- or EGFR-negative, and inflammation may lead to expression of VEGF further limiting these potential targets [64].

Proflavine

Topically applied proflavine has also been used as an agent to detect colonic dysplasia (see Fig. 9.4). Using the HRME system that can highlight subcellular features, Parikh et al. prospectively evaluated 171 polyps and found that real-time HRME performed significantly better compared to conventional endoscopy in terms of accuracy (94 % vs. 65 %), specificity (95 % vs. 39 %), and positive predictive value (87 % vs. 55 %). Moreover, these differences persisted in polyps less than 10 mm and diminutive (less than 5 mm) polyps (all $p < 0.001$) [66]. And with the system costing 2000 US dollars and requiring minimal (~5 min) training [67], the future of this technology is promising.

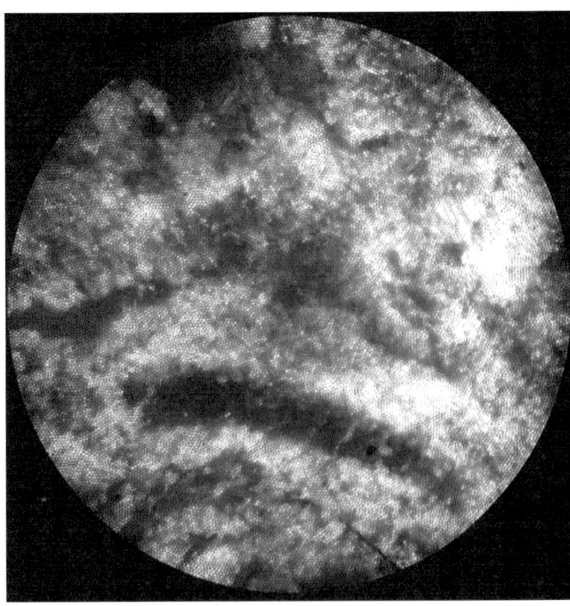

Fig. 9.4 This high-resolution microendoscopy image shows high-grade dysplasia and cancer in the colon. There is no apparent glandular architecture and the cell nuclei are crowded

- Although still in prototype format and not commercially available, HRME with topical proflavine is significantly more accurate than WLE in predicting neoplasia. Whether it will replace standard biopsy is yet to be seen.

Future Directions

The implementation of MCE into standard practice has already taken shape in Japan, replacing tissue biopsy and unnecessary polypectomy [52, 54]. In the USA, a cost–benefit analysis of foregoing biopsy of diminutive polyps (less than 5 mm), showed an upfront savings over a billion US dollars. While foregoing pathology would lead to incorrect management in 11.8 % instead of just 1.9 % of patients, the number needed to harm would exceed 11,000 people and the resulting cost of managing the 10 % of cases that were misdiagnosed would be less than 10 % of the billion dollars initially saved. Moreover, with the assistance of newer technologies including MCE, ECS, and CLE, in vivo diagnosis would be more efficacious than the 90 % estimate used by this study. Thus, as imaging technology continues to improve, there will be more accurate initial management and less downstream consequences and subsequently more net cost–savings. In short, it is only a matter of time before in vivo diagnosis becomes the norm in the USA [68].

Colon: Infectious Disease

At times it is difficult to diagnose infectious causes of gastrointestinal disease. In hopes of improving in vivo diagnosis of microscopic organisms, there has been research into the utilization of contrast agents in endomicroscopy.

Fluorescein and Acriflavine

Clostridium difficile can alter colonic mucosa and cause pseudomembranes and linear ulcers, but at other times, these macroscopic features do not exist and there is only slight erythema. As such, Neumann et al. prospectively studied 80 patients with suspected *C. difficile* infection using CLE. They gave fluorescein intravenously and occasionally applied topical acriflavine and found that CLE was 96.25 % accurate in identifying histologic changes. As opposed to fluorescein, which only stained human mucosa, acriflavine was absorbed by the bacteria and could be visualized as a white spot. Thus, in the ex vivo portion of the study, acriflavine was able to identify *C. difficile* in culture with CLE imaging [69].

IBD: Cancer Screening

The risk of colorectal cancer in patients with IBD is increased relative to the general population and thus additional screening is warranted. In the recent past, random 4-quadrant biopsies taken every ten centimeters plus sampling suspicious lesions was the standard of care. Not only did random biopsy have lower yield, but also conventional white-light endoscopy had lower sensitivity compared to other imaging modalities including chromoendoscopy and CLE [70].

Methylene Blue and Indigo Carmine

The use of topical vital-dyes paired with chromoendoscopy has seen a revolution in cancer detection in IBD patients. In a meta-analysis of six studies totaling nearly 1300 IBD patients, chromoendoscopy with topical dye was compared to WLE in screening for dysplasia. They found that chromoendoscopy had a 7 % higher yield for dysplasia and also detected 44 % more lesions via targeted biopsy and 27 % more flat lesions (see Fig. 9.5) [71].

- It is now recommended that chromoendoscopy with methylene blue or indigo carmine be paired with high-definition WLE for targeted biopsy in cancer surveillance for IBD patients [70].

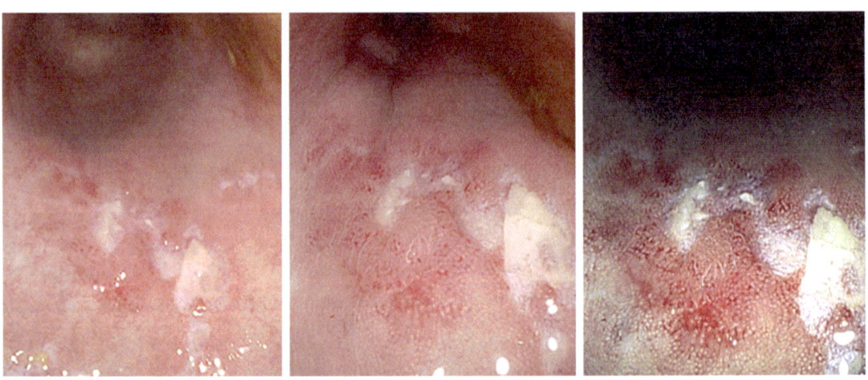

Fig. 9.5 This triptych image shows low-grade dysplasia in a patient with ulcerative colitis. In comparison to white-light endoscopy shown on the *left*, the iScan images (*center* and *right*) demonstrate greater resolution of the glandular architecture and enhancement of the vascular pattern. Photo Courtesy of Steven Naymagon, MD, with permission

Fluorescein

CLE has shown added benefit to chromoendoscopy with studies finding sensitivity and specificity measures greater than 90 %. While promising, CLE adds about 30 min to endoscopic time and currently there is not enough data to support the use of CLE in routine cancer screening of IBD patients [72].

IBD: Diagnosis and Monitoring Disease Activity

Because mucosal healing is strongly predictive of IBD remission, activity, and ultimate need for bowel resection, accurately determining mucosal healing is of high clinical importance. Therefore, because WLE has been shown to be false negative nearly half of the time, other imaging agents are needed in this subset of patients [73].

Fluorescein

With CLE and systemic fluorescein, endoscopists are able to visualize histologic characteristics of ulcerative colitis. Li et al. found that in real-time three individual features, fluorescein leakage into crypts, microvascular changes, and crypt architecture, all correlated strongly ($p<0.001$) with histology. Notably, of the 28 patients WLE read as normal, 16 had histological diagnoses of active disease. By comparison, of the 21 patients CLE (based on crypt architecture) read as having normal or chronic inflammation, zero had histology reads indicating active ulcerative colitis [74].

CLE has also been able to identify markers of disease activity in patients with Crohn's disease. In compiling information from patients with active Crohn's, quiescent Crohn's and a control group, Neumann et al. developed a CLE activity scoring system based on six parameters including crypt number, crypt distortion, goblet cell number, microerosions, cellular infiltrate, and vascularity. This grading system was able to differentiate between the three aforementioned groups. Moreover, it correlated strongly with serum CRP levels (an established marker of disease activity) in Crohn's patients with quiescent versus active disease [75]. While more studies are needed to evaluate real-time efficacy, CLE and fluorescein in IBD patients may develop into an efficacious imaging device.

Antibodies

Imaging Crohn's patients with fluorescently labelled antibodies under CLE has been shown to predict therapeutic response. After topically applying membrane-bound tumor necrosis factor (mTNF) with fluorescently labelled adalimumab, Atreya et al. imaged the bowel mucosa and counted the number of cells per confocal image that were mTNF-positive. Afterwards, they treated all patients with adalimumab therapy for 12 weeks. They found that those who had a clinical response were significantly more likely to have had more mTNF-positive cells on imaging 12 weeks prior ($p=0.02$). And, by selecting a cut-off point of 20 mTNF-positive cells per field, they showed an 84.6 % sensitivity and 91.7 % specificity for predicting therapeutic response to adalimumab, which continued through a follow-up period of 1 year [76]. While this study included just 25 patients, it manifests how advanced imaging can aid in the development of personalized medicine in IBD patients.

Methylene Blue

Endocytoscopic imaging of ulcerative colitis with methylene blue has also shown clinical utility. Specifically, Bessho et al. created a grading system and found that shape, microvasculature, and crypt spacing each were significantly correlated to histopathology ($p<0.001$) and that interobserver agreement for each characteristic was moderate to substantial ($0.52<k<0.73$) [77].

Because disease activity is also largely based on histopathological analysis of inflammatory cells, in vivo diagnosis of these inflammatory markers would be useful. To this end, Neumann et al. demonstrated that ECS was reliable in discriminating various types of inflammatory cells, including neutrophils (Sn = 60 %, Sp = 95 %), lymphocytes (Sn = 89 %, Sp = 93 %), basophils (Sn = 71 %, Sp = 94 %), and eosinophils (Sn = 75 %, Sp = 90 %). Also, inter- and intraobserver agreement between the two endoscopists was substantial to almost perfect for each cell type. And final grading of disease activity was 100 % concordant between ECS and histopathology [78]. Though it takes more than 20 min to perform and is limited to imaging the superficial layer, ECS shows great potential (Table 9.2).

Conclusion

With the continued development of new imaging agents and devices, the diagnostic capacity of endoscopy is expanding. Some of these advancements provide the endoscopist with a wide-field view of the mucosa and act as red-flagging tools while others provide optical biopsies that are similar to histology. Clinically, the ability to identify infections, monitor chronic inflammatory bowel disease, and better target gastrointestinal neoplasia can decrease the need for histology, thereby saving healthcare dollars, and simultaneously provide more effective medical care. At this time, these agents have broadened the field of endoscopy from macroscopic screening to one that includes targeted biopsy; in the future, with continued research into these technologies, the breadth of endoscopy may go on to encompass in vivo diagnosis and immediate management and therapy.

Table 9.2 Endoscopic imaging of GI disease

Disease	Imaging system	Agent
ESCC	ECS	Methylene blue + crystal violet
BE/EAC	ECS	Methylene blue + crystal violet
	HRME, MDM	Acriflavine/proflavine
	CLE	Fluorescein*
	Chromoendoscopy	Acetic acid
	Confocal microscopy	ASYNYDA peptide
BE/EAC (ex vivo)	Confocal microscopy	2-NBDG
	Conventional endoscopy	Lectin
Gastric cancer	CLE	Fluorescein*
		Fluorescein* + acriflavine
		MG7
	High-Definition Endoscope	Indigo carmine + acetic acid
	ECS	Methylene blue + crystal violet
Colon cancer	CLE	Fluorescein*
		Fluorescein* + acriflavine
		Heptapeptide
	HRME	Proflavine
	ECS	Methylene blue + crystal violet
	Chromoendoscopy	Indigo carmine + crystal violet
Colon cancer (ex vivo)	Near-Infrared	Octapeptide
	CLE	VEGF*, EGF-R*
Colon cancer in IBD patients	CLE	Fluorescein*
	Chromoendoscopy	Methylene blue or Indigo carmine
IBD	CLE	Fluorescein*
		mTNF
C. difficile Colitis	CLE	Fluorescein* + acriflavine

This table highlights the clinical research in luminal GI diseases in terms of imaging systems and the in vivo agent utilized. The individual studies are discussed throughout the chapter. Studies that were exclusively performed ex vivo are identified in the left column. Agents marked with an asterisk (*) were given intravenously while all others were given topically

2-NBDG 2-[*N*-(7-nitrobenz-2-oxa-1,3-diaxol-4-yl) amino]-2-deoxyglucose, *BE/EAC* Barrett's esophagus/esophageal adenocarcinoma, *CLE* confocal laser endomicroscopy, *ECS* endocytoscopy, *ESCC* esophageal squamous cell carcinoma, *HRME* high-resolution microendoscopy, *IBD* inflammatory bowel disease, *MDM* multispectral digital microscope, *mTNF* membrane-bound tumor necrosis factor

References

1. Goetz M. Endomicroscopy and targeted imaging of gastric neoplasia. Gastrointest Endosc Clin N Am [Internet]. 2013 [cited 2015 Jan 25];23(3):597–606. http://www.sciencedirect.com/science/article/pii/S1052515713000226
2. Choi K-S, Jung H-Y. Confocal laser endomicroscopy and molecular imaging in barrett esophagus and stomach. Clin Endosc [Internet]. 2014 [cited 2015 Jan 21];47(1):23–30. http://www.pubmedcentral.nih.gov/articlerender.fcgi?artid=3928487&tool=pmcentrez&rendertype=abstract

3. Kodashima S, Fujishiro M, Takubo K, Kammori M, Nomura S, Kakushima N, et al. Ex-vivo study of high-magnification chromoendoscopy in the gastrointestinal tract to determine the optimal staining conditions for endocytoscopy. Endoscopy [Internet]. 2006 [cited 2015 Feb 11];38(11):1115–21. http://www.ncbi.nlm.nih.gov/pubmed/17111333
4. Inoue H, Yokoyama A, Kudo S. [Ultrahigh magnifying endoscopy: development of CM double staining for endocytoscopy and its safety]. Nihon Rinsho [Internet]. 2010 [cited 2015 Jan 27];68(7):1247–52. http://www.ncbi.nlm.nih.gov/pubmed/20662202
5. Neumann H, Kudo S-E, Kiesslich R, Neurath MF. Advanced colonoscopic imaging using endocytoscopy. Dig Endosc [Internet]. 2014 [cited 2014 Dec 18];27(2):232–8. http://www.ncbi.nlm.nih.gov/pubmed/25311804
6. Peitz U, Malfertheiner P. Chromoendoscopy: from a research tool to clinical progress. Dig Dis [Internet]. 2002 [cited 2015 Feb 5];20(2):111–9. http://www.karger.com/Article/FullText/67480
7. Li M, Wang TD. Targeted endoscopic imaging. Gastrointest Endosc Clin N Am [Internet]. 2009 [cited 2015 Jan 25];19(2):283–98. http://www.pubmedcentral.nih.gov/articlerender.fcgi?artid=3217463&tool=pmcentrez&rendertype=abstract
8. O'Neil RG, Wu L, Mullani N. Uptake of a fluorescent deoxyglucose analog (2-NBDG) in tumor cells. Mol Imaging Biol [Internet]. [cited 2015 Jan 25];7(6):388–92. http://www.ncbi.nlm.nih.gov/pubmed/16284704
9. Bird-Lieberman EL, Neves AA, Lao-Sirieix P, O'Donovan M, Novelli M, Lovat LB, et al. Molecular imaging using fluorescent lectins permits rapid endoscopic identification of dysplasia in Barrett's esophagus. Nat Med [Internet]. 2012 [cited 2015 Jan 25];18(2):315–21. http://www.ncbi.nlm.nih.gov/pubmed/22245781
10. Yagi K, Aruga Y, Nakamura A, Sekine A, Umezu H. The study of dynamic chemical magnifying endoscopy in gastric neoplasia. Gastrointest Endosc [Internet]. 2005 [cited 2015 Feb 5];62(6):963–9. http://www.ncbi.nlm.nih.gov/pubmed/16301045
11. Sharma P, Bansal A, Mathur S, Wani S, Cherian R, McGregor D, et al. The utility of a novel narrow band imaging endoscopy system in patients with Barrett's esophagus. Gastrointest Endosc [Internet]. 2006 [cited 2015 Mar 4];64(2):167–75. http://www.sciencedirect.com/science/article/pii/S0016510705031676
12. Saxena P, Canto MI. Red flag imaging techniques in Barrett's esophagus. Gastrointest Endosc Clin N Am [Internet]. 2013 [cited 2015 Jan 25];23(3):535–47. http://www.sciencedirect.com/science/article/pii/S1052515713000202
13. Leggett CL, Gorospe EC. Application of confocal laser endomicroscopy in the diagnosis and management of Barrett's esophagus. Ann Gastroenterol Q Publ Hell Soc Gastroenterol [Internet]. 2014 [cited 2015 Jan 25];27(3):193–9. http://www.pubmedcentral.nih.gov/articlerender.fcgi?artid=4073013&tool=pmcentrez&rendertype=abstract
14. Kiesslich R, Gossner L, Goetz M, Dahlmann A, Vieth M, Stolte M, et al. In vivo histology of Barrett's esophagus and associated neoplasia by confocal laser endomicroscopy. Clin Gastroenterol Hepatol [Internet]. 2006 [cited 2015 Jan 25];4(8):979–87. http://www.cghjournal.org/article/S1542356506004757/fulltext
15. Canto MI, Anandasabapathy S, Brugge W, Falk GW, Dunbar KB, Zhang Z, et al. In vivo endomicroscopy improves detection of Barrett's esophagus-related neoplasia: a multicenter international randomized controlled trial (with video). Gastrointest Endosc [Internet]. 2014 [cited 2015 Jan 25];79(2):211–21. http://www.ncbi.nlm.nih.gov/pubmed/24219822
16. Pech O, Rabenstein T, Manner H, Petrone MC, Pohl J, Vieth M, et al. Confocal laser endomicroscopy for in vivo diagnosis of early squamous cell carcinoma in the esophagus. Clin Gastroenterol Hepatol [Internet]. 2008 [cited 2015 Jan 25];6(1):89–94. http://www.cghjournal.org/article/S1542356507009743/fulltext
17. Sharma P, Meining AR, Coron E, Lightdale CJ, Wolfsen HC, Bansal A, et al. Real-time increased detection of neoplastic tissue in Barrett's esophagus with probe-based confocal laser endomicroscopy: final results of an international multicenter, prospective, randomized, controlled trial. Gastrointest Endosc [Internet]. 2011 [cited 2015 Jan 25];74(3):465–72. http://www.pubmedcentral.nih.gov/articlerender.fcgi?artid=3629729&tool=pmcentrez&rendertype=abstract

18. Gupta A, Attar BM, Koduru P, Murali AR, Go BT, Agarwal R. Utility of confocal laser endomicroscopy in identifying high-grade dysplasia and adenocarcinoma in Barrett's esophagus: a systematic review and meta-analysis. Eur J Gastroenterol Hepatol [Internet]. 2014 [cited 2015 Jan 25];26(4):369–77. http://www.ncbi.nlm.nih.gov/pubmed/24535597
19. Muldoon TJ, Anandasabapathy S, Maru D, Richards-Kortum R. High-resolution imaging in Barrett's esophagus: a novel, low-cost endoscopic microscope. Gastrointest Endosc [Internet]. 2008 [cited 2015 Jan 25];68(4):737–44. http://www.pubmedcentral.nih.gov/articlerender.fcgi?artid=2869299&tool=pmcentrez&rendertype=abstract
20. Muldoon TJ, Thekkek N, Roblyer D, Maru D, Harpaz N, Potack J, et al. Evaluation of quantitative image analysis criteria for the high-resolution microendoscopic detection of neoplasia in Barrett's esophagus. J Biomed Opt [Internet]. [cited 2015 Jan 25];15(2):026027. http://www.pubmedcentral.nih.gov/articlerender.fcgi?artid=2874050&tool=pmcentrez&rendertype=abstract
21. Perl DP, Parikh N, Chang S, Peng P, Thekkek N, Lee MH, et al. Diagnosis of neoplasia in Barrett's esophagus using vital-dye enhanced fluorescence imaging. J Vis Exp [Internet]. 2014 [cited 2015 Jan 27];(87):e50992. http://www.jove.com/video/50992/diagnosis-neoplasia-barretts-esophagus-using-vital-dye-enhanced
22. Roblyer D, Richards-Kortum R, Sokolov K, El-Naggar AK, Williams MD, Kurachi C, et al. Multispectral optical imaging device for in vivo detection of oral neoplasia. J Biomed Opt [Internet]. [cited 2015 Jan 27];13(2):024019. http://www.pubmedcentral.nih.gov/articlerender.fcgi?artid=3970814&tool=pmcentrez&rendertype=abstract
23. Neumann H, Fuchs FS, Vieth M, Atreya R, Siebler J, Kiesslich R, et al. Review article: in vivo imaging by endocytoscopy. Aliment Pharmacol Ther [Internet]. 2011 [cited 2015 Jan 28];33(11):1183–93. http://www.ncbi.nlm.nih.gov/pubmed/21457290
24. Kumagai Y, Kawada K, Yamazaki S, Iida M, Momma K, Odajima H, et al. Endocytoscopic observation for esophageal squamous cell carcinoma: can biopsy histology be omitted? Dis Esophagus [Internet]. 2009 [cited 2015 Mar 4];22(6):505–12. http://www.ncbi.nlm.nih.gov/pubmed/19302209
25. Minami H, Inoue H, Yokoyama A, Ikeda H, Satodate H, Hamatani S, et al. Recent advancement of observing living cells in the esophagus using CM double staining: endocytoscopic atypia classification. Dis Esophagus [Internet]. 2012 [cited 2015 Jan 27];25(3):235–41. http://www.ncbi.nlm.nih.gov/pubmed/21895852
26. Tomizawa Y, Iyer PG, Wongkeesong LM, Buttar NS, Lutzke LS, Wu T-T, et al. Assessment of the diagnostic performance and interobserver variability of endocytoscopy in Barrett's esophagus: a pilot ex-vivo study. World J Gastroenterol [Internet]. 2013 [cited 2015 Jan 27];19(46):8652–8. http://www.pubmedcentral.nih.gov/articlerender.fcgi?artid=3870511&tool=pmcentrez&rendertype=abstract
27. Fortun PJ, Anagnostopoulos GK, Kaye P, James M, Foley S, Samuel S, et al. Acetic acid-enhanced magnification endoscopy in the diagnosis of specialized intestinal metaplasia, dysplasia and early cancer in Barrett's oesophagus. Aliment Pharmacol Ther [Internet]. 2006 [cited 2015 Jan 28];23(6):735–42. http://www.ncbi.nlm.nih.gov/pubmed/16556175
28. Longcroft-Wheaton G, Duku M, Mead R, Poller D, Bhandari P. Acetic acid spray is an effective tool for the endoscopic detection of neoplasia in patients with Barrett's esophagus. Clin Gastroenterol Hepatol [Internet]. 2010 [cited 2015 Jan 28];8(10):843–7. http://www.cghjournal.org/article/S1542356510006609/fulltext
29. Bhandari P, Kandaswamy P, Cowlishaw D, Longcroft-Wheaton G. Acetic acid enhanced chromoendoscopy is more cost-effective than protocol-guided biopsies in a high-risk Barrett's population. Dis Esophagus [Internet]. 2012 [cited 2015 Jan 28];25(5):386–92. http://www.ncbi.nlm.nih.gov/pubmed/21981061
30. Thekkek N, Maru DM, Polydorides AD, Bhutani MS, Anandasabapathy S, Richards-Kortum R. Pre-clinical evaluation of fluorescent deoxyglucose as a topical contrast agent for the detection of Barrett's-associated neoplasia during confocal imaging. Technol Cancer Res Treat [Internet]. 2011 [cited 2015 Jan 25];10(5):431–41. http://www.pubmedcentral.nih.gov/articlerender.fcgi?artid=3193280&tool=pmcentrez&rendertype=abstract

31. Sturm MB, Joshi BP, Lu S, Piraka C, Khondee S, Elmunzer BJ, et al. Targeted imaging of esophageal neoplasia with a fluorescently labeled peptide: first-in-human results. Sci Transl Med [Internet]. 2013 [cited 2015 Jan 8];5(184):184ra61. http://www.pubmedcentral.nih.gov/articlerender.fcgi?artid=3859345&tool=pmcentrez&rendertype=abstract
32. Choi KS, Suh M. Screening for gastric cancer: the usefulness of endoscopy. Clin Endosc [Internet]. 2014 [cited 2015 Jan 29];47(6):490–6. http://www.pubmedcentral.nih.gov/articlerender.fcgi?artid=4260095&tool=pmcentrez&rendertype=abstract
33. Guo Y-T, Li Y-Q, Yu T, Zhang T-G, Zhang J-N, Liu H, et al. Diagnosis of gastric intestinal metaplasia with confocal laser endomicroscopy in vivo: a prospective study. Endoscopy [Internet]. 2008 [cited 2015 Jan 25];40(7):547–53. http://www.ncbi.nlm.nih.gov/pubmed/18618938
34. Zhang J-N, Li Y-Q, Zhao Y-A, Yu T, Zhang J-P, Guo Y-T, et al. Classification of gastric pit patterns by confocal endomicroscopy. Gastrointest Endosc [Internet]. 2008 [cited 2015 Jan 25];67(6):843–53. http://www.ncbi.nlm.nih.gov/pubmed/18440377
35. Ji R, Li Y-Q, Gu X-M, Yu T, Zuo X-L, Zhou C-J. Confocal laser endomicroscopy for diagnosis of Helicobacter pylori infection: a prospective study. J Gastroenterol Hepatol [Internet]. 2010 [cited 2015 Jan 25];25(4):700–5. http://www.ncbi.nlm.nih.gov/pubmed/20492325
36. Wang P, Ji R, Yu T, Zuo X-L, Zhou C-J, Li C-Q, et al. Classification of histological severity of Helicobacter pylori-associated gastritis by confocal laser endomicroscopy. World J Gastroenterol [Internet]. 2010 [cited 2015 Jan 25];16(41):5203–10. http://www.pubmedcentral.nih.gov/articlerender.fcgi?artid=2975091&tool=pmcentrez&rendertype=abstract
37. Lim LG, Yeoh KG, Srivastava S, Chan YH, Teh M, Ho KY. Comparison of probe-based confocal endomicroscopy with virtual chromoendoscopy and white-light endoscopy for diagnosis of gastric intestinal metaplasia. Surg Endosc [Internet]. 2013 [cited 2015 Jan 25];27(12):4649–55. http://www.ncbi.nlm.nih.gov/pubmed/23892761
38. Li Z, Zuo X-L, Yu T, Gu X-M, Zhou C-J, Li C-Q, et al. Confocal laser endomicroscopy for in vivo detection of gastric intestinal metaplasia: a randomized controlled trial. Endoscopy [Internet]. 2014 [cited 2015 Jan 30];46(4):282–90. http://www.ncbi.nlm.nih.gov/pubmed/24473908
39. Li W-B, Zuo X-L, Zuo F, Gu X-M, Yu T, Zhao Y-A, et al. Characterization and identification of gastric hyperplastic polyps and adenomas by confocal laser endomicroscopy. Surg Endosc [Internet]. 2010 [cited 2015 Jan 25];24(3):517–24. http://www.ncbi.nlm.nih.gov/pubmed/19597774
40. Li W-B, Zuo X-L, Li C-Q, Zuo F, Gu X-M, Yu T, et al. Diagnostic value of confocal laser endomicroscopy for gastric superficial cancerous lesions. Gut [Internet]. 2011 [cited 2015 Jan 25];60(3):299–306. http://www.ncbi.nlm.nih.gov/pubmed/21193460
41. Jeon SR, Cho WY, Jin SY, Cheon YK, Choi SR, Cho JY. Optical biopsies by confocal endomicroscopy prevent additive endoscopic biopsies before endoscopic submucosal dissection in gastric epithelial neoplasias: a prospective, comparative study. Gastrointest Endosc [Internet]. 2011 [cited 2015 Jan 25];74(4):772–80. http://www.giejournal.org/article/S0016510711016646/fulltext
42. Sakai Y, Eto R, Kasanuki J, Kondo F, Kato K, Arai M, et al. Chromoendoscopy with indigo carmine dye added to acetic acid in the diagnosis of gastric neoplasia: a prospective comparative study. Gastrointest Endosc [Internet]. 2008 [cited 2015 Feb 5];68(4):635–41. http://www.ncbi.nlm.nih.gov/pubmed/18561923
43. Lee BE, Kim GH, Park DY, Kim DH, Jeon TY, Park SB, et al. Acetic acid-indigo carmine chromoendoscopy for delineating early gastric cancers: its usefulness according to histological type. BMC Gastroenterol [Internet]. 2010 [cited 2015 Feb 2];10(1):97. http://www.biomedcentral.com/1471-230X/10/97
44. Eberl T, Jechart G, Probst A, Golczyk M, Bittinger M, Scheubel R, et al. Can an endocytoscope system (ECS) predict histology in neoplastic lesions? Endoscopy [Internet]. 2007 [cited 2015 Jan 27];39(6):497–501. http://www.ncbi.nlm.nih.gov/pubmed/17554643
45. Recognition of goblet cells upon endocytoscopy indicates the presence of gastric intestinal metaplasia [Internet]. [cited 2015 Feb 2]. file:///Users/katalinbanki/Downloads/540ecdb40cf2d8daaacdccb1.pdf

46. Kaise M, Ohkura Y, Iizuka T, Kimura R, Nomura K, Kuribayashi Y, Yamada A, Yamashita S, Furuhata T, Kikuchi D, Ogawa O, Matsui A, Mitani T, Hoteya S. Endocytoscopy is a promising modality with high diagnostic accuracy for gastric cancer. Endoscopy [Internet]. 2015 [cited 2015 Jan 28];47:19–25. file:///Users/katalinbanki/Desktop/In Vivo Agents Chapter - Papers/endocyscopy gastric.pdf
47. Li Z, Zuo XL, Li CQ, Zhou CJ, Liu J, Goetz M, et al. In vivo molecular imaging of gastric cancer by targeting MG7 antigen with confocal laser endomicroscopy. Endoscopy [Internet]. 2013 [cited 2015 Jan 25];45(2):79–85. http://www.ncbi.nlm.nih.gov/pubmed/23364839
48. Van Rijn JC, Reitsma JB, Stoker J, Bossuyt PM, van Deventer SJ, Dekker E. Polyp miss rate determined by tandem colonoscopy: a systematic review. Am J Gastroenterol [Internet]. The American College of Gastroenterology; 2006 [cited 2015 Jan 25];101(2):343–50. http://dx.doi.org/10.1111/j.1572-0241.2006.00390.x
49. Tung SY, Wu CS, Su MY. Magnifying colonoscopy in differentiating neoplastic from nonneoplastic colorectal lesions. Am J Gastroenterol [Internet]. 2001 [cited 2015 Feb 8];96(9):2628–32. http://www.ncbi.nlm.nih.gov/pubmed/11569686
50. Hurlstone DP, Cross SS, Adam I, Shorthouse AJ, Brown S, Sanders DS, et al. Efficacy of high magnification chromoscopic colonoscopy for the diagnosis of neoplasia in flat and depressed lesions of the colorectum: a prospective analysis. Gut [Internet]. 2004 [cited 2015 Feb 8];53(2):284–90. http://www.pubmedcentral.nih.gov/articlerender.fcgi?artid=1774917&tool=pmcentrez&rendertype=abstract
51. Ichimasa K, Kudo S, Mori Y, Wakamura K, Ikehara N, Kutsukawa M, et al. Double staining with crystal violet and methylene blue is appropriate for colonic endocytoscopy: an in vivo prospective pilot study. Dig Endosc [Internet]. 2014 [cited 2015 Jan 27];26(3):403–8. http://www.pubmedcentral.nih.gov/articlerender.fcgi?artid=4232925&tool=pmcentrez&rendertype=abstract
52. Kudo S-E, Wakamura K, Ikehara N, Mori Y, Inoue H, Hamatani S. Diagnosis of colorectal lesions with a novel endocytoscopic classification—a pilot study. Endoscopy [Internet]. 2011 [cited 2015 Jan 27];43(10):869–75. http://www.ncbi.nlm.nih.gov/pubmed/21837586
53. Mori Y, Kudo S, Ikehara N, Wakamura K, Wada Y, Kutsukawa M, et al. Comprehensive diagnostic ability of endocytoscopy compared with biopsy for colorectal neoplasms: a prospective randomized noninferiority trial. Endoscopy [Internet]. 2013 [cited 2015 Feb 8];45(2):98–105. http://www.ncbi.nlm.nih.gov/pubmed/23307149
54. Kudo S, Mori Y, Wakamura K, Ikehara N, Ichimasa K, Wada Y, et al. Endocytoscopy can provide additional diagnostic ability to magnifying chromoendoscopy for colorectal neoplasms. J Gastroenterol Hepatol [Internet]. 2014 [cited 2015 Feb 8];29(1):83–90. http://www.ncbi.nlm.nih.gov/pubmed/23980563
55. Mori Y, Kudo S-E, Wakamura K, Misawa M, Ogawa Y, Kutsukawa M, et al. Novel computer-aided diagnostic system for colorectal lesions by using endocytoscopy (with videos). Gastrointest Endosc [Internet]. 2014 [cited 2015 Feb 8]. http://www.sciencedirect.com/science/article/pii/S0016510714021713
56. Kiesslich R, Burg J, Vieth M, Gnaendiger J, Enders M, Delaney P, et al. Confocal laser endoscopy for diagnosing intraepithelial neoplasias and colorectal cancer in vivo. Gastroenterology [Internet]. 2004 [cited 2015 Jan 25];127(3):706–13. http://www.ncbi.nlm.nih.gov/pubmed/15362025
57. Sanduleanu S, Driessen A, Gomez-Garcia E, Hameeteman W, de Bruïne A, Masclee A. In vivo diagnosis and classification of colorectal neoplasia by chromoendoscopy-guided confocal laser endomicroscopy. Clin Gastroenterol Hepatol [Internet]. 2010 [cited 2015 Jan 25];8(4):371–8. http://www.cghjournal.org/article/S1542356509007630/fulltext
58. Shahid MW, Buchner AM, Coron E, Woodward TA, Raimondo M, Dekker E, et al. Diagnostic accuracy of probe-based confocal laser endomicroscopy in detecting residual colorectal neoplasia after EMR: a prospective study. Gastrointest Endosc [Internet]. 2012 [cited 2015 Jan 25];75(3):525–33. http://www.ncbi.nlm.nih.gov/pubmed/22051243

59. Wang TD, Friedland S, Sahbaie P, Soetikno R, Hsiung P-L, Liu JTC, et al. Functional imaging of colonic mucosa with a fibered confocal microscope for real-time in vivo pathology. Clin Gastroenterol Hepatol [Internet]. 2007 [cited 2015 Jan 25];5(11):1300–5. http://www.pubmedcentral.nih.gov/articlerender.fcgi?artid=2104519&tool=pmcentrez&rendertype=abstract
60. Hsiung P-L, Wang T. In vivo biomarkers for targeting colorectal neoplasms. Cancer Biomark [Internet]. 2008 [cited 2015 Jan 25];4(6):329–40. http://www.pubmedcentral.nih.gov/articlerender.fcgi?artid=3232019&tool=pmcentrez&rendertype=abstract
61. Liu Z, Miller SJ, Joshi BP, Wang TD. In vivo targeting of colonic dysplasia on fluorescence endoscopy with near-infrared octapeptide. Gut [Internet]. 2013 [cited 2015 Jan 14];62(3):395–403. http://www.pubmedcentral.nih.gov/articlerender.fcgi?artid=3563943&tool=pmcentrez&rendertype=abstract
62. Qiu Z, Liu Z, Duan X, Khondee S, Joshi B, Mandella MJ, et al. Targeted vertical cross-sectional imaging with handheld near-infrared dual axes confocal fluorescence endomicroscope. Biomed Opt Express [Internet]. 2013 [cited 2015 Feb 13];4(2):322–30. http://www.pubmedcentral.nih.gov/articlerender.fcgi?artid=3567718&tool=pmcentrez&rendertype=abstract
63. Hsiung P-L, Hsiung P-L, Hardy J, Friedland S, Soetikno R, Du CB, et al. Detection of colonic dysplasia in vivo using a targeted heptapeptide and confocal microendoscopy. Nat Med [Internet]. 2008 [cited 2015 Jan 15];14(4):454–8. http://www.pubmedcentral.nih.gov/articlerender.fcgi?artid=3324975&tool=pmcentrez&rendertype=abstract
64. Foersch S, Kiesslich R, Waldner MJ, Delaney P, Galle PR, Neurath MF, et al. Molecular imaging of VEGF in gastrointestinal cancer in vivo using confocal laser endomicroscopy. Gut [Internet]. 2010 [cited 2015 Feb 14];59(8):1046–55. http://www.ncbi.nlm.nih.gov/pubmed/20639250
65. Goetz M, Ziebart A, Foersch S, Vieth M, Waldner MJ, Delaney P, et al. In vivo molecular imaging of colorectal cancer with confocal endomicroscopy by targeting epidermal growth factor receptor. Gastroenterology [Internet]. 2010 [cited 2015 Jan 25];138(2):435–46. http://www.ncbi.nlm.nih.gov/pubmed/19852961
66. Parikh ND, Perl D, Lee MH, Shah B, Young Y, Chang SS, et al. In vivo diagnostic accuracy of high-resolution microendoscopy in differentiating neoplastic from non-neoplastic colorectal polyps: a prospective study. Am J Gastroenterol [Internet]. 2014 [cited 2015 Jan 25];109(1):68–75. http://www.pubmedcentral.nih.gov/articlerender.fcgi?artid=3947255&tool=pmcentrez&rendertype=abstract
67. Chang SS, Shukla R, Polydorides AD, Vila PM, Lee M, Han H, et al. High resolution microendoscopy for classification of colorectal polyps. Endoscopy [Internet]. 2013 [cited 2015 Feb 14];45(7):553–9. http://www.ncbi.nlm.nih.gov/pubmed/23780842
68. Kessler WR, Imperiale TF, Klein RW, Wielage RC, Rex DK. A quantitative assessment of the risks and cost savings of forgoing histologic examination of diminutive polyps. Endoscopy [Internet]. 2011 [cited 2015 Feb 10];43(8):683–91. http://www.ncbi.nlm.nih.gov/pubmed/21623556
69. Neumann H, Günther C, Vieth M, Grauer M, Wittkopf N, Mudter J, et al. Confocal laser endomicroscopy for in vivo diagnosis of Clostridium difficile associated colitis—a pilot study. PLoS One [Internet]. 2013 [cited 2015 Feb 11];8(3):e58753. http://www.pubmedcentral.nih.gov/articlerender.fcgi?artid=3602426&tool=pmcentrez&rendertype=abstract
70. Desai D, Desai N. Colorectal cancer surveillance in inflammatory bowel disease: a critical analysis. World J Gastrointest Endosc [Internet]. 2014 [cited 2015 Jan 25];6(11):541–8. http://www.pubmedcentral.nih.gov/articlerender.fcgi?artid=4231493&tool=pmcentrez&rendertype=abstract
71. Subramanian V, Mannath J, Ragunath K, Hawkey CJ. Meta-analysis: the diagnostic yield of chromoendoscopy for detecting dysplasia in patients with colonic inflammatory bowel disease. Aliment Pharmacol Ther [Internet]. 2011 [cited 2015 Jan 25];33(3):304–12. http://www.ncbi.nlm.nih.gov/pubmed/21128987

72. De Palma GD, Rispo A. Confocal laser endomicroscopy in inflammatory bowel diseases: dream or reality? World J Gastroenterol [Internet]. 2013 [cited 2015 Jan 25];19(34):5593–7. http://www.pubmedcentral.nih.gov/articlerender.fcgi?artid=3769894&tool=pmcentrez&rendertype=abstract
73. Liu J, Dlugosz A, Neumann H. Beyond white light endoscopy: the role of optical biopsy in inflammatory bowel disease. World J Gastroenterol [Internet]. 2013 [cited 2015 Jan 25];19(43):7544–51. http://www.pubmedcentral.nih.gov/articlerender.fcgi?artid=3837252&tool=pmcentrez&rendertype=abstract
74. Li C-Q, Xie X-J, Yu T, Gu X-M, Zuo X-L, Zhou C-J, et al. Classification of inflammation activity in ulcerative colitis by confocal laser endomicroscopy. Am J Gastroenterol [Internet]. 2010 [cited 2015 Jan 25];105(6):1391–6. http://www.ncbi.nlm.nih.gov/pubmed/19935787
75. Neumann H, Vieth M, Atreya R, Grauer M, Siebler J, Bernatik T, et al. Assessment of Crohn's disease activity by confocal laser endomicroscopy. Inflamm Bowel Dis [Internet]. 2012 [cited 2015 Jan 25];18(12):2261–9. http://www.ncbi.nlm.nih.gov/pubmed/22344873
76. Atreya R, Neumann H, Neufert C, Waldner MJ, Billmeier U, Zopf Y, et al. In vivo imaging using fluorescent antibodies to tumor necrosis factor predicts therapeutic response in Crohn's disease. Nat Med [Internet]. 2014 [cited 2014 Nov 20];20(3):313–8. http://dx.doi.org/10.1038/nm.3462
77. Bessho R, Kanai T, Hosoe N, Kobayashi T, Takayama T, Inoue N, et al. Correlation between endocytoscopy and conventional histopathology in microstructural features of ulcerative colitis. J Gastroenterol [Internet]. 2011 [cited 2015 Feb 11];46(10):1197–202. http://www.ncbi.nlm.nih.gov/pubmed/21805068
78. Neumann H, Vieth M, Neurath MF, Atreya R. Endocytoscopy allows accurate in vivo differentiation of mucosal inflammatory cells in IBD: a pilot study. Inflamm Bowel Dis [Internet]. 2013 [cited 2015 Jan 25];19(2):356–62. http://www.ncbi.nlm.nih.gov/pubmed/22644957

Chapter 10
Spectroscopy

Tian Gao and Hemant K. Roy

Technology Overview

One of the major advances in gastrointestinal endoscopy is the use of biomedical optics to enhance mucosal examination by traditional white light endoscopy. Until recently, biopsy for histologic examination has been the primary modality to examine tissue on a microscopic level. Numerous imaging enhancing technologies have been developed to provide additional information about targeted tissue of interest. These advances include modifications directly to the endoscope, including high definition and narrow band imaging, fiberoptic probes that provide microscope like images, including optical coherence tomography, confocal endomicroscopy, as well as various spectroscopic approaches that provide microarchitectural quantification. These enhanced imaging techniques offer an additional advantage over conventional biopsies in that they all produce real-time characterization of target tissue.

Spectroscopy characterizes objects based on how they interact with light. The incident light directed toward targeted tissue can be scattered in different patterns. Light scattering can be elastic, where there is no change energy and thus wavelength with scattering represents the dominant process of light transport in tissue. Many elastic scattering spectroscopy systems use white light as the incident light. Interpretation of the scattered light typically utilizes harnessed light scattered in the backward direction, towards the incident light and encompasses a wide range of wavelengths, as light may be shifted to another wavelength. Elastic scattering is driven by spatial variations of tissue refractive index, which is determined by local macromolecular density and thus provides fundamental insights into the size

T. Gao, M.D. (✉) • H.K. Roy, M.D.
Boston University Medical Center, 85 E Concord Avenue, Boston, MA 02118, USA
e-mail: Tian.gao@bmc.org

V.J.A. Konda, I. Waxman (eds.), *Endoscopic Imaging Techniques and Tools*,
DOI 10.1007/978-3-319-30053-5_10

distribution of these tissue structures (e.g., organelles, chromatin structures, enlarged nuclei, and so forth). These characterizations provide essential insights into the histopathology as normal tissue scatters light differently than neoplastic tissue. Additionally, depending on the technique, length scales from a few tens of nanometers to as large as a few micrometers can be assessed. In addition, light absorption spectra can also be used to measure tissue blood concentration, oxygen saturation, and size of blood vessels as absorption which occurs as light propagates through the tissue is mainly due to hemoglobin. One example is low-coherence-enhanced backscattering spectroscopy, which allows for depth selective interrogation of superficial mucosa [1]. This technology has been utilized to detect field changes in the rectum for detection ranging from advanced adenomas and colorectal cancer, to sampling the duodenal mucosa for pancreatic cancer, as well as buccal mucosa for lung cancer detection [2–4]. Additional examples of elastic spectroscopy technology include polarized gated spectroscopy, partial wave spectroscopy, angle-resolved low coherence interferotomy, diffuse reflectance spectroscopy, and polarized scanning spectroscopy system [5].

Light scattering can also be inelastic where the incident light undergoes wavelength shifts as a result of either gain or loss of energy from the incident excitation photons, a phenomenon referred to as the Raman effect [6]. The changes in reflected wavelengths are caused by different vibrational and rotational frequencies of molecules. Raman spectroscopy has wide applications in science and biomedicine where it has applications including revelation of molecular structures of chemicals, to identification of pathological cell states, and more recently integrated into a probe-based system utilized for targeted early detection of dysplasia in Barrett's esophagus [7].

Fluorescence spectroscopy is based on the principle that when light of an appropriate wavelength hits a molecule (fluorophore), it may reach an excited electronic state causing fluorescence to occur. As the molecule relaxes back to its ground state, the molecule emits light of lower energy and thus longer wavelength than incident light, which generates an optical signature directly related to the wavelength and intensity of the emitted fluorescence. Fluorescence spectroscopy has been utilized to differentiate dysplastic tissue from non-dysplastic tissue as normal esophageal tissue, Barrett's metaplasia, and dysplasia have been demonstrated to have different optical signals [8, 9].

Key Clinical Indications

Colon Cancer Screening

Screening for colorectal cancer (CRC) is one of the most commonly recommended screening tests in the United States since first recommended in 1997 [10]. Colonoscopy with polypectomy is associated with a 53 % reduction in mortality from CRC [11]. However, colon cancer remains the third most common cancer diagnosed in both men and women with incidence of roughly 93,000 new cases of colon cancer each year and 40,000 cases of rectal cancer each year. The mortality rate has been declining over the past 20 years likely due to increased screening efforts as well as improvement in treatment for CRC. Despite these modest improvements, there is still considerable work remaining to improve outcomes.

One area where spectroscopy has been shown to be promising is risk stratification through field carcinogenesis detection. Field carcinogenesis (also known as field effect, field change, field defect) is the biological concept that the genetic/environmental milieu that results in a permissive environment for a focal cancer to develop is diffuse and pervasive throughout an organ and nearby associated tissue. These changes in tissue ultrastructure encompass all structures smaller than the diffraction limit of conventional light microscopy (smaller than 200 nm). The ultimate tumor location is determined likely by a combination stochastic events including genomic, proteomic, cellular, and epigenetic disruptions, which in essence is the rationale for surveillance colonoscopy as the risk of recurrent adenoma can occur anywhere in the colon. An advantage of spectroscopy then gives possibility to harness understanding of the entire organ through less invasive means of sampling readily accessible surrogate measurement locations. Although such changes are heterogeneous, they may share common downstream microarchitectural aberrations that can be detected via spectroscopy. Current efforts in spectroscopy utilize this advantage in that these technologies can risk stratify patients who harbor advanced adenomas or carcinomas based on analysis of "normal" tissue away from the primary site.

Current limitations of colonoscopy include inconsistent protection against CRC incidence and death occurring within the proximal colon [12–14]. Perhaps the most significant factor is the operator dependence of colonoscopy, since adenoma detection rates vary widely among even well-trained endoscopists, from 2.5 to 8 fold which likely mirrors the variation in cancer protection [15, 16]. Furthermore, patient factors such as tumor biology, quality of bowel preparation, as well as environmental factors (such as diet and smoking) can all influence CRC protection after colonoscopy. Other challenges include patient discomfort, procedure complications, as well as cost and endoscopic capacity to accommodate the entire average-risk population (~100 million Americans older than 50 years). This is juxtaposed with the low prevalence of advanced neoplasia on screening colonoscopy (~5 %), resulting in more than 90 % of colonoscopies being unproductive from a cancer prevention perspective. Methods of non-endoscopy-based CRC screening including stool-based tests as well as virtual colonoscopy have also been implemented, but they suffer from poor diagnostic performance or difficulty being applied in the clinic.

Fecal occult blood testing is well-tolerated, but has poor sensitivity for clinically significant lesions (~10 % for advanced adenomas and ~33 % for CRC) [17]. Other stool-based tests include fecal immunochemical test (FIT) and multitarget stool DNA test. Sensitivity for detecting colorectal cancer is ~90 % for DNA testing and ~70 % for FIT, decreasing to ~40 % with DNA testing and ~25 % for FIT for advanced precancerous lesions [18]. Virtual colonoscopy has been approved for average risk screening with 90 % sensitivity and 85 % specificity for adenomas ≥10 mm and cancers, but carries with it an inconvenience of colon purge as well as risk of radiation exposure [19].

Low Coherence Enhanced Backscattering Spectroscopy

Low coherence enhanced backscattering spectroscopy (LEBS) introduces a major advance for this application by providing quantitative insights into the mucosal microarchitecture. A proof-of-concept study for colonic risk stratification analyzed biopsies from endoscopically normal-appearing rectal mucosa of 219 patients undergoing either screening or surveillance colonoscopy. LEBS signals were recorded through a bench-top instrument. Rectal LEBS marker was able to discriminate between patients who harbored no neoplasia vs those with advanced adenomas (size, >10 mm; >25 % villous features; or high-grade dysplasia) with 100 % sensitivity and 80 % specificity (AUROC, 0.89) [20]. A subsequent in situ validation trial used a fiberoptic LEBS probe to take five rectal readings (each reading requiring 250 ms) immediately prior to screening/surveillance colonoscopy. Within this cohort of 414 patients, the sensitivity for advanced adenoma was 92 % and specificity was 74 % (AUROC 0.87) [21]. A small pilot study of the LEBS marker in patients with unprepped colons showed similar progressive increase in the LEBS marker for patients with increasing levels of dysplasia. Compared to healthy controls, the LEBS marker was significantly increased ($P=0.04$) [2].

Early Increase in Blood Supply

The development of a polarization-gated fiber-optic probe has allowed for in vivo measurement of rectal microvascular content. Rectal microvascular blood content is elevated in the presence of neoplastic lesions anywhere in the colon such that an early increase in blood supply (EIBS) has also been demonstrated to be a powerful marker of field carcinogenesis. Similar to the LEBS system, EIBS readings were taken from normal appearing rectal mucosa during time of colonoscopy. In a study of 216 patients undergoing screening colonoscopy, microvascular blood content was increased by approximately 50 % of the endoscopically normal rectal mucosa of patients with advanced adenomas. Logistic regression using mucosal oxyhemoglobin concentration and patient age resulted in a sensitivity of 83 %, a specificity of 82 %, and an AUROC of 0.88 for the detection of advanced adenomas [22].

Partial Wave Spectroscopic Microscopy

Similarly, results from partial wave spectroscopic microscopy (PWS) have been shown to correlate with risk of developing colorectal cancer, again utilizing the concept of field carcinogenesis to identify high-risk patients [23]. In this case, nanocytology performed on rectal biopsies via PWS, which is sensitive to nanoscale cellular architecture, demonstrated an AUROC 0.85. The findings in LEBS, EIBS, and PWS parameters were not confounded by site of adenomas, presence of non-neoplastic lesions, demographics, medications, bowel preparation, time of procedure, nor removal of adenoma, suggesting that these technologies all have further potential to be developed into a screening and risk stratification tool for CRC.

Esophagus

Current screening recommendations are ineffective in capturing all patients who are at risk of developing Barrett's esophagus. Estimates of prevalence of Barrett's esophagus have ranged from 0.4 to more than 20 %, depending on the population and definitions used. Furthermore, the rate of progression from non-dysplastic Barrett's esophagus to esophageal adenocarcinoma is quite low, at a rate of 0.12–0.5 % per year. Endoscopic surveillance methods have not been proven to be cost-effective accurate as current recommendations include random biopsies every 2 cm performed every 3–5 years. This approach generates a vast number of negative biopsies and remains clinically labor-intensive and time-consuming. As such, the limitations of this method are associated with sampling of tissue less than 5 % in an area of potential interest [24] as well as considerable variations in techniques and biopsy intervals when applied in practice by endoscopists [25]. Furthermore, histological diagnosis can be extremely subjective with possibly poor level of inter-observer agreement even among expert histopatholgists to distinguish low-grade dysplasia from high-grade dysplasia [26]. In addition, 10–50 % of cancers were missed using this technique when biopsies were taken from patients with high-grade dysplasia [27–29]. Thus, additional diagnostic tests, especially those that can provide real-time data regarding tissue which may harbor pre-cancerous change, are needed.

A study utilizing elastic scattering spectroscopy measured spectra from 181 matched biopsy sites from 81 patients with consensus histopathology. ESS detected high-grade dysplasia with a sensitivity of 92 % and a specificity of 60 % and was able to differentiate these sites from inflammation with a sensitivity and specificity of 79 %. The number of low-risk biopsies was decreased by 60 % when ESS was used to target biopsy during endoscopy. Furthermore, a negative spectroscopy result excluded high-grade dysplasia or cancer with an accuracy >99.5 % [30].

Pancreas

Pancreatic cancer (PC) is the fourth leading cause of US cancer deaths and carries the highest mortality rate of all major cancers with an overall 5-year survival of approximately 6 % over the past decade [31]. A major reason for this grim prognosis is due in a large part to the advanced stage of disease at time of diagnosis as there is no current available screening technique available for PC. Currently used imaging modalities such as computed tomography (CT), positron emission tomography (PET), and magnetic resonance imaging can only detect larger and more advanced lesions. In addition, CT and PEt also pose risk of ionizing radiation to the patient, making it an undesirable screening technique. Endoscopic techniques such as endoscopic ultrasound is limited by ability to detect lesions smaller than a few millimeters in size and endoscopic retrograde cholangiopancreatography is too invasive and risky from a complication perspective to allow for population-wide implementation. As mucosal biopsies are standard practice for colon cancer surveillance in patients with inflammatory bowel disease and esophageal biopsies performed in patients with Barrett's esophagus for esophageal cancer surveillance, assessment of duodenal mucosa adjacent to the ampulla presents as an attractive screening target given its accessibility.

An ex vivo study of 203 patients using LEBS on biopsy samples from periampullary duodenal mucosa demonstrated a 95 % sensitivity, 71 % specificity, and 85 % AUROC and performance was uncompromised for detecting potentially curable stages of disease. Additionally, optical markers in higher risk populations such as family history and history of pancreatitis had values between those of healthy control and cancer patients, thus allowing for future investigations of screening from these high-risk groups [32]. An in vivo study of 203 patients demonstrated significant changes in LEBS markers between control patients and those with adenocarcinoma but not between control and patients with mucinous cysts, thus demonstrating a step-wise progression in LEBS markers from normal to malignancy.

Identification of Polyps

Polypectomy during colonoscopy incurs time, cost, and risk of bleeding and perforation. The need for polyp histological examination contributes substantially to medical and economic resources, especially since one in every two patients undergoing screening or diagnostic colonoscopy is diagnosed with at least one polyp [33, 34]. Additionally, the majority of these polyps are diminutive ($\leq$5 mm) with very low prevalence of advanced neoplasia, thus making the argument for further costly histopathological examination almost negligible for providing further clinical impact [33, 34] leading to a proposed predict-resect-and-discard approach or diagnose and leave behind strategy especially for these types of polyps. A myriad of technologies including chromo-endoscopy, autofluorescence, electronic chromoendoscopy such as narrow band imaging (NBI), and confocal endomicroscopy and spectroscopy techniques are currently being evaluated for "optical biopsy" with the main goal of differentiating between hyperplastic vs. neoplastic polyps as well as noninvasive and invasive neoplastic lesions.

Standard white light endoscopy fails to accurately predict in vivo the histological diagnosis with a wide range of sensitivity between 60 and 90 % with specificity between 40 and 90 % without much improvement with introduction of high-definition endoscopy [35–37]. There is a similar trend of sensitivity and specificity with the use of NBI [38, 39].

Elastic scattering spectroscopy appears promising in distinguishing polyp histology between hyperplastic vs. adenomatous tissue. In one series of 218 polyps from 83 patients, spectral data were correlated with classification of biopsy samples by 3 GI pathologists. The diagnostic performance of ESS resulted in a sensitivity of 92 %, specificity of 92 %, and accuracy of 92 %. These numbers were reduced slightly with polyps smaller than 1 cm ($n = 179$), with a sensitivity of 87 %, specificity of 92 %, and accuracy of 91 %. When analysis was limited to polyps 5 mm or smaller ($n = 157$), sensitivity remained similar at 87 %, specificity 91 %, and accuracy of 90 % [40].

Techniques

Each spectroscopy instrument system will vary in set up and location of intended use will dictate technique as well. The instrumentation generally consists of a light source, a probe, and processor to record and process data. As an example, the LEBS probe consists of four optical fibers arranged in a linear array (shown in Fig. 10.1). One of these fibers carries the incident white light for illumination onto the tissue surface and the remaining three fibers acquire LEBS signal intensities at three backscattering angles: –0.6°, 0.6°, and 1.12°. A 9 mm glass rod spacer is placed between the optical fibers and tissue surface to control the spatial coherence length of the illumination. Each collection fiber is connected to a spectrometer, which collects the backscattered light as a function of wavelength, from 500 to 700 nm. The fibers are bundled into a probe that is 3.4 mm in diameter, allowing it to be inserted into the accessory channel of commercially available endoscopes. Patient measurements are then managed through a point-of-care optical system with custom data acquisition software and instrumentation [3].

Assessment

Safety and Cost Considerations

In studies to date, spectroscopy techniques have had a favorable safety profile. There is potential to induce thermal injury from exposure to the incident light, although the energy involved is quite modest. Compared to endomicroscopic techniques such as confocal microscopy and optical coherence tomography,

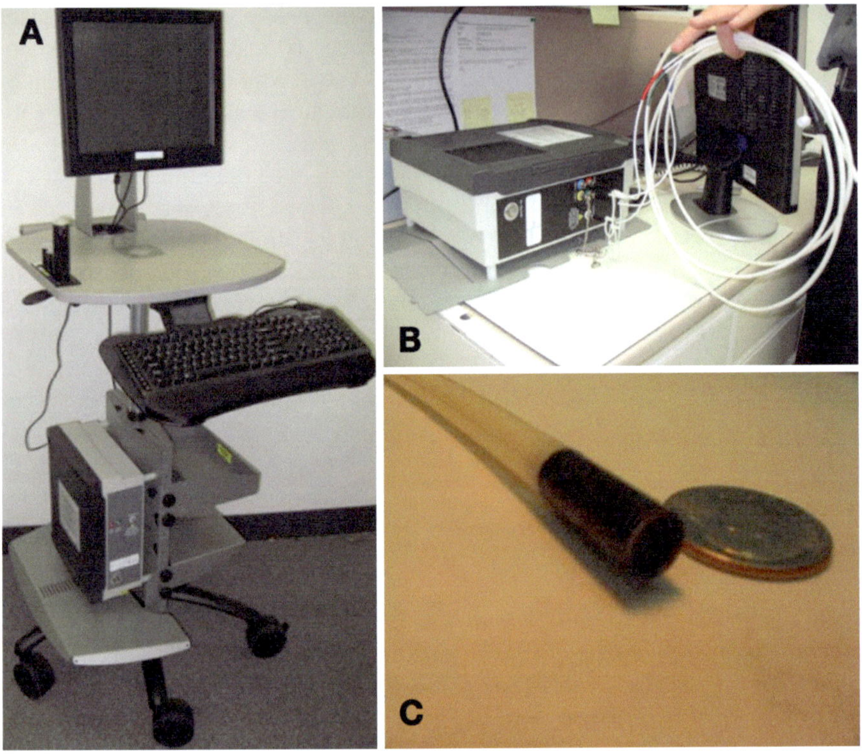

Fig. 10.1 (**a**) Spectroscopy processor, monitor, and keyboard of polarization gating spectroscopy unit. (**b**, **c**) Fiberoptic probe of polarization gating spectroscopy measurement unit

spectroscopy is potentially more cost-effective and more accessible. There is also no need for any IV medications such as the IV fluorescent dye required for confocal endomicroscopy, which may trigger an allergic response. A true cost-benefit analysis cannot be done using the present data, but need to be further addressed in larger trials where equipment costs are weighed against the costs of endoscopy and histopathology. The biggest attraction of these technologies is the potential to reduce the number of "random" biopsies, such as those taken for surveillance in Barrett's esophagus and potentially even surveillance for colonic dysplasia in inflammatory bowel disease. The goal for integrating these optic techniques would be aimed at increasing targeted biopsies to optimize detection yield, which in return would decrease the overall cost of dysplasia surveillance. However, many of the technologies described above are still in early phases of research and development and may take years before any may be widely available and utilized by the general GI community.

Conclusion and Future Directions

Ongoing research is currently being conducted to improve the current described spectroscopic devices. The goal of spectroscopy is to provide real-time optical biopsy at the time of endoscopy so that lesions can be identified and targeted for high-risk tissue targets (i.e., high-grade dysplasia) with noninvasive or minimally invasive techniques, which greatly reduce random biopsy sampling errors as well as decrease healthcare expenses. Another advantage is that these techniques require no further endoscopic training. Further work is needed for all spectroscopy to optimize diagnostic accuracy to approach 100 % in vivo, particularly for high-grade dysplasia or early cancer. Much work still needs to be done prior to routine clinical practice including large scale clinical trials to demonstrate multi-center, multi-operator, and cross-system reliability as well as ensuring reproducibility and transferability of data across platforms. Future directions could aim to combine any of these technologies with other endoscopic imaging technologies for functional imaging at the tissue, cellular, molecular, and organ levels with an ultimate goal of improving early diagnosis of dysplastic lesions, cancers, identifying flat dysplasia while improving cost and efficiency.

Helpful Hints

- Spectroscopy may be utilized to aid in resect and discard approach or diagnose and leave behind strategy.
- Spectroscopy can help better target biopsies.
- Spectroscopy can be utilized for long-term risk stratification and thus targeting screening.

Disclosure Dr. Roy is a co-founder of Nanocytomics LLC and American BioOptics LLC.

References

1. Radosevich AJ, Turzhitsky VM, Mutyal NN, Rogers JD, Stoyneva V, Tiwari AK, et al. Depth-resolved measurement of mucosal microvascular blood content using low-coherence enhanced backscattering spectroscopy. Biomed Opt Express. 2010;1(4):1196–208.
2. Radosevich AJ, Mutyal NN, Eshein A, Nguyen TQ, Gould B, Rogers JD, et al. Rectal optical markers for in-vivo risk stratification of premalignant colorectal lesions. Clin Cancer Res. 2015;21(19):4347–55.
3. Mutyal NN, Radosevich AJ, Bajaj S, Konda V, Siddiqui UD, Waxman I, et al. In vivo risk analysis of pancreatic cancer through optical characterization of duodenal mucosa. Pancreas. 2015;44(5):735–41.
4. Radosevich AJ, Mutyal NN, Rogers JD, Gould B, Hensing TA, Ray D, et al. Buccal spectral markers for lung cancer risk stratification. PLoS One. 2014;9(10):e110157.

5. Committee AT. Enhanced imaging in the GI tract: spectroscopy and optical coherence tomography. Gastrointest Endosc. 2013;78(4):568–73.
6. Nima ZA, Biswas A, Bayer IS, Hardcastle FD, Perry D, Ghosh A, et al. Applications of surface-enhanced Raman scattering in advanced bio-medical technologies and diagnostics. Drug Metab Rev. 2014;46(2):155–75.
7. Almond LM, Hutchings J, Lloyd G, Barr H, Shepherd N, Day J, et al. Endoscopic Raman spectroscopy enables objective diagnosis of dysplasia in Barrett's esophagus. Gastrointest Endosc. 2014;79(1):37–45.
8. Kara MA, DaCosta RS, Streutker CJ, Marcon NE, Bergman JJ, Wilson BC. Characterization of tissue autofluorescence in Barrett's esophagus by confocal fluorescence microscopy. Dis Esophagus. 2007;20(2):141–50.
9. Bourg-Heckly G, Blais J, Padilla JJ, Bourdon O, Etienne J, Guillemin F, et al. Endoscopic ultraviolet-induced autofluorescence spectroscopy of the esophagus: tissue characterization and potential for early cancer diagnosis. Endoscopy. 2000;32(10):756–65.
10. Winawer SJ, Fletcher RH, Miller L, Godlee F, Stolar MH, Mulrow CD, et al. Colorectal cancer screening: clinical guidelines and rationale. Gastroenterology. 1997;112(2):594–642.
11. Zauber AG, Winawer SJ, O'Brien MJ, Lansdorp-Vogelaar I, van Ballegooijen M, Hankey BF, et al. Colonoscopic polypectomy and long-term prevention of colorectal-cancer deaths. N Engl J Med. 2012;366(8):687–96.
12. Baxter NN, Warren JL, Barrett MJ, Stukel TA, Doria-Rose VP. Association between colonoscopy and colorectal cancer mortality in a US cohort according to site of cancer and colonoscopist specialty. J Clin Oncol. 2012;30(21):2664–9.
13. Singh H, Nugent Z, Demers AA, Kliewer EV, Mahmud SM, Bernstein CN. The reduction in colorectal cancer mortality after colonoscopy varies by site of the cancer. Gastroenterology. 2010;139(4):1128–37.
14. Brenner H, Chang-Claude J, Jansen L, Knebel P, Stock C, Hoffmeister M. Reduced risk of colorectal cancer up to 10 years after screening, surveillance, or diagnostic colonoscopy. Gastroenterology. 2014;146(3):709–17.
15. Imperiale TF, Glowinski EA, Juliar BE, Azzouz F, Ransohoff DF. Variation in polyp detection rates at screening colonoscopy. Gastrointest Endosc. 2009;69(7):1288–95.
16. Shaukat A, Oancea C, Bond JH, Church TR, Allen JI. Variation in detection of adenomas and polyps by colonoscopy and change over time with a performance improvement program. Clin Gastroenterol Hepatol. 2009;7(12):1335–40.
17. Imperiale TF, Ransohoff DF, Itzkowitz SH, Turnbull BA, Ross ME. Fecal DNA versus fecal occult blood for colorectal-cancer screening in an average-risk population. N Engl J Med. 2004;351(26):2704–14.
18. Imperiale TF, Ransohoff DF, Itzkowitz SH, Levin TR, Lavin P, Lidgard GP, et al. Multitarget stool DNA testing for colorectal-cancer screening. N Engl J Med. 2014;370(14):1287–97.
19. Johnson CD, Chen MH, Toledano AY, Heiken JP, Dachman A, Kuo MD, et al. Accuracy of CT colonography for detection of large adenomas and cancers. N Engl J Med. 2008;359(12):1207–17.
20. Roy HK, Turzhitsky V, Kim Y, Goldberg MJ, Watson P, Rogers JD, et al. Association between rectal optical signatures and colonic neoplasia: potential applications for screening. Cancer Res. 2009;69(10):4476–83.
21. Roy HK, Mutyal NN, Goldberg MJ, Du H, Radosevich A, Bianchi LK, et al. 545 In situ rectal spectral markers for colonic neoplasia risk stratification—a blinded validation study. Gastroenterology. 2012;142(5):S-109.
22. Gomes AJ, Roy HK, Turzhitsky V, Kim Y, Rogers JD, Ruderman S, et al. Rectal mucosal microvascular blood supply increase is associated with colonic neoplasia. Clin Cancer Res. 2009;15(9):3110–7.
23. Damania D, Roy HK, Subramanian H, Weinberg DS, Rex DK, Goldberg MJ, et al. Nanocytology of rectal colonocytes to assess risk of colon cancer based on field cancerization. Cancer Res. 2012;72(11):2720–7.

24. Isenberg G, Chak A. Should there be light in the esophageal tunnel? An appraisal of optical coherence tomography in Barrett's esophagus. Gastrointest Endosc. 2007;65(1):57–9.
25. Singh M, Gupta N, Gaddam S, Balasubramanian G, Wani S, Sinh P, et al. Practice patterns among U.S. gastroenterologists regarding endoscopic management of Barrett's esophagus. Gastrointest Endosc. 2013;78(5):689–95.
26. Kerkhof M, van Dekken H, Steyerberg EW, Meijer GA, Mulder AH, de Bruine A, et al. Grading of dysplasia in Barrett's oesophagus: substantial interobserver variation between general and gastrointestinal pathologists. Histopathology. 2007;50(7):920–7.
27. Falk GW, Rice TW, Goldblum JR, Richter JE. Jumbo biopsy forceps protocol still misses unsuspected cancer in Barrett's esophagus with high-grade dysplasia. Gastrointest Endosc. 1999;49(2):170–6.
28. Cameron AJ, Carpenter HA. Barrett's esophagus, high-grade dysplasia, and early adenocarcinoma: a pathological study. Am J Gastroenterol. 1997;92(4):586–91.
29. Reid BJ, Blount PL, Feng Z, Levine DS. Optimizing endoscopic biopsy detection of early cancers in Barrett's high-grade dysplasia. Am J Gastroenterol. 2000;95(11):3089–96.
30. Lovat LB, Johnson K, Mackenzie GD, Clark BR, Novelli MR, Davies S, et al. Elastic scattering spectroscopy accurately detects high grade dysplasia and cancer in Barrett's oesophagus. Gut. 2006;55(8):1078–83.
31. Siegel R, Ma J, Zou Z, Jemal A. Cancer statistics, 2014. CA Cancer J Clin. 2014;64(1):9–29.
32. Turzhitsky V, Liu Y, Hasabou N, Goldberg M, Roy HK, Backman V, et al. Investigating population risk factors of pancreatic cancer by evaluation of optical markers in the duodenal mucosa. Dis Markers. 2008;25(6):313–21.
33. Gupta N, Bansal A, Rao D, Early DS, Jonnalagadda S, Wani SB, et al. Prevalence of advanced histological features in diminutive and small colon polyps. Gastrointest Endosc. 2012;75(5):1022–30.
34. Hassan C, Pickhardt PJ, Kim DH, Di Giulio E, Zullo A, Laghi A, et al. Systematic review: distribution of advanced neoplasia according to polyp size at screening colonoscopy. Aliment Pharmacol Ther. 2010;31(2):210–7.
35. Longcroft-Wheaton G, Brown J, Cowlishaw D, Higgins B, Bhandari P. High-definition vs. standard-definition colonoscopy in the characterization of small colonic polyps: results from a randomized trial. Endoscopy. 2012;44(10):905–10.
36. Chiu HM, Chang CY, Chen CC, Lee YC, Wu MS, Lin JT, et al. A prospective comparative study of narrow-band imaging, chromoendoscopy, and conventional colonoscopy in the diagnosis of colorectal neoplasia. Gut. 2007;56(3):373–9.
37. Su MY, Hsu CM, Ho YP, Chen PC, Lin CJ, Chiu CT. Comparative study of conventional colonoscopy, chromoendoscopy, and narrow-band imaging systems in differential diagnosis of neoplastic and nonneoplastic colonic polyps. Am J Gastroenterol. 2006;101(12):2711–6.
38. Gupta N, Bansal A, Rao D, Early DS, Jonnalagadda S, Edmundowicz SA, et al. Accuracy of in vivo optical diagnosis of colon polyp histology by narrow-band imaging in predicting colonoscopy surveillance intervals. Gastrointest Endosc. 2012;75(3):494–502.
39. Ladabaum U, Fioritto A, Mitani A, Desai M, Kim JP, Rex DK, et al. Real-time optical biopsy of colon polyps with narrow band imaging in community practice does not yet meet key thresholds for clinical decisions. Gastroenterology. 2013;144(1):81–91.
40. Rodriguez-Diaz E, Huang Q, Cerda SR, O'Brien MJ, Bigio IJ, Singh SK. Endoscopic histological assessment of colonic polyps by using elastic scattering spectroscopy. Gastrointest Endosc. 2015;81(3):539–47.

Chapter 11
Endosonography, Contrast Agents, and Elastography

Masayuki Kitano, Kosuke Minaga, and Masatoshi Kudo

Abbreviations

AUC	Area under ROC curve
CP	Chronic pancreatitis
CT	Computed tomography
EUS	Endoscopic ultrasonography
FNA	Fine-needle aspiration
GISTs	Gastrointestinal stromal tumors
NPV	Negative predictive value
PEI	Pancreatic exocrine insufficiency
PPV	Positive predictive value
PSC	Primary sclerosing cholangitis
ROI	Region of interest
SETs	Subepithelial tumors
SR	Strain ratio
TIC	Time–intensity curve
UCAs	Ultrasound contrast agents

Electronic supplementary material: The online version of this chapter (doi:10.1007/978-3-319-30053-5_11) contains supplementary material, which is available to authorized users. Videos can also be accessed at http://link.springer.com/chapter/10.1007/978-3-319-30053-5_11.

M. Kitano, M.D., Ph.D. (✉) • K. Minaga, M.D. • M. Kudo, M.D., Ph.D.
Department of Gastroenterology and Hepatology, Kinki University Faculty of Medicine,
377-2 Ohno-Higashi, Osaka-Sayama 589-8511, Japan
e-mail: m-kitano@med.kindai.ac.jp

V.J.A. Konda, I. Waxman (eds.), *Endoscopic Imaging Techniques and Tools*,
DOI 10.1007/978-3-319-30053-5_11

Introduction

In endoscopic ultrasonography (EUS), the ultrasonic transducer at the tip of the echoendoscope can be placed into the esophagus, stomach, and duodenum. This yields high spatial and contrast resolution images of lesions within and adjacent to the digestive tract wall. As a result, EUS is superior to other imaging techniques, including conventional transabdominal ultrasound, computed tomography (CT), and magnetic resonance imaging, in terms of the reliability and efficiency with which it detects and stages various benign and malignant conditions in the upper and lower gastrointestinal tract and the pancreatobiliary system [1–3]. However, the ability of conventional fundamental B-mode EUS to characterize the lesions in digestive organs is limited. Recent developments that aim to overcome this limitation of conventional EUS have led to the evolution of several upcoming EUS imaging techniques, including contrast enhancement [4–6] and tissue elastography [7, 8] techniques. These techniques provide detailed information on the structure of the tissue and thus greatly improve the diagnostic capabilities of conventional EUS. This chapter focuses on these new imaging techniques in the field of EUS.

Technology Overview

Contrast-Enhanced EUS

Ultrasound Contrast Agents

Intravenous ultrasound contrast agents (UCAs) are microbubbles consisting of a gas core that is stabilized by a shell [9, 10]. A certain range of acoustic power induces the microbubble to oscillate or break [10–12]. Contrast-enhanced harmonic ultrasonography selectively depicts the signals produced by microbubble oscillation or breakage. The first generation of air-filled UCAs was Levovist®, which is composed of microbubbles of air covered by galactose and palmitic acid. Levovist® requires high acoustic power to oscillate or break its microbubbles [9]. In recent years, a new class of more stable and longer lasting UCAs has been manufactured. These second-generation UCAs include SonoVue®, Sonazoid®, and Definity® and employ the heavy gas perfluorocarbon, which has a lower diffusibility and blood solubility than room air. They can be oscillated or broken by lower acoustic powers [9–12], making them more suitable for EUS because the small EUS transducer produces limited acoustic power [13].

Principle of Contrast-Enhanced EUS

Intravenous UCAs enhance EUS images by depicting the vessels. Contrast-enhanced EUS includes contrast-enhanced Doppler EUS and contrast-enhanced harmonic EUS. The former modality is based on the principle that the phase shift of the signals received from the UCA produces pseudo-Doppler signals [12]. The detection of these pseudo-Doppler signals by contrast-enhanced Doppler EUS increases the sensitivity with which color and power Doppler imaging depict the Doppler signals from vessels [14–19]. However, this modality remains limited in terms of real-time vessel imaging because of artifacts such as blooming; it is also not sensitive enough to detect the slow and low-volume flow at the tissue perfusion level [20].

The other contrast-enhanced EUS modality, namely contrast-enhanced harmonic EUS, selectively depicts harmonic components that are integer multiples of the fundamental frequency [4–6, 11–13]. When microbubbles oscillate or break after receiving a certain range of acoustic power, harmonic components are produced. The harmonic component derived from microbubbles is higher than that from tissues; thus, by selectively detecting the harmonic components, contrast-harmonic imaging depicts the signals from the microbubbles more intensely than the signals from the tissue (Fig. 11.1) [4, 5, 11–13]. Contrast-enhanced harmonic EUS can be performed by using a wide-band transducer that is equipped with EUS and the second-generation UCAs that are oscillated or broken by low acoustic powers [4, 5, 13].

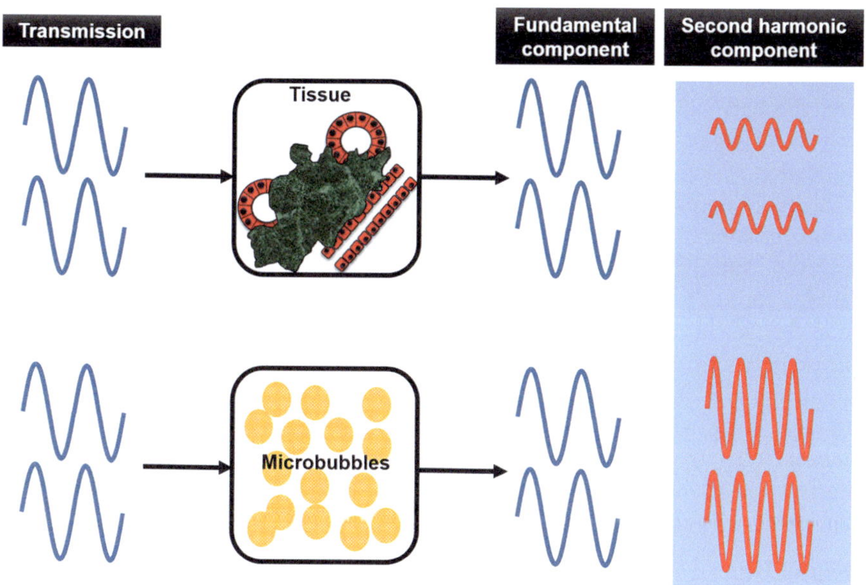

Fig. 11.1 Principle of contrast-enhanced harmonic technique. When microbubbles oscillate or break after receiving a certain range of acoustic power, harmonic components are produced. The second harmonic component derived from microbubbles is higher than that from tissues; thus, by selectively detecting the second harmonic components, contrast-harmonic imaging depicts the signals from the microbubbles more intensely than the signals from the tissue

EUS Elastography

Principle of EUS Elastography

Ultrasound elastography is a diagnostic technique that measures tissue elasticity. This novel upcoming technique is based on low-frequency compression of the tissue, which is applied manually via gentle compression with the ultrasound transducer or by using a physiological body movement such as respiration or pulsation [21, 22]. The main principle of tissue elastography is that the compressive force on the tissue causes axial tissue deformation (strain), which is then calculated by comparing the echo sets before and after the compression [23, 24]. The degree of deformation serves as an indicator of the stiffness of the tissue: the deformation is smaller in hard tissue than in soft tissue. Thus, the method compares the strain of one tissue to that of another [23, 24].

Techniques

Techniques of Contrast-Enhanced EUS

Immediately before performing contrast enhancement, the UCA is reconstituted with sterile water. After images of the ideal scanning plane are displayed on the specific mode for contrast enhancement, a bolus injection of the UCA is administered through a 22-gauge cannula placed in the antecubital vein. This was followed by a 10-mL saline solution flush to ensure that all contrast was administered into the circulation system. Enhancement of the target lesions with selective depiction of circulating microbubbles (UCA) is observed in a real-time or intermittent fashion. Before infusion of the UCA, neither signals from the tissue nor microbubbles can be observed. Approximately 10–15 s after infusion of UCA, spotty signals from microbubbles appear, followed by branching vessels (Videos 11.1 and 11.2). The maximum changes in echo intensity were seen 15–35 s after the injection of UCA, when diffuse parenchymal perfusion of microbubbles is observed (Videos 11.1 and 11.2). For quantitative analysis, a time–intensity curve of echo intensity in the target tissue after infusion of UCA was made for each patient [5]. After positioning a region-of-interest (ROI), the echo intensity was taken from the histogram of the ROI. A time course of the changes in echo intensity observed in the ROI was created from scans taken up to 60 s after the infusion of UCA.

Helpful Hints

1. Before infusion of the UCA, neither signals from the tissue nor microbubbles can be observed. Approximately 10–15 s after infusion of UCA, spotty signals from microbubbles appear, followed by branching vessels. The maximum changes in echo intensity were seen 15–35 s after the injection of UCA, when diffuse parenchymal perfusion of microbubbles is observed.

Techniques of EUS Elastography

EUS elastography is an adjunctive imaging technique that allows the tissue elasticity of a solid mass to be assessed during a conventional EUS examination [7, 8]. In this technique, the strain information is superimposed on the fundamental B-mode image: this yields a strain distribution map that is called an elastogram. For visualization purposes, the map is color coded and displayed next to the fundamental image on the screen (Video 11.3) [7, 8]. Red encodes soft tissues, blue encodes hard tissues, and yellow/green encodes tissues with intermediate stiffness [7, 8]. The elasticity information derived from this method is qualitative or semiquantitative. The strain of each area is compared to the strain of the remaining tissue within the elastogram, which is a relative image that is available for visual comparison only.

Several EUS elastography variables have been used as a measure of tissue elasticity. These include the color patterns [8, 25–29], the strain ratio (SR) [30, 31], hue histogram analysis [32, 33], and artificial neural networks [34, 35]. The color pattern is qualitative; since its subjectivity could lead to differences in interpretation between endosonographers, this variable may be limited in its usefulness. By contrast, the remaining three variables are quantitative and less subjective, and thus may complement the qualitative variable.

Helpful Hints

2. In EUS elastography, tissue elasticity is displayed in color. Red encodes soft tissues, blue encodes hard tissues, and yellow/green encodes tissues with intermediate stiffness.

Key Clinical Indications

Characterization of Conventional EUS-Detected Lesions

In general, contrast-enhanced EUS and EUS elastography are used for characterization of EUS-detected lesions. EUS is limited in its ability to characterize pancreatic masses. Like most carcinomas, endocrine tumors and inflammatory pseudotumors caused by focal pancreatitis are simply depicted as hypoechoic masses. To characterize such hypoechoic masses, elastography or contrast enhancement is needed (Figs. 11.2 and 11.3).

Contrast enhanced EUS may aid the diagnosis of pancreatic cysts by depicting the vascularity of structures such as the cyst wall, septa, or mural nodules. It also discriminates contrast-enhancing mural nodules from non-enhancing mucus clots (Fig. 11.4 and Video 11.1). This is particularly important in the case of intraductal papillary mucinous neoplasm, which can transform from a benign tumor to a malignant tumor.

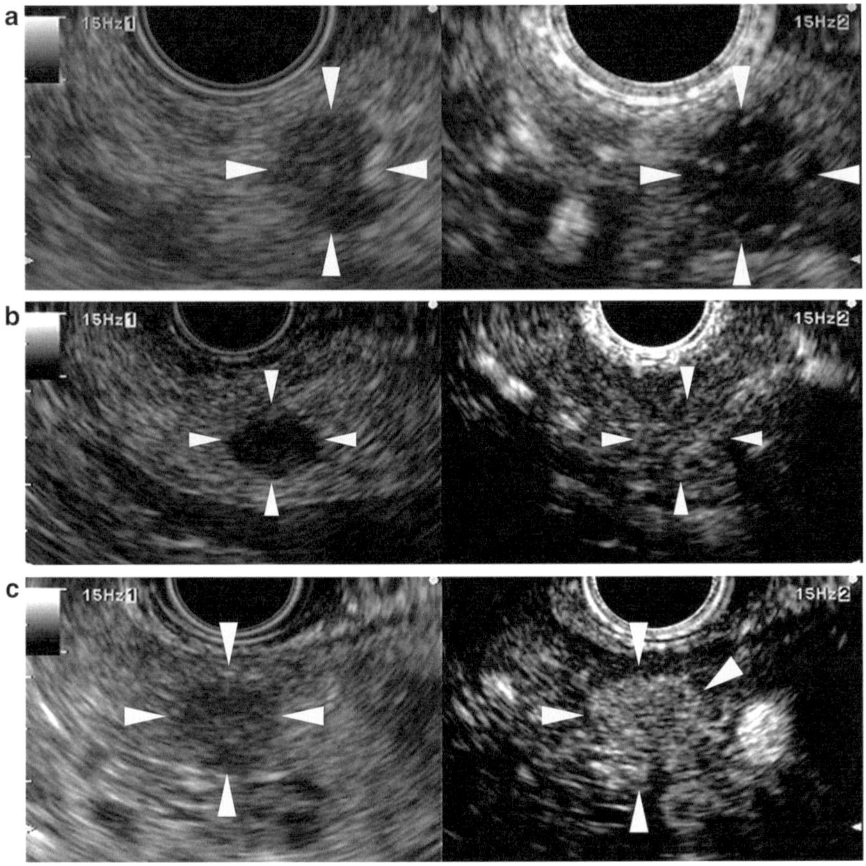

Fig. 11.2 Endoscopic ultrasonography (EUS) images of small solid tumors in the pancreas. Left image shows conventional EUS image, and right image shows contrast-enhanced harmonic EUS image. (**a**) A typical case of small ductal adenocarcinoma in the head of the pancreas. Conventional EUS reveals a low echoic mass lesion (*arrowheads*) of 8 mm in diameter (*left*). Contrast-enhanced harmonic EUS indicates that the lesion exhibits hypoenhancement (*arrowheads*) compared with the surrounding tissue (*right*). (**b**) A typical case of inflammatory pseudotumor in the head of the pancreas. Conventional EUS reveals a low echoic mass lesion (*arrowheads*) of 7 mm in diameter (*left*). Contrast-enhanced harmonic EUS indicates that the lesion exhibits homogeneous iso-enhancement (*arrowheads*) compared with the surrounding tissue (*right*). (**c**) A typical case of small neuroendocrine tumor in the body of the pancreas. Conventional EUS reveals a low echoic mass lesion (*arrowheads*) of 9 mm in diameter (*left*). Contrast-enhanced harmonic EUS indicates that the lesion exhibits hyperenhancement (*arrowheads*) compared with the surrounding tissue (*right*)

The differential diagnosis of benign and malignant lymph nodes is essential for clinically staging patients with cancer. EUS elastography and contrast-enhanced EUS can be used to assess the malignant properties of enlarged lymph nodes that are found during EUS (Figs. 11.5a, b and 11.6; Video 11.4). Also, these techniques are applied to characterization of biliary lesions (Fig. 11.7 and Video 11.2) and gastrointestinal subepithelial tumors (SETs) (Fig. 11.8).

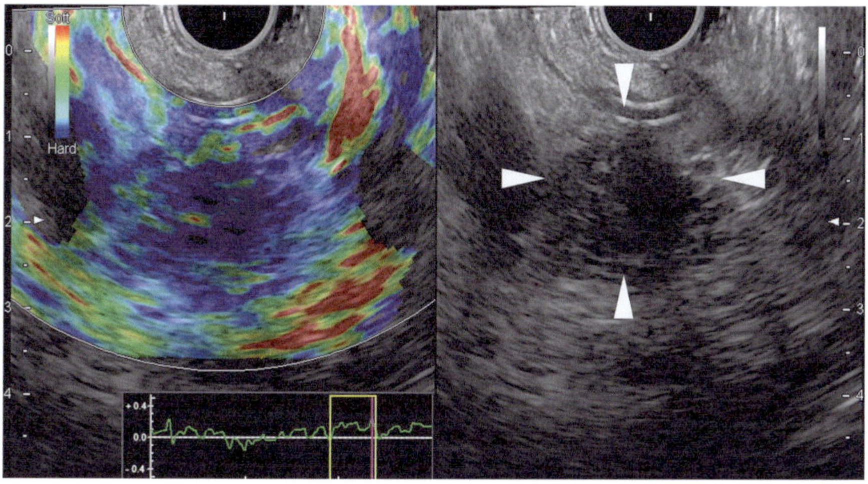

Fig. 11.3 Endoscopic ultrasonography (EUS) images of a ductal adenocarcinoma in the head of the pancreas. Right image shows conventional B-mode EUS image, and left image shows EUS elastography image. Conventional EUS shows a low echoic mass lesion in the body of the pancreas (*arrowheads*) (*right*). EUS elastography reveals relatively homogenous hard pattern (predominant *blue* pattern) at the site of the tumor as compared to the surrounding tissue (*left*)

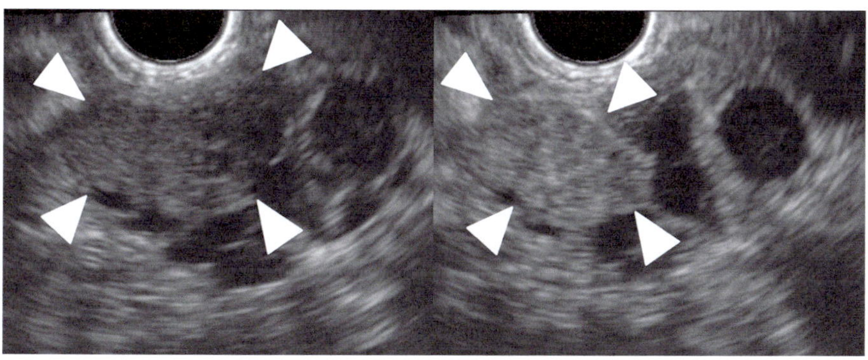

Fig. 11.4 Endoscopic ultrasonography (EUS) images of a branch-duct type malignant intraductal papillary mucinous neoplasm in the head of the pancreas. Left image shows conventional EUS image, and right image shows contrast-enhanced harmonic EUS image. Conventional EUS reveals a multilocular cystic lesion of 40 mm in diameter. A 15 × 12 mm mural nodule (*arrowheads*) is depicted inside the lesion (*left*). Contrast-enhanced harmonic EUS images (*right*) show that the mural nodule has abundant vascularity (*arrowheads*)

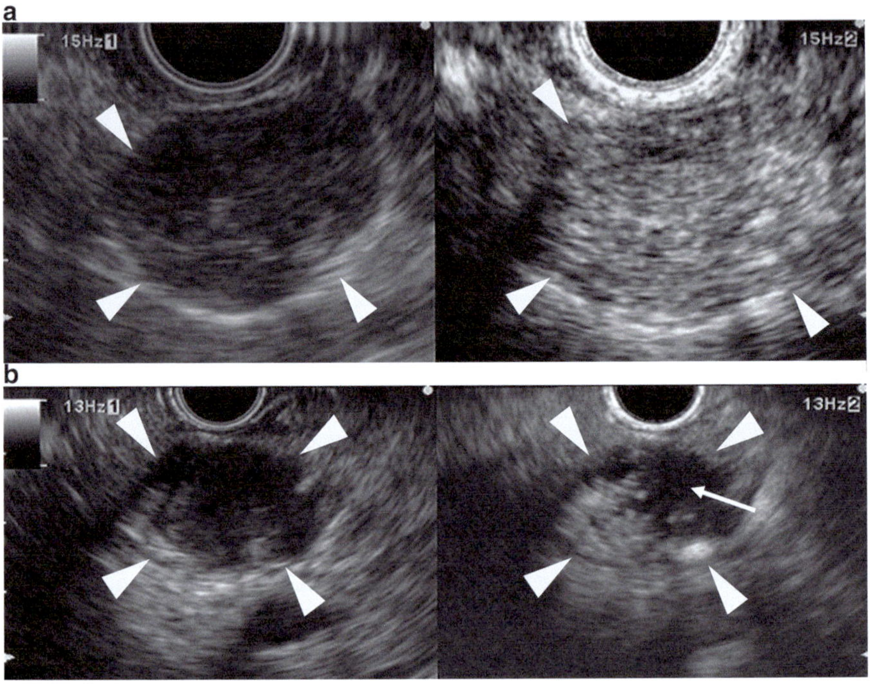

Fig. 11.5 Endoscopic ultrasonography (EUS) images of benign and malignant intra-abdominal lymph nodes (LN). Left image shows conventional EUS image, and right image shows contrast-enhanced harmonic EUS image. (**a**) A typical case of benign intra-abdominal LN. Conventional EUS reveals a low echoic lesion (*arrowheads*) of 25 mm in diameter around the gastric wall (*left*). Contrast-enhanced harmonic EUS indicates that the lesion exhibits homogenous enhancement (*arrowheads*) (*right*). (**b**) A typical case of malignant metastatic intra-abdominal LN. Conventional EUS reveals a low echoic lesion (*arrowheads*) of 14 mm in diameter around the pancreatic body (*left*). Contrast-enhanced harmonic EUS indicates that the lesion exhibits heterogeneous enhancement (*arrowheads*). The lesion includes avascular site with slow flow (*arrow*) (*right*)

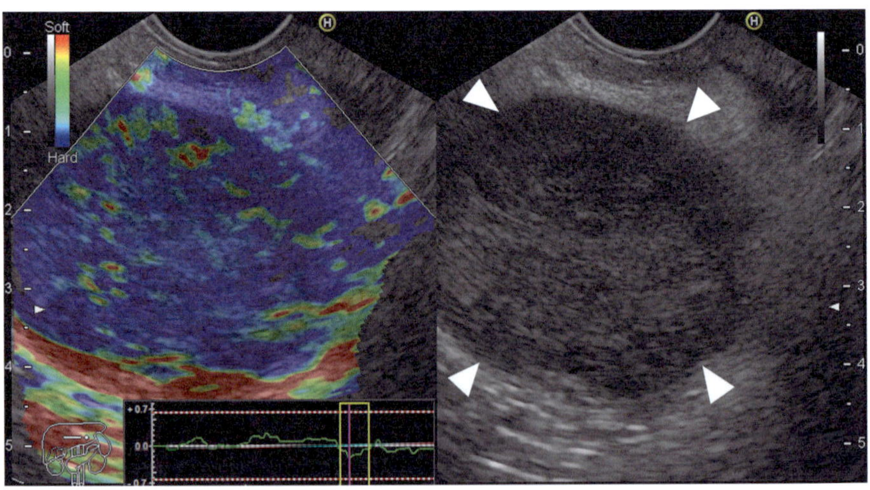

Fig. 11.6 Endoscopic ultrasonography (EUS) images of a malignant intra-abdominal lymph node. Right image shows conventional B-mode EUS image, and left image shows EUS elastography image. Conventional EUS reveals a 46 × 38 mm low echoic lesion (*arrowheads*) of around the pancreatic head (*right*). EUS elastography reveals relatively homogenous hard pattern (predominant *blue* pattern) at the site of the lesion as compared to the surrounding tissue (*left*)

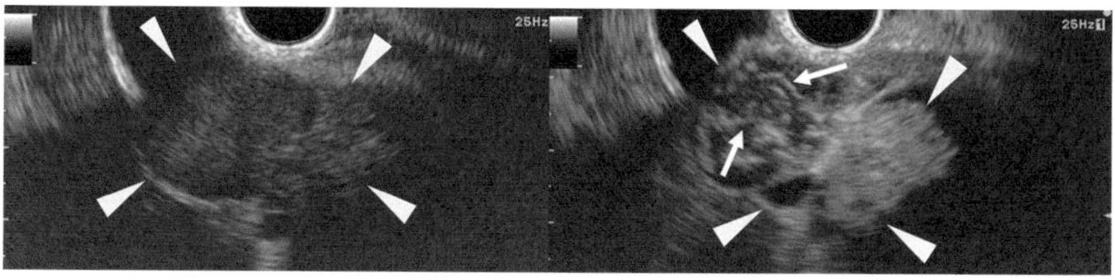

Fig. 11.7 Endoscopic ultrasonography (EUS) images of a gallbladder adenocarcinoma. Left image shows conventional EUS image, and right image shows contrast-enhanced harmonic EUS image. Conventional EUS reveals a 30 × 13 mm low echoic mass lesion in the body of the gallbladder (*arrowheads*) (*left*). Contrast-enhanced harmonic EUS indicates that the lesion exhibits heterogeneous enhancement (*arrowheads*). Contrast-enhanced harmonic EUS could depict intratumoral irregular vessels (*arrows*) (*right*)

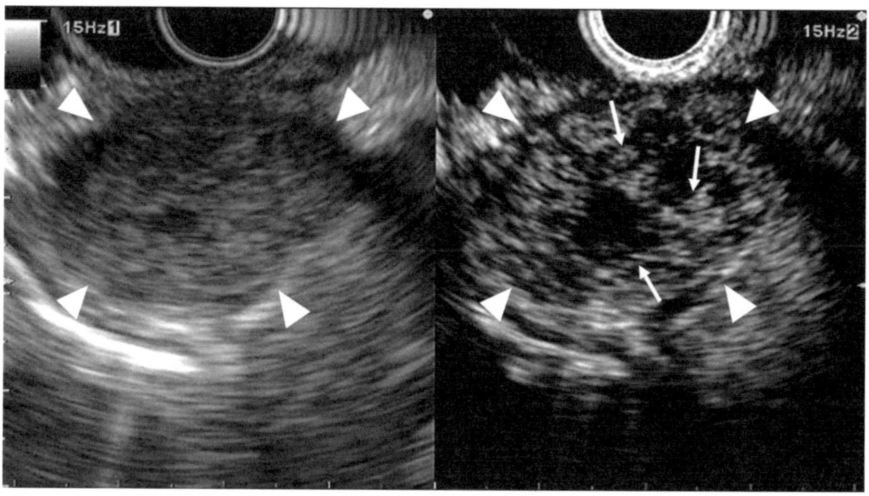

Fig. 11.8 Endoscopic ultrasonography (EUS) images of a high-grade malignant gastrointestinal stromal tumors (GIST) of the stomach. Left image shows conventional EUS image, and right image shows contrast-enhanced harmonic EUS image. Conventional EUS reveals a 30 × 21 mm low echoic mass lesion in the fourth layer of the gastric wall (*arrowheads*) (*left*). Contrast-enhanced harmonic EUS indicates that the lesion exhibits heterogeneous enhancement (*arrowheads*). Irregular vessels are observed in parts of the tumor (*right*)

Identification of the EUS-FNA-Target

Since EUS elastography and contrast-enhanced EUS clearly depict some subtle lesions that conventional EUS cannot identify, they can also be used to identify the target of EUS-FNA (Fig. 11.9 and Video 11.3) [36–38]. Moreover, they can be employed to find specific sites within a lesion that would be more suitable for EUS-FNA than other sites (Fig. 11.10 and Video 11.4). In particular, contrast-enhanced EUS can identify the avascular sites in a lesion; this would also help to prevent EUS-FNA sampling of necrotic areas and improve the sensitivity with which

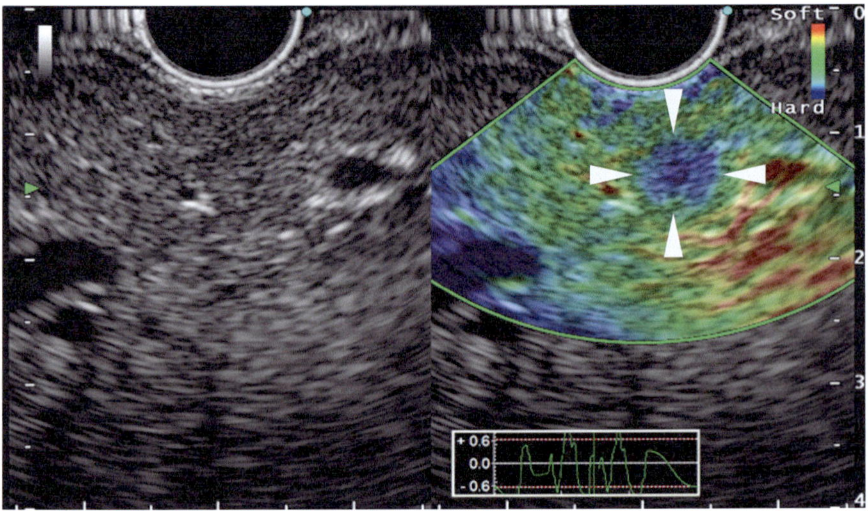

Fig. 11.9 Endoscopic ultrasonography (EUS) images of a liver metastasis of a pancreatic carcinoma. Left image shows conventional B-mode EUS image, and right image shows EUS elastography image. EUS elastography depicts a nodule of 6 mm in diameter which shows relatively homogenous hard pattern (predominant *blue* pattern) in the liver (*arrowheads*) (*right*). However, conventional EUS cannot identify the nodule (*left*). EUS-guided fine-needle aspiration of this nodule confirms a liver metastasis of pancreatic adenocarcinoma

EUS-FNA diagnoses pancreatic tumors (Fig. 11.10 and Video 11.4) [11]. EUS elastography and contrast-enhanced EUS may also be helpful in terms of identification of suspicious lymph nodes for which pathological diagnosis with EUS-FNA is required (Figs. 11.5 and 11.6). Finally, these techniques can eliminate the need to perform EUS-FNA at a second site, which in turn saves time and reduces risk [38].

Helpful Hints

3. Since EUS elastography and contrast-enhanced EUS clearly depict some subtle lesions that conventional EUS cannot identify, they can be used to identify the target of EUS-FNA.
4. Contrast-enhanced EUS can identify the avascular sites in a lesion, which helps to prevent EUS-FNA sampling of necrotic areas.

Assessment

Assessment of Pancreatic Solid Masses

Contrast-Enhanced EUS for Pancreatic Solid Masses

On contrast-enhanced EUS, solid pancreatic lesions can be characterized on the basis of their enhancement patterns relative to their surrounding tissue. There are three main enhancement patterns, namely, hypo-, iso- or hyperenhancement

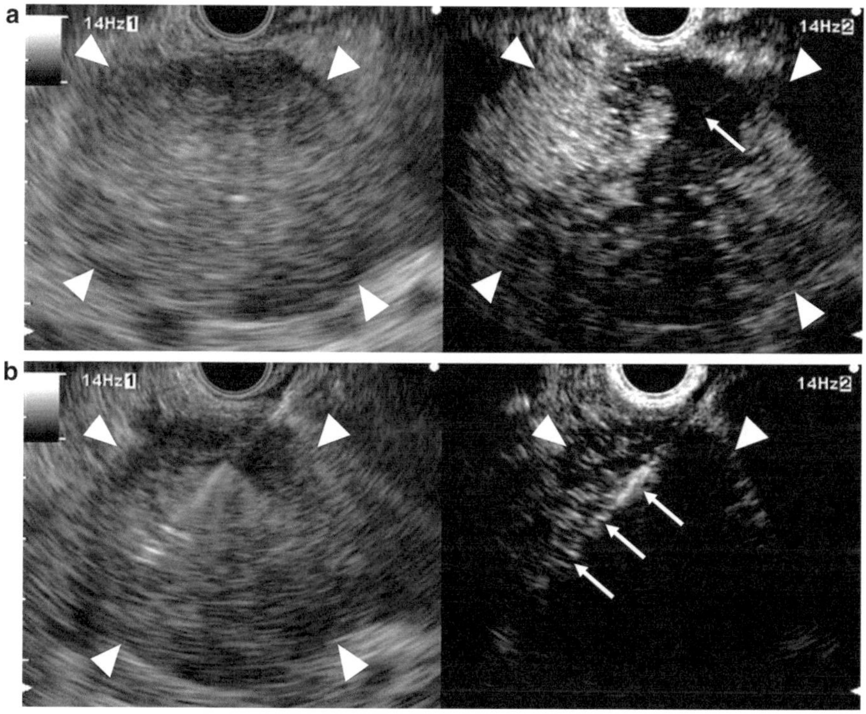

Fig. 11.10 Endoscopic ultrasonography (EUS) images and contrast-enhanced harmonic EUS-guided fine-needle aspiration of a malignant intra-abdominal lymph node. Left image shows conventional EUS image, and right image shows contrast-enhanced harmonic EUS image. (**a**) EUS images before EUS-FNA. Conventional EUS reveals a low echoic lesion (*arrowheads*) of 40 mm in diameter around the aorta (*left*). Contrast-enhanced harmonic EUS indicates that the lesion exhibits heterogeneous enhancement (*arrowheads*) with avascular area (*arrows*) (*right*). (**b**) EUS images during EUS-FNA. On real-time imaging with contrast-enhancement EUS, the site with hyperenhancement in the lesion (*arrowheads*) is punctured with a 22-gauge EUS-FNA needle (*arrows*), which revealed a lymph node metastasis of neuroendocrine carcinoma

(Fig. 11.2) [36, 37, 39, 40]. Contrast-enhanced harmonic EUS depicts pancreatic ductal carcinomas as nodules with hypoenhancement that mostly have irregular vessels (Fig. 11.2a) [36, 37, 39, 40]. By contrast, most pancreatitis-associated masses exhibit iso-enhancement (Fig. 11.2b) while most neuroendocrine tumors display hyperenhancement (Fig. 11.2c) [36, 37, 39, 40]. When using Sonazoid®, which is the most sensitive UCA in contrast-enhanced harmonic EUS, all pancreatic carcinomas exhibit some enhancement; nevertheless, they can still be distinguished from pancreatitis-associated masses and neuroendocrine tumors, which exhibit more enhancement than pancreatic carcinomas. The use of Sonazoid® means that pancreatic carcinomas can be distinguished from benign necrotic tissues, which exhibit non-enhancement [37]. A recently published meta-analysis showed that hypoenhancement in contrast-enhanced harmonic EUS diagnoses pancreatic adenocarcinomas with a pooled diagnostic sensitivity and specificity of 94 % and 89 %, respectively [41]. Moreover, contrast-enhanced harmonic EUS detects pancreatic adenocarcinomas (defined as hypoenhanced lesions) with better sensitivity and specificity (96 % and 64 %, respectively) than conventional fundamental B-mode EUS where pancreatic adenocarcinomas are defined as hypoechoic lesions (sensitivity and specificity of 86 % and 18 %, respectively) [36]. Contrast-enhanced harmonic EUS also improves the depiction of the outline of ductal carcinomas whose conventional EUS findings are uncertain [36–38].

Compared to contrast-enhanced CT, contrast-enhanced harmonic EUS differentiates ductal carcinomas from other masses with comparable sensitivity and specificity. However, contrast-enhanced harmonic EUS (91 % sensitivity and 94 % specificity) is superior to contrast-enhanced CT (71 % sensitivity and 92 % specificity) in diagnosing small (≤2 cm) ductal carcinomas [37]. In particular, contrast-enhanced harmonic EUS is useful for characterizing small neoplasms that contrast-enhanced CT cannot identify [37]. Fusaroli et al. also indicated that contrast-enhanced EUS may play an important role in compensating for the tendency of conventional EUS to return uncertain findings in cases with biliary stents or chronic pancreatitis (CP) [36].

Contrast-enhanced EUS can complement EUS-FNA in terms of identifying pancreatic ductal carcinomas that have false-negative EUS–FNA findings [37, 39, 40]. For example, a report showed that when ductal carcinomas were defined as tumors with hypoenhancement on contrast-enhanced harmonic EUS and/or a positive EUS–FNA, the ductal carcinomas in the patient cohort were detected with a sensitivity and specificity of 100 % and 92.6 %, respectively: adding contrast-enhanced EUS to EUS–FNA increased the sensitivity of EUS–FNA from 92.2 to 100 % [37]. A French multicenter study also showed that all five false-negative EUS–FNA cases in their cohort were correctly classified by contrast-enhanced EUS [40].

Helpful Hints

5. Contrast-enhanced harmonic EUS detects most pancreatic adenocarcinomas as hypoenhanced lesions. By contrast, most pancreatitis-associated masses exhibit iso-enhancement while most neuroendocrine tumors display hyperenhancement.

Quantitative Assessment of Parenchymal Perfusion with Contrast-Enhanced EUS

The classification of pancreatic lesions based on their enhancement patterns on contrast-enhanced EUS is a convenient way to characterize conventional EUS-depicted lesions. However, the classification system depends on subjective assessment, which means that different readers can differ in their interpretations. This problem may be overcome by using time–intensity curves (TICs) to quantitatively analyze contrast-enhanced EUS images. Several TIC variables are useful for the differential diagnosis of pancreatic masses. In particular, a low ratio of the uptake inside the mass relative to the uptake of the surrounding parenchyma [42], a low median intensity [43], a low maximum intensity [44], a long time to peak uptake [44], a high area under the curve [44], and a high echo intensity reduction rate [45] have been found to be predictive of ductal adenocarcinomas. Recently, Săftoiu et al. performed a prospective multicenter trial to assess the ability with which quantitative contrast-enhanced EUS can differentially diagnose focal pancreatic masses. This study showed that the TIC variables accurately differentiated CP from pancreatic carcinoma and could be used in an automated computer-aided diagnostic system with good diagnostic results [6].

EUS Elastography for Pancreatic Solid Masses

EUS elastography is increasingly being used to improve the characterization of the benign or malignant nature of a lesion because more elastic (soft) tumors are more likely to be benign while less elastic (hard) tumors are more likely to be malignant [7, 8]. Iglesias-Garcia et al. extended the field further by using four patterns, as follows: homogeneous green, heterogeneous green-predominant, homogeneous blue, and heterogeneous blue-predominant patterns [27]. They found that this method diagnosed pancreatic malignancy as blue-predominant patterns (Fig. 11.3) with a sensitivity, specificity, and overall accuracy of 100 %, 85.5 %, and 94 %, respectively.

Meta-analyses assessing the ability of EUS elastography to differentiate between benign and malignant pancreatic masses were published. One was by Pei et al., whose meta-analysis identified 1042 patients with solid pancreatic masses. EUS elastography differentiated benign from malignant masses with a pooled sensitivity and specificity of 95 % (93–96 %) and 69 % (63–75 %), respectively [46]. The meta-analysis of Mei et al., which consisted of 1044 cases, yielded similar results: EUS elastography discriminated between benign and malignant masses with a pooled sensitivity of 95 % (94–97 %) and a pooled specificity of 67 % (61–73 %) [47].

Quantitative analysis using strain ratio, huc histogram, and neural artificial neural networks may overcome the limitations in the subjective analysis. Three studies assessing the accuracy with which SR-based EUS elastography diagnoses pancreatic malignancies found that the sensitivity and specificity ranged from 93 to 100 % and from 17 to 95 %, respectively [31–33]. In European multicenter study, real-time EUS elastography using computer-aided diagnosis of pancreatic adenocarcinomas by artificial neural network analysis revealed that the sensitivity and specificity were 88 % and 83 %, respectively [35].

Helpful Hints

6. EUS elastography detects most pancreatic adenocarcinomas as hard tumors (predominantly blue).

Combination of Contrast-Enhanced EUS and EUS Elastography

It is unclear whether combining contrast-enhanced EUS and EUS elastography yields a better diagnostic ability than each individual method. However, when Săftoiu et al. assessed the diagnostic accuracy of contrast-enhanced EUS and/or EUS elastography for solid masses in the pancreas, they found that contrast-enhanced Doppler EUS and EUS elastography had comparable sensitivity (91 % and 85 %, respectively). However, they both had low specificities (less than 70 %). By contrast, when hypoenhancement on contrast-enhanced Doppler EUS and hard elasticity on EUS elastography were used to diagnose these masses, this combination was highly specific (95 %). Thus, a combination of the two methods may be useful for reducing the number of false-positive cases [33]. However, Hocke et al. reported that the combination of fundamental B-mode, elastography, and contrast-enhanced Doppler imaging (90 % sensitivity and 64 % specificity) did not improve the result of contrast-enhanced Doppler EUS alone (90 % sensitivity and 92 % specificity) [29]. Further studies are needed to establish the contrast-enhanced EUS and EUS elastography criteria that can be applied together to diagnose pancreatic tumors with superior accuracy.

Assessment of Pancreatic Cystic Lesions

Contrast-Enhanced EUS for Pancreatic Cystic Tumors

Pancreatic cystic tumors encompass a wide variety of lesions that have similar conventional EUS images but different biological behaviors. The key internal structural features of cystic tumors include their lobularity, cystic component, appearance, and/or whether a thick wall and/or mural nodules are present. These features play an important role in the differential diagnosis of cystic lesions in the pancreas [48–50]. Conventional EUS occasionally misdiagnoses the mucus clots in these tumors as a mural nodule, which can lead to unnecessary surgical resection. This problem is avoided by using contrast-enhanced harmonic EUS to determine whether the mural nodule or mucous clot exhibits vascularity. In contrast-enhanced EUS, the mural nodules exhibit enhancement suggestive of positive vascularity (Fig. 11.4 and Video 11.1) while the mucous clots do not. This approach is supported by the recent study by Yamashita et al., which showed that contrast-enhanced EUS distinguishes the mural nodules from mucous clots in intraductal papillary mucinous neoplasms with an excellent sensitivity, specificity, positive predictive value (PPV), negative predictive value (NPV), and accuracy (100 %, 80 %, 92 %, 100 % and 94 %, respectively) [51]. Furthermore, relative to conventional EUS, contrast-enhanced EUS improves the diagnosis of intraductal papillary mucinous neoplasms and mucinous cystic neoplasms by more accurately identifying mural nodules [52]. Also, when the presence of a mural nodule was considered indicative of a malignant cyst, contrast-enhanced EUS was significantly more accurate than conventional EUS (sensitivity,

97 % vs. 97 %; specificity, 75 % vs. 40 %; accuracy, 84 % vs. 64 %, $p=0.0001$) [52]. Contrast-enhanced EUS can also be used to classify mural nodules into four classes, namely, low papillary, polypoid, papillary, and invasive. The papillary and invasive nodules associate frequently with malignancy. When intraductal papillary mucinous neoplasms were defined to be malignant when they had papillary or invasive nodules, the diagnostic sensitivity, specificity, and accuracy of this approach were 60 %, 92.9 %, and 75.9 %, respectively [53].

Helpful Hints

7. Contrast-enhanced EUS distinguishes the mural nodules (presence of vessels) from mural clots (absence of vessels) in intraductal papillary mucinous neoplasms.

Diagnosis of Chronic Pancreatitis

EUS Elastography for Diagnosing Chronic Pancreatitis

EUS elastography can also be used to diagnose chronic pancreatitis (CP) because the color map of CP is more heterogeneous and more predominantly blue than that of normal pancreatic parenchyma. Several studies on the usefulness of EUS elastography in diagnosing this condition have been performed. Iglesias-Garcia et al. reported that there is a significant linear correlation between the SR and the number of EUS criteria for CP ($r=0.813$; $P<0.0001$) [54]. The study of Jansen et al. sought to identify a pancreatic elasticity that would allow patients with CP to be discriminated from subjects with normal pancreas. In this analysis, subjects with normal pancreas were divided according to age into younger (≤60 years) or older (>60 years) groups, after which these two groups were compared to a third group of patients with CP [55]. Histogram analysis of the elastograms (where 0 indicates the hardest tissue and 255 indicates the softest tissue) showed that the younger, older, and CP groups had mean strains of 110.2 ± 23.9, 80.0 + 16.4, and 32.4 ± 11.9, respectively. The cut-off value of 50 distinguished between CP and healthy people who were older than 60 years with an AUC of 0.993. Itoh et al. evaluated the ability of EUS elastography to quantify the fibrosis in the parenchyma surrounding pancreatic tumors. In their analysis of 58 patients undergoing pancreatectomy, the mean EUS elastography value (as measured by software analysis) distinguished between normal and mild fibrosis with an AUC of 0.90. It also diagnosed marked fibrosis and severe fibrosis with AUCs of 0.90 and 0.90, respectively [56]. Recently, the prospective study of Dominguez-Muñoz et al. on 115 patients with CP who were undergoing EUS showed that EUS elastography SR (a measure of pancreatic fibrosis) associated significantly with pancreatic exocrine insufficiency (PEI): the patients with PEI (30 % of the entire population) had significantly higher SRs than those without PEI (4.89 vs. 2.99; $P<0.001$). They also estimated that in patients with SR <2.5 and >5.5, the probability of PEI was <5 % and >90 %, respectively [57].

Assessment of Gallbladder and Biliary Lesions

Contrast-Enhanced EUS for Biliary Tree and Gallbladder Lesions

In terms of gallbladder lesions, Imazu et al. reported recently that when contrast-enhanced EUS is used to assess the thickened walls of the gallbladder, an inhomogeneous enhancement pattern is indicative of malignancy [58]. When this variable was used in contrast-enhanced EUS with the second-generation UCA Sonazoid®, it detected gallbladder malignancy with a sensitivity, specificity, PPV, NPV, and accuracy of 89.6 %, 98 %, 97.7 %, 92.2 %, and 94.4 %, respectively. These values were all superior to the values for conventional EUS. With respect to gallbladder polyps, Choi et al. showed that the presence of irregular intratumoral vessels and perfusion defects on contrast-enhanced harmonic EUS (Fig. 11.7 and Video 11.2) are both sensitive and accurate predictors of malignant gallbladder polyps [59]. Specifically, their study of 93 patients with gallbladder polyps larger than 10 mm in diameter revealed that an irregular vessel pattern (as determined by contrast-enhanced EUS) diagnosed malignant polyps with a sensitivity and specificity of 90.3 % and 96.6 %, respectively. Moreover, the presence of perfusion defects (as detected by contrast-enhanced EUS) diagnosed malignant polyps with a sensitivity and specificity of 90.3 % and 94.9 %, respectively. Thus, contrast-enhanced EUS can be used to diagnose malignant gallbladder lesions on the basis of their inhomogeneous enhancement and/or irregular vessels [58]. In another small series, Park et al. found that contrast-enhanced EUS also helped differentiate cholesterol polyps from gallbladder adenomas [60]: their study of 87 patients with gallbladder polyps showed that on the basis of the enhancement patterns on contrast-enhanced EUS, gallbladder adenomas could be discriminated from cholesterol polyps with a sensitivity and specificity of 75.0 % and 66.6 %, respectively [60]. Thus, contrast-enhanced EUS may be useful for the differential diagnosis of gallbladder lesions. However, it remains unclear whether this modality has sufficient clinical efficacy to determine the treatment strategy for gallbladder lesions. Moreover, the visual assessment of the contrast-enhanced EUS images of gallbladder lesions is subjective; additional quantitative analyses that allow more objective measurements of the features of these lesions on contrast-enhanced EUS are required.

EUS Elastography for Evaluating Biliary Tree Lesion

There are relatively few reports on the usefulness of EUS elastography for evaluating biliary tree and gallbladder lesions. Since the common bile duct is a hollow organ, the application of EUS elastography may be limited when the bile duct is not completely blocked and the mass does not infiltrate beyond the wall. Rustemovic et al. evaluated whether EUS elastography could be used to screen patients with suspected primary sclerosing cholangitis (PSC). Analysis of patients with and without PSC ($n=20$ and 21, respectively) revealed that the PSC group was significantly more likely to have a hard or mixed Elasto Score than the non-PSC group ($p<0.001$). This suggests that EUS elastography may be a useful noninvasive method for diagnosing PSC [61]. Nevertheless, further studies are needed to validate this notion.

Assessment of Gastrointestinal Subepithelial Tumors

Contrast-Enhanced EUS for Gastrointestinal Subepithelial Tumors

Gastrointestinal Subepithelial tumors (SETs) encompass both non-neoplastic and neoplastic conditions of various etiologies. They include benign tumors, such as leiomyoma, lipoma or schwannoma, and potentially malignant tumors such as gastrointestinal stromal tumors (GISTs), which constitute the overwhelming majority of the mesenchymal tumors in the gastrointestinal tract. After the introduction of EUS, the evaluation of SETs improved significantly. However, poor interobserver agreement in terms of the subjective interpretation of conventional EUS images has limited the analysis of the characteristic EUS features of SETs, thus hampering the differential diagnosis of SETs on the basis of conventional EUS.

A contrast-enhanced harmonic EUS study of SETs in the upper gastrointestinal tract showed that GISTs have a significantly higher echo intensity than benign tumors such as lipomas [62]. In addition, contrast-enhanced harmonic EUS visualizes the vessels flowing from the periphery to the center of GISTs [63]. By contrast, contrast-enhanced CT cannot identify most of these vessels. All high-grade malignant GISTs possess these contrast-enhanced harmonic EUS-depicted irregular vessels (Fig. 11.8). When contrast-enhanced harmonic EUS is used to diagnose high-grade malignancy GISTs on the basis of higher echo intensity and the presence of irregular vessels, it is more sensitive than when conventional EUS variables (i.e., large size, lobular border, and heterogeneous structure) are employed [63]. These results suggest that contrast-enhanced harmonic EUS can be used to identify GISTs and estimate their malignant potential. Indeed, Yamashita et al. reported recently that the presence of intratumoral vessels in GISTs on contrast-enhanced EUS correlated significantly with a higher risk classification [64].

Helpful Hints

8. Depiction of intratumoral irregular vessels with contrast-enhanced EUS can be used to identify GISTs and estimate their malignant potential.

EUS Elastography for Evaluating Gastrointestinal Subepithelial Tumors

Two reports evaluated a diagnostic potential of SETs of EUS elastography [7, 65]. Săftoiu et al. indicated that EUS elastography can add valuable information and enhance diagnostic accuracy in patients with gastric SETs [7]. Gheorghe et al.

reported that neither conventional EUS nor EUS elastography can accurately differentiate between benign and malignant GISTs, leiomyomas, and schwannomas; they stated that it is essential to continue performing biopsy and/or EUS-FNA with histological examination and immunochemistry when gastrointestinal SETs are detected [65]. However, although the ability of EUS elastography to diagnose SETs is at present not fully defined and established, it is likely that EUS elastography will decrease the number of unnecessary EUS-FNA procedures for gastrointestinal SETs in the future.

Tumor Staging and Lymph Nodes Assessment

Contrast-Enhanced EUS for Tumor Staging and Lymph Node Assessment

Contrast-enhanced harmonic EUS is superior to conventional EUS in terms of the preoperative T-staging of pancreatobiliary tumors [66]. It is also much better at diagnosing portal invasion by pancreatobiliary adenocarcinomas [66]. With respect to lymph node metastases, the presence of a filling defect is a typical characteristic of malignant lymphadenopathy (Figs. 11.5b and 11.10; Video 11.4) [67]. When this property is used, contrast-enhanced Doppler EUS distinguishes benign from malignant lymph nodes with a sensitivity and specificity of 100 % and 86 %, respectively. By contrast, when conventional EUS using other variables is employed, it discriminates benign from malignant lymph nodes with a sensitivity and specificity of 88 % and 77 %, respectively [67]. Contrast-enhanced EUS is also useful for diagnosing intra-abdominal lesions of unknown origin. When it is used, 96.3 % of malignant lesions exhibit heterogeneous enhancement, whereas 75 % of benign lesions exhibit homogeneous enhancement [68].

EUS Elastography for Evaluating Lymph Nodes

On EUS elastography, the predominant red–green and predominant blue patterns (Fig. 11.6) diagnose benign and malignant lymph nodes, respectively, with high sensitivity and specificity [69]. A recent meta-analysis that included seven studies, involving 368 patients with 431 lymph nodes, showed that EUS elastography differentially diagnosed benign and malignant lymph nodes with a pooled sensitivity and specificity of 88 % and 85 %, respectively [70]. Knabe et al. evaluated the lymph nodes of 40 patients with esophageal cancer and found that fundamental B-mode EUS criteria diagnosed malignant lymph nodes with a sensitivity and specificity of 91.3 % and 64.7 %, respectively; adding qualitative (color patterns) EUS elastography data to this analysis increased the sensitivity to 100 % while not changing the specificity markedly (64.1 %) [71]. Larsen et al. reported that qualitative (color patterns) EUS elastography and EUS elastography SR on their own diagnosed malignant lymph nodes with a worse sensitivity but better specificity than EUS B-mode criteria: the sensitivity and specificity of EUS B-mode criteria were 86 % and 71 %, respectively, while these values for qualitative EUS elastography were 55 % and 82 %, respectively. EUS elastography SR associated with a sensitivity and specificity of 59 % and 85 %, respectively [72].

Conclusion and Future Directions

Recent technological progress in EUS has yielded modalities such as contrast-enhanced EUS and EUS elastography that have enabled EUS to detect, characterize, and stage tumors in the upper gastrointestinal tract and pancreatobiliary system. Moreover, they complement EUS-FNA by correctly diagnosing lesions with EUS-FNA false-negative findings and by identifying the most appropriate target site of EUS-FNA.

Although they have limitations in depiction of real histopathological structures such as tumor microvessels and fibrotic stroma, further improvement of these technologies may lead to their clear depiction. Also, in the future perspective, development of UCA combined with a neoplasm-specific antibody would lead to molecular imaging of neoplasms. Depiction of these tumor-specific structures may improve the diagnostic ability of EUS imaging and possibly replace EUS-FNA in some difficult cases.

References

1. Rösch T, Lightdale CJ, Botet JF, et al. Localization of pancreatic endocrine tumors by endoscopic ultrasonography. N Engl J Med. 1992;326:1721–6.
2. DeWitt J, Devereaux B, Chriswell M, et al. Comparison of endoscopic ultrasonography and multidetector computed tomography for detecting and staging pancreatic cancer. Ann Intern Med. 2004;141:753–63.
3. Khashab MA, Yong E, Lennon AM, et al. EUS is still superior to multidetector computed tomography for detection of pancreatic neuroendocrine tumors. Gastrointest Endosc. 2011;7:691–6.
4. Dietrich CF, Ignee A, Frey H. Contrast-enhanced endoscopic ultrasound with low mechanical index: a new technique. Z Gastroenterol. 2005;43:1219–23.
5. Kitano M, Sakamoto H, Matsui U, et al. A novel perfusion imaging technique of the pancreas: contrast-enhanced harmonic EUS (with video). Gastrointest Endosc. 2008;67:141–50.
6. Săftoiu A, Vilman P, Dietrich CF, et al. Quantitative contrast-enhanced harmonic EUS in differential diagnosis of focal pancreatic masses. Gastrointest Endosc. 2015;82:59–69.
7. Săftoiu A, Vilman P. Endoscopic ultrasound elastography—a new imaging technique for the visualization of tissue elasticity distribution. J Gastrointestin Liver Dis. 2006;15:161–5.
8. Giovannini M, Hookey LC, Bories E, et al. Endoscopic ultrasound elastography: the first step towards virtual biopsy? Preliminary results in 49 patients. Endoscopy. 2006;38:344–8.
9. Quaia E. Classification and safety of microbubble-based contrast agents. In: Quaia E, editor. Contrast media in ultrasonography. basic principles and clinical applications. Berlin: Springer; 2005. p. 1–14.
10. Sontum PC. Physiochemical characteristics of Sonazoid, a new contrast agent for ultrasound imaging. Ultrasound Med Biol. 2008;34:824–33.

11. Kitano M, Kamata K, Imai H, et al. Contrast-enhanced harmonic endoscopic ultrasonography for pancreatobiliary diseases. Dig Endosc. 2015;27 Suppl 1:60–7.
12. Whittingham TA. Contrast-specific imaging techniques; technical perspective. In: Quaia E, editor. Contrast media in ultrasonography. Basic principles and clinical applications. Berlin: Springer; 2005. p. 43–84.
13. Kitano M, Kudo M, Sakamoto H, et al. Preliminary study of contrast-enhanced harmonic endosonography with second-generation contrast agents. J Med Ultrason. 2008;35:11–8.
14. Becker D, Strobel D, Bernatik T, et al. Echo-enhanced color and power-Doppler EUS for the discrimination between focal pancreatitis and pancreatic carcinoma. Gastrointest Endosc. 2001;53:784–9.
15. Hocke M, Schulze E, Gottschalk P, et al. Contrast-enhanced endoscopic ultrasound in discrimination between focal pancreatitis and pancreatic cancer. World J Gastroenterol. 2006;12:246–50.
16. Sakamoto H, Kitano M, Suetomi Y, et al. Utility of contrastenhanced endoscopic ultrasonography for diagnosis of small pancreatic carcinomas. Ultrasound Med Biol. 2008;34:525–32.
17. Das K, Kudo M, Kitano M, et al. Diagnostic value of endoscopic ultrasound-guided directional eFLOW in solid pancreatic lesions. J Med Ultrason. 2013;40:211–8.
18. Dietrich CF, Ignee A, Braden B, et al. Improved differentiation of pancreatic tumors using contrast-enhanced endoscopic ultrasound. Clin Gastroenterol Hepatol. 2008;6:590–7.
19. Ishikawa T, Itoh A, Kawashima H, et al. Usefulness of EUS combined with contrast-enhancement in the differential diagnosis of malignant versus benign and preoperative localization of pancreatic endocrine tumors. Gastrointest Endosc. 2010;71:951–9.
20. Wilson SR, Greenbaum LD, Goldberg BB. Contrast-enhanced ultrasound: what is the evidence and what are the obstacles? AJR Am J Roentgenol. 2009;193:55–60.
21. Ophir J, Cespedes I, Ponnekanti H, Yazdi Y, Li X. Elastography: a quantitative method for imaging the elasticity of biological tissues. Ultrason Imaging. 1991;13:111–34.
22. Lerner RM, Huang SR, Parker KJ. "Sonoelasticity" images derived from ultrasound signals in mechanically vibrated tissues. Ultrasound Med Biol. 1990;16:231–9.
23. Ophir J, Cespedes EI, Garra BS, et al. Elastography: ultrasonic imaging of tissue strain and elastic modulus in vivo. Eur J Ultrasound. 1996;3:49–70.
24. Doyley MM, Meaney PM, Bamber JC. Evaluation of an iterative reconstruction method for quantitative elastography. Phys Med Biol. 2000;45:1521–40.
25. Janssen J, Schlorer E, Greiner L, et al. EUS elastography of the pancreas: feasibility and pattern description of the normal pancreas, chronic pancreatitis, and focal pancreatic lesions. Gastrointest Endosc. 2007;65:971–8.
26. Giovannini M, Thomas B, Erwan B, et al. Endoscopic ultrasound elastography for evaluation of lymph nodes and pancreatic masses: a multicenter study. World J Gastroenterol. 2009;15:1587–93.
27. Iglesias-Garcia J, Larino-Noia J, Abdulkader I, et al. EUS elastography for the characterization of solid pancreatic masses. Gastrointest Endosc. 2009;70:1101–8.
28. Itokawa F, Itoi T, Sofuni A, et al. EUS elastography combined with the strain ratio of tissue elasticity for diagnosis of solid pancreatic masses. J Gastroenterol. 2011;46:843–53.
29. Hocke M, Ignee A, Dietrich CF. Advanced endosonographic diagnostic tools for discrimination of focal chronic pancreatitis and pancreatic carcinoma-elastography, contrast enhanced high mechanical index (CEHMI) and low mechanical index (CELMI) endosonography in direct comparison. Z Gastroenterol. 2012;50:199–203.
30. Mayerle J, Simon P, Dickson EJ, et al. The role of EUS guided elastography to diagnose solid pancreatic mass lesions. Pancreas. 2010;39:1334.
31. Iglesias-Garcia J, Larino-Noia J, Abdulkader I, et al. Quantitative endoscopic ultrasound elastography: an accurate method for the differentiation of solid pancreatic masses. Gastroenterology. 2010;139:1172–80.
32. Dawwas MF, Taha H, Leeds JS, et al. Diagnostic accuracy of quantitative EUS elastography for discriminating malignant from benign solid pancreatic masses: a prospective, single-center study. Gastrointest Endosc. 2012;76:953–61.

33. Săftoiu A, Iordache SA, Gheonea DI, et al. Combined contrast-enhanced power Doppler and real-time sonoelastography performed during EUS, used in the differential diagnosis of focal pancreatic masses (with videos). Gastrointest Endosc. 2010;72:739–47.
34. Săftoiu A, Vilmann P, Gorunescu F, et al. Neural network analysis of dynamic sequences of EUS elastography used for the differential diagnosis of chronic pancreatitis and pancreatic cancer. Gastrointest Endosc. 2008;68:1086–94.
35. Săftoiu A, Vilmann P, Gorunescu F, et al. Efficacy of an artificial neural network-based approach to endoscopic ultrasound elastography in diagnosis of focal pancreatic masses. Clin Gastroenterol Hepatol. 2012;10:84–90.
36. Fusaroli P, Spada A, Mancino MG, et al. Contrast harmonic echo-endoscopic ultrasound improves accuracy in diagnosis of solid pancreatic masses. Clin Gastroenterol Hepatol. 2010;8:629–34.
37. Kitano M, Kudo M, Yamao K, et al. Characterization of small solid tumors in the pancreas: the value of contrast enhanced harmonic endoscopic ultrasonography. Am J Gastroenterol. 2012;107:303–10.
38. Romagnuolo J, Hoffman B, Vela S, et al. Accuracy of contrast enhanced harmonic EUS with a second-generation perflutren lipid microsphere contrast agent (with video). Gastrointest Endosc. 2011;73:52–63.
39. Napoleon B, Alvarez-Sanchez MV, Gincoul R, et al. Contrast enhanced harmonic endoscopic ultrasound in solid lesions of the pancreas: results of a pilot study. Endoscopy. 2010;42:564–70.
40. Gincul R, Palazzo M, Pujol B, et al. Contrast-harmonic endoscopic ultrasound for the diagnosis of pancreatic adenocarcinoma: a prospective multicenter trial. Endoscopy. 2014;46:373–9.
41. Gong TT, Hu DM, Zhu Q. Contrast-enhanced EUS for differential diagnosis of pancreatic mass lesions: a meta-analysis. Gastrointest Endosc. 2012;76:301–9.
42. Seicean A, Badea R, Stan-Iuga R, Mocan T, Gulei I, Pascu O. Quantitative contrast-enhanced harmonic endoscopic ultrasonography for the discrimination of solid pancreatic masses. Ultraschall Med. 2010;31:571–6.
43. Imazu H, Kanazawa K, Mori N, et al. Novel quantitative perfusion analysis with contrast-enhanced harmonic EUS for differentiation of autoimmune pancreatitis from pancreatic carcinoma. Scand J Gastroenterol. 2012;47:853–60.
44. Gheonea DI, Streba CT, Ciurea T, Săftoiu A. Quantitative low mechanical index contrast enhanced endoscopic ultrasound for the differential diagnosis of chronic pseudotumoral pancreatitis and pancreatic cancer. BMC Gastroenterol. 2013;13:2.
45. Matsubara H, Itoh A, Kawashima H, et al. Dynamic quantitative evaluation of contrast enhanced endoscopic ultrasonography in the diagnosis of pancreatic diseases. Pancreas. 2011;40:1073–9.
46. Pei Q, Zou X, Zhang X, et al. Diagnostic value of EUS elastography in differentiation of benign and malignant solid pancreatic masses: a meta-analysis. Pancreatology. 2012;12:402–8.
47. Mei M, Ni J, Liu D, et al. EUS elastography for diagnosis of solid pancreatic masses: a meta-analysis. Gastrointest Endosc. 2013;77:578–89.
48. Koito K, Namieno T, Nagakawa T, et al. Solitary cystic tumor of the pancreas: EUS-pathologic correlation. Gastrointest Endosc. 1997;45:268–76.
49. Kubo H, Nakamura K, Itaba S, et al. Differential diagnosis of cystic tumors of the pancreas by endoscopic ultrasonography. Endoscopy. 2009;41:684–9.
50. Hocke M, Cui XW, Domagk D, et al. Pancreatic cystic lesions: the value of contrast-enhanced endoscopic ultrasound to influence the clinical pathway. Endosc Ultrasound. 2014;3:123–30.
51. Yamashita Y, Ueda K, Itonaga M, et al. Usefulness of contrast-enhanced endoscopic ultrasonography for discriminating mural nodules from mucous clots in intraductul papillary mucinous neoplasms; a single-center prospective study. J Ultrasound Med. 2013;32:61–8.
52. Kamata K, Kitano M, Omoto S, et al. Contrast-enhanced harmonic endoscopic ultrasonography for differential diagnosis of pancreatic cysts. Endoscopy. 2016;48(1):35–41.
53. Ohno E, Hirooka Y, Itoh A, et al. Intraductal papillary mucinous neoplasms of the pancreas: differentiation of malignant and benign tumors by endoscopic ultrasound findings of mural nodules. Ann Surg. 2009;249:628–34.

54. Iglesias-Garcia J, Domínguez-Muñoz JE, Castiñeira-Alvariño M, et al. Quantitative elastography associated with endoscopic ultrasound for the diagnosis of chronic pancreatitis. Endoscopy. 2013;45:781–8.
55. Janssen J, Papavassiliou I. Effect of aging and diffuse chronic pancreatitis on pancreas elasticity evaluated using semiquantitative EUS elastography. Ultraschall Med. 2014;35:253–8.
56. Itoh Y, Itoh A, Kawashima H, et al. Quantitative analysis of diagnosing pancreatic fibrosis using EUS-elastography (comparison with surgical specimens). J Gastroenterol. 2014;49:1183–92.
57. Dominguez-Muñoz JE, Iglesias-Garcia J, Castiñeira Alvariño M, et al. EUS elastography to predict pancreatic exocrine insufficiency in patients with chronic pancreatitis. Gastrointest Endosc. 2015;81:136–42.
58. Imazu H, Mori N, Kanazawa K, et al. Contrast-enhanced harmonic endoscopic ultrasonography in the differential diagnosis of gallbladder wall thickening. Dig Dis Sci. 2014;59:1909–16.
59. Choi JH, Seo DW, Choi JH, Park do H, Lee SS, Lee SK, Kim MH. Utility of contrast-enhanced harmonic EUS in the diagnosis of malignant gallbladder polyps (with videos). Gastrointest Endosc 2013; 78: 484–93
60. Park CH, Chung MJ, Oh TG, Park JY, Bang S, Park SW, Kim H, Hwang HK, Lee WJ, Song SY. Differential diagnosis between gallbladder adenomas and cholesterol polyps on contrast-enhanced harmonic endoscopic ultrasonography. Surg Endosc. 2013;27:1414–21.
61. Rustemovic N, Cukovic-Cavka S, Opacic M, et al. Endoscopic ultrasound elastography as a method for screening the patients with suspected primary sclerosing cholangitis. Eur J Gastroenterol Hepatol. 2010;22:748–53.
62. Kannengiesser K, Mahlke R, Petersen F, et al. Contrast enhanced harmonic endoscopic ultrasound is able to discriminate benign submucosal lesions from gastrointestinal stromal tumors. Scand J Gastroenterol. 2012;47:1515–20.
63. Sakamoto H, Kitano M, Matsui S, et al. Estimation of malignant potential of GIST by contrast-enhanced harmonic EUS (with video). Gastrointest Endosc. 2011;73:27–237.
64. Yamashita Y, Kato J, Ueda K, et al. Contrast-enhanced endoscopic ultrasonography can predict a higher malignant potential of gastrointestinal stromal tumors by visualizing large newly formed vessels. J Clin Ultrasound. 2015;43:89–97.
65. Gheorghe L, Gheorghe C, Cotruta B, Carabela A. CT aspects of gastrointestinal stromal tumors: adding EUS and EUS elastography to the diagnostic tools. J Gastrointestin Liver Dis. 2007;16:346–7.
66. Imazu H, Uchiyama Y, Matsunaga K, et al. Contrast-enhanced harmonic EUS with novel ultrasonographic contrast (Sonazoid) in the preoperative T-staging for pancreaticobiliary malignancies. Scand J Gastroenterol. 2010;45:732–8.
67. Kanamori A, Hirooka Y, Itoh A, et al. Usefulness of contrast enhanced endoscopic ultrasonography in the differentiation between malignant and benign lymphadenopathy. Am J Gastroenterol. 2006;101:45–51.
68. Xia Y, Kitano M, Kudo M, et al. Characterization of intra-abdominal lesions of undetermined origin by contrast-enhanced harmonic EUS (with video). Gastrointest Endosc. 2010;72:637–42.
69. Okasha HH, Mansour M, Attia KA, et al. Role of high resolution ultrasound/endosonography and elastography in predicting lymph node malignancy. Endosc Ultrasound. 2014;3:58–62.
70. Xu W, Shi J, Zeng X, et al. EUS elastography for the differentiation of benign and malignant lymph nodes: a meta-analysis. Gastrointest Endosc. 2011;74:1001–9.
71. Knabe M, Günter E, Ell C, et al. Can EUS elastography improve lymph node staging in esophageal cancer? Surg Endosc. 2013;27:1196–202.
72. Larsen MH, Fristrup C, Hansen TP, et al. Endoscopic ultrasound, endoscopic sonoelastography, and strain ratio evaluation of lymph nodes with histology as gold standard. Endoscopy. 2012;44:759–66.

Chapter 12
Cholangioscopy and Biliary Confocal Laser Endomicroscopy

Kunal Karia, Angela Saul, Amy Tyberg, Monica Gaidhane, and Michel Kahaleh

Cholangioscopy

Technology Overview

Cholangioscopy is an endoscopic platform allowing direct visualization of the bile duct (Video 12.1). Since the first description of a cholangioscope in 1941 [1] and its clinical introduction in 1975 [2], many improvements have been made resulting in improved functionality and maneuverability. These include smaller diameter scopes with high-resolution imaging, tip deflection, and a working channel to perform biopsies and/or lithotripsy [2, 3].

There are two ways of performing cholangioscopy: peroral and percutaneous. The peroral approach can be done with a slim gastroscope directly inserted into the common bile duct or with a cholangioscope passed through the 4.2 mm working channel of a standard therapeutic duodenoscope. The latter can be done by two systems: an endoscope-based system, referred to as the "mother–daughter" system (Olympus America, Center Valley, PA; Pentax, Montvale, NJ) and a catheter-based system referred to as single operator cholangioscopy (SOC) in the literature (SpyGlass Direct Visualization System, Boston Scientific Endoscopy, Marlboro, MA). The SpyGlass system, which is strapped just below the duodenoscope's working channel by a silicone rubber belt (Silastic, Dow Corning, Midland,

---

Electronic supplementary material: The online version of this chapter (doi:10.1007/978-3-319-30053-5_12) contains supplementary material, which is available to authorized users. Videos can also be accessed at http://link.springer.com/chapter/10.1007/978-3-319-30053-5_12.

K. Karia, M.D. • A. Saul, M.D. • A. Tyberg, M.D. • M. Gaidhane, M.D.
M. Kahaleh, M.D., A.G.A.F., F.A.C.G., F.A.S.G.E. (✉)
Division of Gastroenterology and Hepatology, Weill Cornell Medical College,
New York, NY 10021, USA
e-mail: mkahaleh@gmail.com

V.J.A. Konda, I. Waxman (eds.), *Endoscopic Imaging Techniques and Tools*,
DOI 10.1007/978-3-319-30053-5_12

Michigan), consists of a reusable optical probe inserted via a multi-lumen disposable catheter. Technical aspects of the cholangioscopes available are described in Table 12.1 [2, 4–7].

A new digital SpyGlass platform is currently under trial in some centers in the United States and expected to become publicly available in the near future. The newer platform offers improved imaging resolution, is slightly more flexible, contains a wider working channel to facilitate biopsy, and will consist of a single catheter with built in optical probe.

Cholangioscopy is a challenging procedure that should be performed by an experienced biliary endoscopist. There is a lack of consensus, but at least 50 cholangioscopies are required to become competent [8]. There is no evidence to support which cholangioscope system is better. To date the only two systems approved by the FDA in the United States are the SpyGlass and the Mother-daughter system (MDS). Table 12.2 shows the mayor advantages and disadvantages of each system [3, 5, 9–12].

Key Clinical Indications

The most common indications for cholangioscopy are the evaluation of indeterminate biliary strictures and treatment of choledocholithiasis. Less common indications include guide wire placement during endoscopic retrograde cholangiography (ERC), assessment of post-liver transplantation biliary strictures, differentiation of indeterminate intraductal filling defects of the bile duct seen on radiographic studies, staging and ablation of biliary neoplasms, surveillance of primary sclerosing cholangitis (PSC), guidance of advanced biliary imaging techniques such as confocal laser endomicroscopy, and rarely evaluation of hemobilia of unknown etiology [4, 5, 8, 9].

Due to the technical differences, the percutaneous approach is indicated in patients who are not able to tolerate a peroral procedure due to comorbidities, have altered gastrointestinal anatomy due to a previous surgery, or for targeting inaccessible intrahepatic stones or strictures. Currently, this approach is performed in few parts of the world in centers with considerably experience in the technique (200 procedures/year), like in some countries of eastern Asia where the incidence of intrahepatic stones and cholangiocarcinoma is higher [2, 5, 9, 13].

There is a lack of standardized criteria in the assessment of bile duct pathology via cholangioscopy. Ramachandran et al. found an overall accuracy of 89 % distinguishing malignant from benign lesions based on the presence or absence of the following: mass, dilated tortuous vessels, papillary or villous projections and intraductal nodules [14]. Nishikawa et al. demonstrated an accuracy of 97 % in distinguishing malignant versus benign lesions based on degree of friability, irregular or smooth surface, the presence or absence of dilated tortuous vessels, mass and papillogranular mucosa [15]. However, there is a slight overall interobserver agreement between experts for a presumed final diagnosis based on imaging (growth, stricture, ulceration and hyperplasia) with a Kappa = 0.18, SE 0.022, supporting the need of a validated and standardized criteria [8].

Table 12.1 Technical aspects of available cholangioscopes

	Catheter-based system	Endoscope-based system		
	SpyGlass	"Mother-daughter"	Ultraslim gastroscope	Percutaneous cholangioscope
Outer diameter (mm)	3.4	3.1–3.4	4.9–5.9	4.8–6.0
Working length (cm)	190–220	187–200	110	35–67
Working channel diameter (mm)	1.2 plus two additional of 0.6[a]	1.2	2.0	2.0–2.6
Accessories introduced	Biopsy forceps, 1.9–3.0 F electrohydraulic LF	Miniature biopsy forceps and intraductal LF	5 Fr instruments, larger biopsy forceps, APC probes and LF	Retrieval forceps, baskets, larger intraductal LF
Tip deflection	Four directions: up-down, left-right	Two directions	Four directions: up-down, left-right	Two directions
Operators required	Single	Two	Single	Single
Technology	Optical probe[b] (6000 pixels)	Fiberoptic Digital with NBI Videoscope	Videoscope with HR-CCD and NBI	Fiberoptic Videoscope with NBI

LF lithotripsy fibers, *APC* Argon plasma coagulation, *HR-CCD* high-resolution charge-coupled devices, *NBI* narrow band imaging
[a]For irrigation
[b]Outer diameter of 0.77 mm introduced through the 0.9 mm optical probe lumen channel

Table 12.2 Advantages and disadvantages of available cholangioscopes

	SpyGlass system	Mother–daughter system	Ultraslim gastroscope	Percutaneous cholangioscope
Advantages	Higher irrigation flow rates	Allows NBI (the digital scope)	Allows NBI	Allows NBI
	Tip maneuverability		High-quality image	Allows visualization of IH and far distal CBD stricture
	Allows simultaneous irrigation and instrumentation		Larger working channel	Easy maneuverability
			Lower cost	
Disadvantages	Expensive	More expensive	More challenging procedure	More invasive
	Difficulty in accessing the intrahepatic ducts or crossing a stricture	Fragile	Too flexible	Inability to visualize the opposite segment
		Requires 2 endoscopists	Easy to loop in the stomach	Risk of tumor seeding along the tract (unusual)
		Limited maneuverability	Requires a widely opened ampulla	Higher complication rate
		Insufficient irrigation system		
Availability	USA/Europe/Asia	USA/Europe/Asia	Asia/Europe	Asia

IH intrahepatic, *CBD* common bile duct

Table 12.3 The performance of the different cholangioscopic systems and the alternative approaches available to evaluate undetermined strictures and differentiate a malignant stricture

	Accuracy (%)	Sensitivity (%)	Specificity (%)	PPV (%)	NPV (%)	Procedure success rate
ERC	53	51	54	88	77	
Brushing	35.5	30–57	100		36	
Standard BX	30–54	43–65			42.8	
Brush + Standard BX	50					
SpyGlass VI	80–87	78–100	82–90	80–90	80–100	89–97
SpyGlass BX	25–84	69	98		69.2	
SpyGlass VI + BX	75	49–88	94–100	96–100	65–85	
MDVC VI	92–97	96–100	80–92	95	100	
MDVC BX	60–85	38–81	100	100	48	
MDDC VI		73	100			
Ultraslim						70–95
PC VI + BX	88.4					

PPV positive predictive value, *NPV* negative predictive value, *ERC* endoscopic retrograde cholangiography, *VI* visual impression, *BX* biopsy, *PC* percutaneous cholangioscopy, *MDVC* mother–daughter videocholangioscope, *MDD* mother–daughter digital cholangioscope

Currently, the ERC remains the gold standard for therapy of biliary diseases but the degree to which cholangioscopy improves the ERC's diagnostic yield and the clinical management remains unclear. There are no randomized controlled trials that directly compare ERC with the different cholangioscopic approaches available or between them. A recent meta-analysis of eight studies (335 patients with undetermined strictures) shows that visual impression is useful for detecting malignant lesion, whereas targeted biopsies are better at confirming a malignancy diagnosis, but none is perfect in excluding cancer and their negative results should be interpreted with caution [16]. Based on one meta-analysis and several multicentric studies and cohorts, Table 12.3 summarizes the performance of the different cholangioscopic systems and the alternative approaches available to evaluate indeterminate strictures [15–22].

As previously mentioned, cholangioscopy can be used in evaluation of strictures due to PSC, a common cause of both inflammatory and malignant strictures. In fact, its diagnostic yield increases compared to ERC alone [4]. The technical success with SpyGlass is 96 %, with the ability to target the lesion in 91 %, and accuracy, sensitivity, specificity, and negative predictive value of 96 %, 33 %, 100 %, and 95 %, respectively [23].

Another common indication for cholangioscopy is treatment of choledocholithiasis. The overall success rate of cholangioscopy-guided lithotripsy (electrohydraulic or laser lithotripsy) is between 70 and 100 % with a mean number of sessions of 1.6. The success rate for each type of cholangioscopy system is 71–100 %, 76–100 %, 88.9 %, and 80 % for SpyGlass, MDS, ultraslim gastroscope, and percutaneous approach, respectively [9, 17, 19, 24–26].

Techniques

The techniques for performing peroral (POC) and percutaneous cholangioscopy (PCC) are for the most part different and will be described separately. However, both require antibiotic prophylaxis with similar preparation, sedation, and post-procedure care as conventional ERC. Sometimes, stricture dilatation is required prior to cholangioscopy, although this is associated with mucosal changes that alter the appearance, which will be described in detail later in this chapter.

Peroral Cholangioscopy

Before performing a POC, a sphincterotomy is required. A standard cholangiogram can be done to identify the site of the lesion or stones. Excess contrast injection should be avoided as it may interfere with visual clarity. If using the MDS or the SpyGlass system, the dials of the cholangioscope are kept in the unlocked position and the duodenoscope positioned near the papilla to improve the angle of introduction into the duct. Cannulation of the bile duct can be performed using a guide wire previously loaded into a sphincterotome or by using the cholangioscope itself. Once inside the bile duct, the guide wire is removed to permit the use of the accessory channel (MDS) or introduce the optical probe (SpyGlass). The duodenoscope's elevator can be used with the Spyglass, but should be limited or avoided with the MDS to avoid damaging the cholangioscope. In order to achieve a better visualization of the bile duct, frequent water irrigation is required and is achieved by using a foot-controlled water pump attached to the cholangioscope in a coaxial manner [2, 8].

Cholangioscopy being performed with an ultraslim gastroscope requires a bile duct diameter of at least 8 mm and a wide papillary orifice; therefore, a sphincterotomy and/or sphincteroplasty must be performed. The scope can be introduced using a guide wire as described above but due to its wider diameter, this is only accomplished in less than 5 % of the cases. So an intraductal anchoring balloon (MTW Endoskopie, Wesel, Germany or Endo Flex, Voerde, Germany) introduced through the scope is required in order to gain access, stability, and position. This balloon is anchored in an intrahepatic branch or in the proximal edge of a biliary stricture and the scope is advanced while pulling and pushing the balloon and the scope, respectively. In order to achieve good visualization, water irrigation or CO2 insufflation is needed [5, 21].

Percutaneous Cholangioscopy

In PCC, the scope is lubricated and passed into the biliary system through a percutaneous sheath placed through a preexisting mature percutaneous tract. To accomplish this, percutaneous transhepatic biliary drainage is performed using an 8.5 Fr catheter inserted under fluoroscopic guidance. Approximately 2–3 days later, the percutaneous tract is dilated usually by one stage dilatation (from 8.5 Fr to 16–18 Fr). For sinus tract maturation, a 16–18 Fr catheter is left in place and the cholangioscope is introduced 7–8 days after (diagnostic cholangioscopy) or 10–12 days after (therapeutic cholangioscopy). The use of a guide wire is optional. It is worth mentioning that antibiotic prophylaxis is mandatory in the percutaneous tract formation as well as during the cholangioscopic procedure [2, 13].

Assessment

There is a variety of mucosal findings that can be seen at the time of cholangioscopy. For examples of lesions that can be seen on cholangioscopy, see Fig. 12.1.

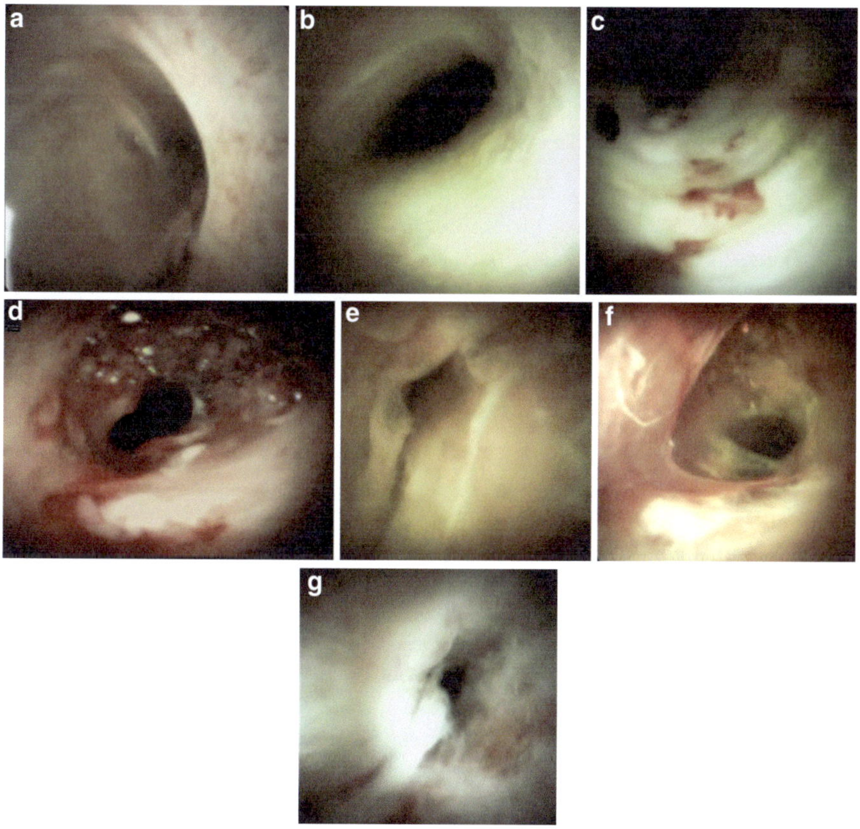

Fig. 12.1 Examples of lesions visible by cholangioscopy. (**a**) Normal bile duct with cystic duct takeoff. (**b**) Extrinsic compression of the common bile duct. (**c**) Bile duct superficial ulceration related to wire-guided trauma and stone extraction. (**d**) Asymmetric malignant stricture involving the common bile duct. (**e**) Malignant biliary stricture with papillary projections. (**f**) Malignant stricture with marginal ulcer in the setting of invasive pancreatic cancer. (**g**) Cystic duct insertion involved by malignancy

Both cholangioscopic and histologic evaluation of the biliary mucosa can be altered by previous stent placement or recent stricture dilatation. In fact, atypical squamous cells can be obtained from tissue around a duct stent representing a metaplastic phenomenon, so caution should be taken when interpreting these findings [4, 27].

As previously mentioned, Nishikawa et al. described criteria for differentiating benign (smooth surface without tumor vessels and papillogranular mucosa without a mass) from malignant lesions (irregular surface, dilated tortuous vessels, and easy oozing of blood) [15]. The presence of a tortuous vessel was found to have a specificity and positive predictive value of 100 % for malignancy [28]. Despite this, there is a lack of standardized criteria. Visual inspection alone is associated with false-negative results, strongly supporting the use of targeted biopsies even when the visual appearance suggests a benign lesion [16].

Cholangioscopy can also be used to diagnose biliary tract intraductal papillary mucinous neoplasm (BT-IPMN), a rare finding recognized as a distinct pathological entity by the World Health Organization (WHO) since 2010. When encountered, the macroscopic appearance of this lesion is an intraluminal mass with papillary proliferation and visible mucin [29]. In patients with BT-IPMN, preoperative assessment prior to resection is essential, with cholangioscopy successfully able to localize and determine the extent of the lesion in 87.5 % and 75 % cases, respectively [30].

Safety and Cost Considerations

Safety

Some studies have shown twofold higher rates of adverse events in ERC combined with POC than with ERC alone [10, 19]. However in a study involving 2087 patients (169 with SpyGlass), the multivariate analysis showed that the POC was not associated with an increased risk of complications. In fact, the risk of bleeding was higher in the ERC group compared to the combined group (2.3 % vs. 0 %, $p=0.05$, respectively) with no difference in the rate of cholangitis. The latter could be due to aggressive ductal irrigation as well as biliary stenting and prophylactic antibiotic use when obstruction was suspected [29].

The overall complication rate for MDS, ultraslim gastroscope, SpyGlass, and percutaneous cholangioscopy is 7.0 %, 1.8–7.7 %, 9.5 %, and 6.9–12.9 %, respectively, with 0 % of mortality for each [10, 13, 21, 29]. This rate differs between a diagnostic cholangiography and a therapeutic cholangioscopy. The incidence of complications is around 7.5 % and 6–20 %, respectively, for the peroral approach, while the percutaneous approach has a incidence of 8 % and 4–40 %, respectively [2, 3, 13, 17].

The most common complications of cholangioscopy are cholangitis, hemobilia, pancreatitis, and bile leak with a higher incidence in the percutaneous approach as shown in Table 12.4 [2, 5, 13, 21]. This incidence is mainly due to the biliary drainage and dilatation more than the cholangioscopy procedure itself and therefore decreases in the second session of a percutaneous cholangioscopy ($p=0.001$) [2, 13].

Table 12.4 Common complications of the different cholangioscopic approaches

	SpyGlass system	Mother–daughter system	Ultraslim gastroscope	Percutaneous cholangioscopy
Cholangitis (%)	0–14	0–14	1.5–14	5.3–35
Hemobilia (%)	0–3	0–3	1.5	1–6

Among other complications associated with the percutaneous approach are loss of tract access, hemoperitoneum, catheter blockage, catheter migration and very unusual, tumor seeding along the tract [2, 12, 13]. The risk factors associated with this high incidence of complications are electrohydraulic lithotripsy (EHL) and balloon dilatation of a bile stricture (OR 2.68, 95 % CI 1.44–4.98, $p=0.002$) [13].

Cholangioscopy via ultraslim gastroscope carries a small risk of air embolism. The probability of this rare and fatal complication is between 0 and 2.3 %, therefore aggressive water irrigation is strongly recommended with complete avoidance or minimal insufflation with CO_2. Minimizing CO_2 insufflation has been associated with a decrease in the risk of air embolism (0.33 vs. 0.0, $p<0.001$) [5, 21]. Other complications associated with this approach are abdominal pain, hypoxia, and bradyarrhythmias [21]. The risk of pancreatitis is very similar between the different approaches including the percutaneous one, especially when the papilla is crossed [5, 13, 29, 31].

Cost

The total cost of a cholangioscope depends on the hospital needs. For the POC using MDS and SpyGlass system, a travel cart and an extra monitor are usually required raising the total cost of the procedure. In the POC using an ultraslim gastroscope as well as in the PCC, there is no need of additional equipment because both scopes use the same monitor as a regular scope. The cost is about $27,900 for the SpyGlass system, $60,000 USD for the MDS.

At this time, there has been no cost-effective analysis of incorporating cholangioscopy in addition to ERC for its various indications.

Conclusion and Future Directions

Cholangioscopy is a useful tool that allows the direct visualization and targeted biopsies and/or treatment of biliary tract lesions. There are different ways of performing cholangioscopy, either peroral or percutaneously the latter being more invasive and associated with a higher complication rate. The choice between them depends on the local availability and local experience. Cholangioscopy is a challenging and advanced procedure that requires an experienced biliary endoscopist in order to avoid complications.

There is a need of specific and standardized criteria to assess biliary lesions and an improvement in the current technology. Studies with the new digital SpyGlass system and a new prototype of a peroral cholangioscope with two accessory channels may show improved outcomes in terms of diagnosis and treatment.

Helpful Hints for Cholangioscopy

1. Cholangioscopy allows the direct visualization of the bile duct, and it is a platform for advanced intraductal imaging and treatment.
2. Cholangioscopy is a challenging procedure that requires an experienced biliary endoscopist.
3. Cholangioscopy may be performed via peroral or percutaneous routes. The latter is associated with a higher complication rate but the choice between them depends on the local availability and expertise.
4. The overall accuracy rate for cholangioscopy in the evaluation of indeterminate strictures is 75–97 %.
5. The overall success rate of cholangioscopic lithotripsy is 70–100 %.
6. The overall complication rate for cholangioscopy is 2–13 % but increases up to 20–40 % for a therapeutic cholangioscopy.

Biliary Confocal Laser Endomicroscopy

Technology Overview

Confocal laser endomicroscopy (CLE is an imaging technique that can provide real-time optical biopsies during endoscopic evaluation, including endoscopic retrograde cholangiopancreatography (ERCP). CLE utilizes a low-power laser beam that is focused onto the tissue through an objective [32]. The same objective gathers the reflected light through a small aperture placed in a conjugate focal plane as the tissue specimen, allowing only the light emitted from a desired focal spot to pass through [32].

Biliary CLE is performed using a probe-based CLE system (pCLE)—the CholangioFlex miniprobe (Cellvizio; Mauna Kea Technologies, Paris, France) (Video 12.2). The CholangioFlex miniprobe, with its outer diameter measuring 0.94 mm, can be introduced into the biliary tree through the working channel of a standard duodenoscope via a biliary catheter, typically either a Boston Scientific SpyScope catheter or Olympus Swing Tip catheter or a cholangioscope [33]. The miniprobe is attached to a laser scanning unit (excitation wavelength 488 nm) and a confocal processor that provides real-time image processing with up to 9–18 images/s with a 325 μm field of view, lateral resolution of 3.5 μm, and depth focus of 40–70 μm [34]. Images can be viewed in real time but are also stored for review on the pCLE system.

CLE employs the use of a fluorophore, which is a dye that fluoresces when stimulated by the excitation light and allows for contrast enhancement [32]. The fluorophore typically used in CLE is fluorescein (AK-Fluor®), which is nontoxic and used routinely in diagnostic angiography of the retina [35]. Other benefits to the use of fluorescein include relative inexpensiveness, better image quality compared to topical agents, and relatively low rate of adverse drug reaction (approximately 1 %) with the vast majority being mild nausea and vomiting [36, 37]. Seven to fourteen seconds after injection, fluorescein diffuses through the capillaries into the extracellular matrix, allowing for detection of neo-angiogenesis within malignancies and providing contrast between surface epithelium and surrounding tissue [33, 35, 36]. Image acquisition can occur for up to 40 min; however, the highest quality images are obtained within 10 min of fluorescein [38].

Clinical Indications

pCLE is indicated for the evaluation of indeterminate biliary strictures. Differentiating between malignant and inflammatory strictures by routine tissue sampling methods remains difficult, leading to repeat procedures and delayed diagnosis and treatment of malignancies. Cytological brushing and biopsy of indeterminate strictures at the time of ERCP have low sensitivities for malignancy, 35 % and 43 %, respectively; when combined the sensitivity is still suboptimal at 63 % [39]. Fluorescence in situ hybridization (FISH) has been evaluated to improve diagnostic yield; however, its sensitivity is only 45 % in patients with known cholangiocarcinoma [40].

After previous studies revealed differing pCLE findings in malignant and inflammatory strictures, the Miami Classification for malignant biliary strictures was created and validated. The four components of the Miami Classification are: thick white bands (>20 μm), thick dark bands (>40 μm), dark clumps, and epithelial structures. The presence of two or more criteria significantly raises the suspicion for malignancy and increases the sensitivity to 98 % [41]. However, due to false-positive findings in the setting inflammation or reactive changes, the specificity of Miami Classification was only 67 %.

The effect of ERCP with recent (<1 month) stent placement or cholangitis on pCLE findings at the time of ERCP was confirmed by in a study by Caillol et al. showing significantly lower diagnostic accuracy (87 % vs. 73 %, $p<0.001$) in this population [42]. To refine pCLE findings, a retrospective review of false-positive cases identified four pCLE findings indicative of benign inflammatory strictures known as the Paris Classification: vascular congestion, dark granular pattern with scales, increased inter-glandular space, and thickened reticular structures [43]. Incorporating both the Miami and Paris Classifications during pCLE of indeterminate strictures raises the specificity to 83 % and furthermore raises the overall accuracy of pCLE to 82 % compared to 75 % for index pathology alone [43].

The diagnostic accuracy of the Miami and Paris Classification has been validated by a prospective study of patients with indeterminate biliary strictures who underwent pCLE at the time of ERCP, revealing pCLE alone was more sensitive (89 % vs. 56 %) and accurate (82 % vs. 72 %) than tissue sampling alone [44]. When both tissue sampling and pCLE were combined, the accuracy improved to 88 % and confirmed the utility of pCLE in this setting [44].

pCLE Technique

ERCP is performed in usual fashion with cannulation of the bile duct and localization of the stricture with contrast injection. If not previously done, the pCLE system should be brought into the procedure room and turned on with subsequent connection of the miniprobe to the pCLE system. While the miniprobe is calibrated, 1.0–5.0 mL of fluorescein should be administered intravenously. Once calibrated, the miniprobe should then be preloaded into a biliary catheter (e.g., Boston Scientific SpyScope, Olympus Swing Tip) and inserted through the working channel of the duodenoscope and advanced into the biliary tree just proximal to the stricture. Under direct visualization via SpyGlass or with fluoroscopic guidance, advance the miniprobe so that distal tip extends past the introducer catheter. Then, retract the catheter and miniprobe simultaneously to evaluate the entire length of the stricture.

There are several important aspects to obtaining high-quality images. First is the timing of image acquisition. Any manipulation of the stricture resulting in trauma or bleeding can alter pCLE findings; therefore, images should be obtained prior to brushing or biopsy of the stricture. Image acquisition is optimal within 10 min of fluorescein administration, after which time there is a decrease in the signal-to-noise ratio leading to reduced image quality [38].

Positioning of the miniprobe is also crucial to obtaining high-quality images. The miniprobe should be placed gently into contact with the stricture with avoidance of trauma to minimize bleeding, the importance of which was highlighted previously. Furthermore, highest quality images are obtained when the probe is placed perpendicular to the mucosa; therefore, the use of a catheter with a flexible tip may help achieve optimal positioning of the probe [36].

Lastly, stability of the miniprobe is important for image acquisition. When feasible, we recommend general intubation for the procedure to minimize patient movement during pCLE. While performing pCLE, it is important that the duodenoscope is in a stable position and that the miniprobe be adjusted with fine movements within the stricture as this will lead to maximal evaluation of the mucosa while minimizing artifactual distortion of the images.

Assessment

The differential diagnosis for biliary pathology is broad. The pCLE findings that may be seen during evaluation of the biliary tree fall into three main categories: normal, malignant, or inflammatory/benign for which there are validated criteria.

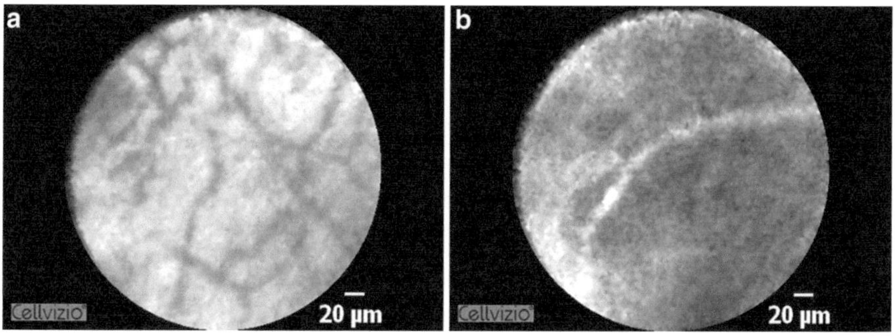

Fig. 12.2 The Miami classification: healthy bile duct [43]. (**a**) Reticular network of thin dark branching bands (<20 µm) with light gray background. (**b**) Vessels < 20 µm

An important thing to remember when reviewing biliary is the pCLE depth of focus is 40–70 µm. As the bile duct is composed of a single layer of thin cuboidal cells, the images obtained via pCLE are submucosal in nature. The presence of epithelial structures is always abnormal but not always indicative of malignancy.

The Miami Classification: Healthy Bile Duct

The Miami Classification for the healthy bile duct has three distinct findings: reticular network of thin dark branching bands (<20 µm), a light gray background, and vessels (<20 µm) (see Fig. 12.2). The proposed histologic correlation for the thin reticular network is normal submucosal collagen bundles.

The Miami Classification: Malignant Bile Duct

As previously mentioned, there are four criteria in the Miami Classification for a malignant biliary stricture: thick white bands (>20 µm), thick dark bands (>40 µm), dark clumps, and epithelial structures (see Fig. 12.3). A fifth pCLE finding suggestive of malignancy is fluorescein leakage. The proposed histologic correlates for thick white bands are blood vessels associated with tumor angiogenesis. The proposed histologic correlate for thick dark bands is thickened collagen bundles.

In the study that created the Miami Classification, the most common finding in malignant strictures is epithelial structures, which is seen in 73 % of cases but also present in 58 % of benign cases, resulting in a sensitivity, specificity, positive predicative value (PPV), and negative predicative value (NPV) of 73 %, 42 %, 77 %, and 36 %, respectively [13]. Thick dark bands (>40 µm) were present in 27 % of malignant cases but only 16 % of benign cases [13]. Thick white bands and dark clumps were seen only in malignant strictures with a frequency of 36 % and 27 %, respectively [13]. The sensitivity increases to greater than 80 % if epithelial structures plus

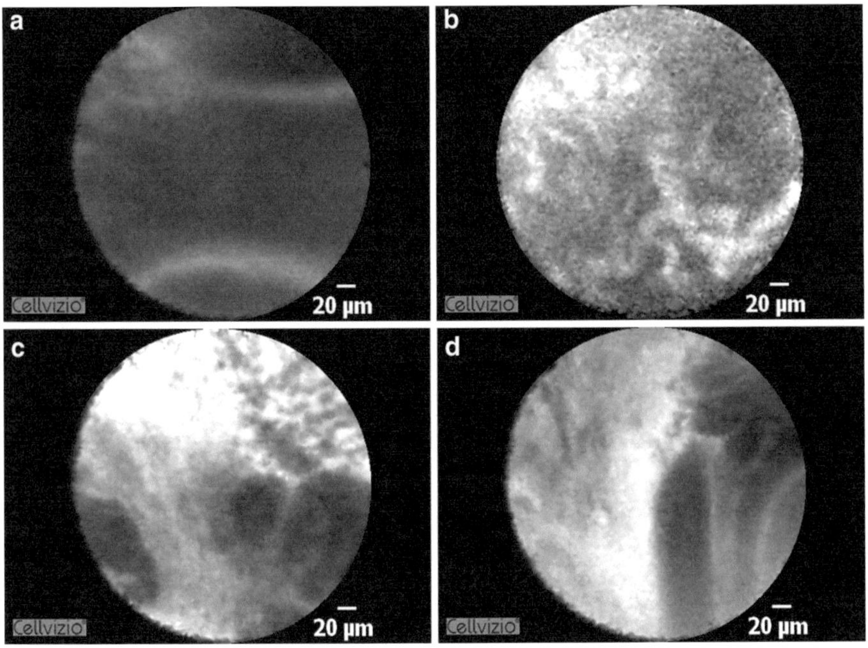

Fig. 12.3 The Miami classification: malignant bile duct [43]. (**a**) Thick dark bands (>40 μm). (**b**) Thick white bands (>20 μm). (**c**) Dark Clumps. (**d**) Epithelial structures

any additional criteria are found simultaneously and greater than 90 % if epithelial structures plus and two additional criteria are present [41]. When assessing pCLE findings, the presence of only one criterion is not sufficient for diagnosis while the presence of multiple criteria makes raises the suspicion for malignancy.

The Paris Classification: Inflammatory Stricture

The four criteria in the Paris Classification for inflammatory strictures: vascular congestion, dark granular pattern with scales, increased inter-glandular space, and thickened reticular structures (see Fig. 12.4). These criteria were developed by a group of expert endoscopists who reviewed false-cases in which the pCLE findings were suggestive of malignancy and subsequently validated in a later study showing improved specificity (83 % vs. 67 %) and accuracy (82.5 % vs. 81 %) when incorporating both the Miami and Paris Classifications during assessment of pCLE findings [43].

When beginning to use pCLE, it should be mentioned that there is an inherent learning curve with performing pCLE and image interpretation. Meining et al. showed improvements in technical aspects of pCLE with continued use. In their study of 89 consecutive patients, the ease of pCLE performance and ease of pCLE image interpretation was significantly improved in the second half (44 patients) of the study population compared to their initial 45 patients with decreased procedure time [45].

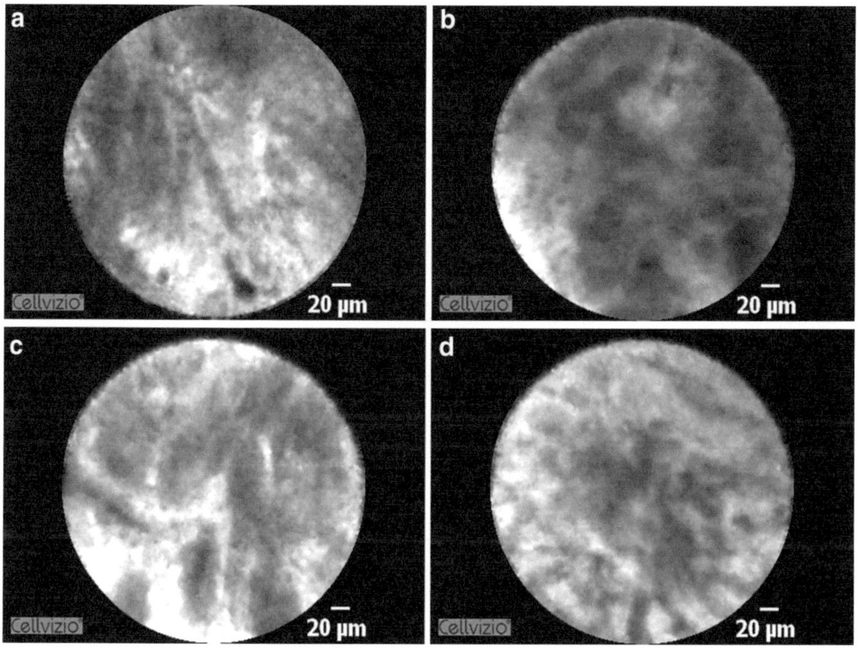

Fig. 12.4 The Paris classification: Inflammatory stricture [43]. (**a**) Vascular congestion. (**b**) Dark granular pattern with scales. (**c**) Increased inter-glandular space. (**d**) Thickened reticular structures

To optimize the utility of pCLE, endoscopists interested in incorporating pCLE into their practice should undergo formal training in pCLE image interpretation. The effect of training was highlighted by Talreja et al. who compared the pre and post-training accuracy among five endoscopists, four of whom had performed <10 pCLE cases prior to training. After a teaching session comprises 20 cases with an expert in pCLE, diagnostic accuracy increased from by 17 % (72 % vs. 89 %, $p=0.007$) [46]. Cellvizio, the pCLE manufacturer, offers training materials that are available on their website (www.cellvizio.net) and as a downloadable application for use on smart devices (i.e., iPhone, Android).

Safety and Cost Considerations

Safety

There has been no published review data on the safety of pCLE. An extensive literature search identified 13 peer-reviewed scientific articles involving >500 pCLE procedures. Only one adverse event (<1 % adverse rate) was identified, which was an episode of pancreatitis in a patient undergoing biliary CLE with the high-definition

GastroFlex^{UHD} miniprobe (UHDp), which has a larger outer diameter compared to the CholangioFlex miniprobe (2.6 mm vs. 0.94 mm) [47]. It is unclear if this adverse event was due to the larger probe or an inherent risk of ERCP in general.

Cost Considerations

In the setting of malignant biliary strictures, the key is early diagnosis. The low sensitivity of cytology and biopsy leads to frequent repeat procedures. By the time most diagnoses of cholangiocarcinoma are made, the tumor is at advanced stages and curative resection is no longer an option. pCLE offers the ability to improve diagnostic yield and minimize delays in treatment.

The cost of purchasing the pCLE system is approximately $100,000–$150,000 depending on the system configuration. The cost of a single CholangioFlex miniprobe (which is reusable up to ten times) is approximately $4000 each or approximately $400 per use. According to the current American Medical Association Current Procedural Terminology (CPT) codes, CLE of the upper GI tract is assigned a value of $1064.

In the current literature, there is little data analyzing the cost-effectiveness of pCLE. A retrospective study by Sharaiha et al. suggests that the institutional cost of performing pCLE for indeterminate strictures with pCLE is negated by findings leading to subsequent procedures [48]. In this study, 14/67 (20.1 %) of patients went on to have further surgical procedures after pCLE. In these cases, the average gross revenue generated per patient was $109,667 while the average net profit per patient was $38,231. The overall profit margin was 34 % per patient.

Conclusion and Future Directions

pCLE has been shown to be a safe and important diagnostic tool in the evaluation of indeterminate biliary strictures with improved sensitivity and accuracy compared to routine sampling alone. Therefore, pCLE has the potential to allow for targeted biopsies of suspicious areas, leading to improved diagnostic yields at the time of initial pCLE, and thereby reducing the need for repeat procedures. However, further studies are needed to evaluate the cost effectiveness of pCLE.

Helpful Hints for Biliary pCLE

1. Biliary pCLE is an imaging modality that provides in vivo, real-time optical biopsies during ERCP.
2. The main indication for pCLE is the evaluation of indeterminate strictures.

3. The Miami and Paris Classifications describe findings of malignant and inflammatory biliary strictures, respectively.
4. When performing pCLE, one should evaluate a stricture with the Miami and Paris Classifications simultaneously, which will provide a sensitivity, specificity, and accuracy of 97 %, 67 %, and 81 %, respectively.
5. There is a learning curve involved with reviewing pCLE images, with improved accuracy after formalized training.
6. The complication rate of pCLE is low (~1 %) with the majority of events associated with intravenous fluorescein administration.
7. Further studies regarding the cost-effectiveness of pCLE are needed.

References

1. McIver MA. An instrument for visualizing the interior of the common ductal operation. Surgery. 1941;9:112.
2. Parsi MA. Peroral cholangioscopy in the new millennium. World J Gastroenterol. 2011;17:1–6.
3. ASGE Technology Committee, Shah RJ, Adler DG, Conway JD, Diehl DL, Farraye FA, Kantsevoy SV, et al. Cholangiopancreatoscopy. Gastrointest Endosc. 2008;68:411–21.
4. Chen YK, Pleskow DK. SpyGlass single-operator peroral cholangiopancreatoscopy system for the diagnosis and therapy of bile-duct disorders: a clinical feasibility study (with video). Gastrointest Endosc. 2007;65:832–41.
5. Brauer BC, Shah RJ. Cholangioscopy in liver disease. Clin Liver Dis. 2014;18:927–44.
6. Moon JH, Choi HJ. The role of direct peroral cholangioscopy using an ultraslim endoscope for biliary lesions: indications, limitations, and complications. Clin Endosc. 2013;46:537–39.
7. Osanai M, Itoi T, Igarashi Y, Tanaka K, Kida M, Maguchi H, et al. Peroral videocholangioscopy to evaluate indeterminate bile duct lesions and preoperative mucosal cancerous extension: a prospective multicenter study. Endoscopy. 2013;45:635–42.
8. Parsi MA, Jang S, Sanaka M, Stevens T, Vargo JJ. Diagnostic and therapeutic cholangiopancreatoscopy: performance of a new digital cholangioscope. Gastrointest Endosc. 2014;79: 936–42.
9. Sethi A, Widmer J, Shah NL, Pleskow DK, Edmundowicz AS, Sejpal DV, et al. Interobserver agreement for evaluation of imaging with single operator choledochoscopy: What are we looking at? Dig Liver Dis. 2014;46:518–22.
10. Oh HC, Lee SK, Lee TY, Kwon S, Lee SS, Seo DW, Kim MH. Analysis of percutaneous transhepatic cholangioscopy related complications and the risk factors for those complications. Endoscopy. 2007;39:731–36.
11. Sethi A, Chen YK, Austin GL, Brown WR, Brauer BC, Fukami NN, et al. ERCP with cholangiopancreatoscopy may be associated with higher rates of complications than ERCP alone: a single-center experience. Gastrointest Endosc. 2011;73:251–56.
12. Itoi T, Moon JH, Waxman I. Current status of direct peroral cholangioscopy. Dig Endosc. 2011;23 Suppl 1:154–57.
13. Choi JH, Lee SK. Percutaneous transhepatic cholangioscopy: does its role still exist? Clin Endosc. 2013;46:529–36.
14. Takahashi Y, Nagino M, Nishio H, Ebata T, Igami T, Nimura Y. Percutaneous transhepatic biliary drainage catheter tract recurrence in cholangiocarcinoma. Br J Surg. 2010;97:1860–66.
15. Ramachandani M, Reddy N, Gupta R, Lakhtakia S, Tandan M, Darisetty S, et al. Role of single operator peroral cholangioscopy in the diagnosis of indeterminate biliary lesions: a single-center, prospective study. Gastrointest Endosc. 2011;74:511–19.

16. Nishikawa T, Tsuyuguchi T, Sakai Y, Sugiyama H, Miyazaki M, Yokosuko O. Comparison of the diagnostic accuracy of peroral video-cholangioscopic visual findings and cholangioscopy-guided forceps biopsy findings for indeterminate biliary lesions: a prospective study. Gastrointest Endosc. 2013;77:219–26.
17. Sun X, Zhou Z, Tian J, Wang Z, Huang Q, Fan K, et al. Is single-operator peroral cholangioscopy a useful tool for the diagnosis of indeterminate biliary lesion? A systematic review and meta-analysis. Gastrointest Endosc. 2015;82(1):79–87.
18. Chen YK, Parsi MA, Binmoeller KF, Hawes RH, Pleskow DK, Slivka A, et al. Single operator cholangioscopy in patients requiring evaluation of bile duct disease or therapy of biliary stones (with videos). Gastrointest Endosc. 2011;74:805–14.
19. de Bellis M, Fogel EL, Sherman S, Watkins JL, Chappo J, Younger C, et al. Influence of stricture dilation and repeat brushing on the cancer detection rate of brush cytology in the evaluation of malignant biliary obstruction. Gastrointest Endosc. 2003;58:176–82.
20. Tieu AH, Kumbhari V, Jakhete N, Onyimba F, Patel Y, Shin EJ, et al. Diagnostic and therapeutic utility of SpyGlass peroral cholangioscopy in intraductal biliary disease: Single-center, retrospective, cohort study. Dig Endosc. 2015;27(4):479–85.
21. Manta R, Frazzoni M, Conigliaro R, Maccio L, Melotti G, Dabizzi E, et al. SpyGlass single-operator peroral cholangioscopy in the evaluation of indeterminate biliary lesions: a single-center, prospective, cohort study. Surg Endosc. 2013;27:1569–72.
22. Farnik H, Weigt J, Malfertheiner P, Grützmann A, Gossner L, Friedrich-Rust M, et al. A multicenter study on the role of direct retrograde cholangioscopy in patients with inconclusive endoscopic retrograde cholangiography. Endoscopy. 2014;46:16–21.
23. Arnelo U, Seth E, Bergquist A. Prospective evaluation of the clinical utility of single-operator peroral cholangioscopy in patients with primary sclerosing cholangitis. Endoscopy. 2015;47(8):696–702.
24. Patel SN, Rosenkranz L, Hooks B, Tarnasky PR, Raijman I, Fishman DS, et al. Holmium-yttrium aluminum garnet laser lithotripsy in the treatment of biliary calculi using single-operator cholangioscopy: a multicenter experience (with video). Gastrointest Endosc. 2014;79:344–8.
25. Arya N, Nelles SE, Haber GB, Kim YI, Kortan PK. Electrohydraulic lithotripsy in 111 patients: a safe and effective therapy for difficult bile duct stones. Am J Gastroenterol. 2004;99:2330–34.
26. Moon JH, Ko BM, Choi HJ, Koo HC, Hong SJ, Cheon YK, et al. Direct peroral cholangioscopy using an ultra-slim upper endoscope for the treatment of retained bile duct stones. Am J Gastroenterol. 2009;104:2729–33.
27. Layfield LJ, Cramer H, Madden J, Gopez E, Lui K. Atypical squamous epithelium in cytologic specimens from the pancreas: cytological differential diagnosis and clinical implications. Diagn Cytopathol. 2000;25:38–42.
28. Kim HJ, Kim MH, Lee SK, Yoo KS, Seo DW, Min YI. Tumor vessel: a valuable cholangioscopic clue of malignant biliary stricture. Gastrointest Endosc. 2000;52:635–38.
29. Tsuyuguchi T, Sakai Y, Sugiyama H, Miyakawa K, Ishihara T, Ohtsuka M, et al. Endoscopic diagnosis of intraductal papillary mucinous neoplasm of the bile duct. J Hepatobiliary Pancreat Sci. 2010;17:230–35.
30. Wang X, Cai YQ, Chen YH, Liu XB. Biliary tract intraductal papillary mucinous neoplasm: Report of 19 cases. World J Gastroenterol. 2015;21(14):4261–67.
31. Woo YS, Lee JK, Oh SH, Kim MJ, Jung JG, Lee KH, et al. Role of SpyGlass peroral cholangioscopy in the evaluation of indeterminate biliary lesions. Dig Dis Sci. 2014;59:2565–70.
32. Nwaneshiudu A, Kuschal C, Sakamoto FH, Anderson RR, Schwarzenberger K, Young RC. Introduction to confocal microscopy. J Invest Dermatol. 2012;132(12):1–5.
33. Smith I, Kline PE, Gaidhane M, Kahaleh M. A review on the use of confocal laser endomicroscopy in the bile duct. Gastroenterol Res Pract. 2012;2012:1–5.
34. Mauna Kea Technologies [Internet]. Cellvizio 100 Series datasheet. 2013 Nov [cited 2015 Mar 3]. www.maunakeatech.com

35. Neumann H, Kiesslich R, Wallace MB, Neurath MF. Confocal laser endomicroscopy: technical advances and clinical applications. Gastroenterology. 2010;139(2):388–92.
36. Wallace M, Lauwers GY, Chen Y, Dekker E, et al. Miami classification for probe-based confocal laser endomicroscopy. Endoscopy. 2011;43(10):882–91.
37. Kwan AS, Barry C, McAllister L, Constable I. Fluorescein angiography and adverse drug reactions revisited: the Lions Eye experience. Clin Experiment Ophthalmol. 2006;34(1):33–8.
38. Becker V, von Delius S, Bajbouj M, et al. Intravenous application of fluorescein for confocal laser scanning microscopy: evaluation of contrast dynamics and image quality with increasing injection-to-imaging time. Gastointest Endosc. 2008;68(2):319–23.
39. Ponchon T, Gagnon P, Berger F, et al. Value of endobiliary brush cytology and biopsies for the diagnosis of malignant bile duct stenosis: results of a prospective study. Gastrointest Endosc. 1995;42:565–72.
40. Bangarulingam SY, Bjornsson E, Enders F, et al. Long-term outcomes of positive fluorescence in situ hybridization tests in primary sclerosing cholangitis. Hepatology. 2010;51:174–80.
41. Meining A, Shah RJ, Slivka A, et al. Classification of probe-based confocal laser endomicroscopy findings in pancreaticobiliary strictures. Endoscopy. 2012;44(3):251–7.
42. Caillol F, Bories E, Poizat F, et al. Endomicroscopy in bile duct: Inflammation interferes with pCLE applied in the bile duct: a prospective study of 54 patients. United European Gastroenterol J. 2013;1(2):120–7.
43. Caillol F, Filoche B, Gaidhane M, Kahaleh M. Refined probe-based confocal laser endomicroscopy classification of biliary strictures: the paris classification. Dig Dis Sci. 2013;58: 1784–9.
44. Slivka A, Gan I, Jamidar P, et al. Validation of the diagnostic accuracy of probe-based confocal laser endomicroscopy for the characterization of indeterminate biliary strictures: results of a prospective multicenter international study. Gastrointest Endosc. 2015;81(2):282–90.
45. Meining A, Chen YK, Pleskow D, et al. Direct visualization of indeterminate pancreaticobiliary strictures with probe-based confocal laser endomicroscopy: a multicenter experience. Gastrointest Endosc. 2011;74(5):961–8.
46. Talreja JP, Turner BG, Gress FG, et al. Pre- and post-training session evaluation for interobserver agreement and diagnostic accuracy of probe-based confocal laser endomicroscopy for biliary strictures. Dig Endosc. 2014;26:577–80.
47. Shieh FK, Drumm H, Nathanson MH, Jamidar PA. High-definition confocal endomicroscopy of the common bile duct. J Clin Gastroenterol. 2012;46(5):401–6.
48. Cellvizio [Internet]. Downstream revenue generated by Probe-based Confocal Laser Endomicroscopy (pCLE) in Undetermined Pancreaticobiliary lesions. http://www.cellvizio.net/sites/default/files/issu_presentation/ICCU2014%20-%20Sharaiha.pdf

Chapter 13
Needle-Based Confocal Microscopy (nCLE)

Marc Giovannini

Introduction

Confocal laser endomicroscopy (CLE) is a newly developed endoscopic technique that enables imaging of the mucosal layer during endoscopy at a subcellular level of resolution. The method can therefore be used for the assessment of changes in vascular architecture, connective tissue, and cellular components in the mucosa, enabling endoscopists to collect real-time in vivo histological images or "optical biopsies" of the gastrointestinal (GI) mucosa during endoscopy [1–3].

The techniques have primarily been applied to the differentiation of colon polyps and for the detection of dysplasia and neoplasia in conditions such as Barrett's esophagus and ulcerative colitis. Since the first visible neoplastic changes in epithelial cancers occur at a cellular level, these imaging techniques may allow for earlier diagnosis and treatment. In addition, confocal laser endomicroscopy may allow for targeted biopsies of abnormal mucosa, thereby decreasing the number of biopsies required to diagnose dysplasia or neoplasia while increasing diagnostic yield.

During the last 5 years, new applications of confocal laser endomicroscopy were developed as pCLE in the bile duct and nCLE for pancreatic cystic tumors, pancreatic masses, and lymph nodes. The aim of this paper would be to give you an update in this new technology and to try to define its place in the diagnosis of cystic and solid pancreatic masses and in the lymph nodes staging.

M. Giovannini, M.D. (✉)
Department of Gastroenterology and Endoscopy, Paoli-Calmettes Institute, Marseille, France
e-mail: giovanninim@ipc.unicancer.fr

V.J.A. Konda, I. Waxman (eds.), *Endoscopic Imaging Techniques and Tools*,
DOI 10.1007/978-3-319-30053-5_13

Material and Technique

Confocal microscopy consists of focusing a laser beam onto the plane of interest and filtering the returned light by means of a small pinhole which rejects out-of-focus light. The illumination and detection systems are in the same focal plane and are termed "confocal." After passing the pinhole, the fluorescent light is detected by a photodetection device transforming the light signal into an electrical one that is recorded by a computer. All detected signals from the illuminated spot are captured and measured. The gray-scale image created is an optical section representing one focal plane within the examined specimen. Because confocal images depend on fluorescence, a fluorescent dye (contrast agent) is required to make objects visible. The contrast agents can be applied systemically (fluorescein, tetracycline) or topically (acriflavine, cresyl violet) by using a spraying catheter. For nCLE, intravenous fluorescein sodium (10 %) was mainly used.

The material used was a 19G EUS-Needle in which the stylet was replaced by the Confocal mini-probe (Fig. 13.1) (AQ-flex Cellvizio Technology, Mauna-Kea company-France). The mini-probe (0.632 mm of diameter) pre-loaded and screwed

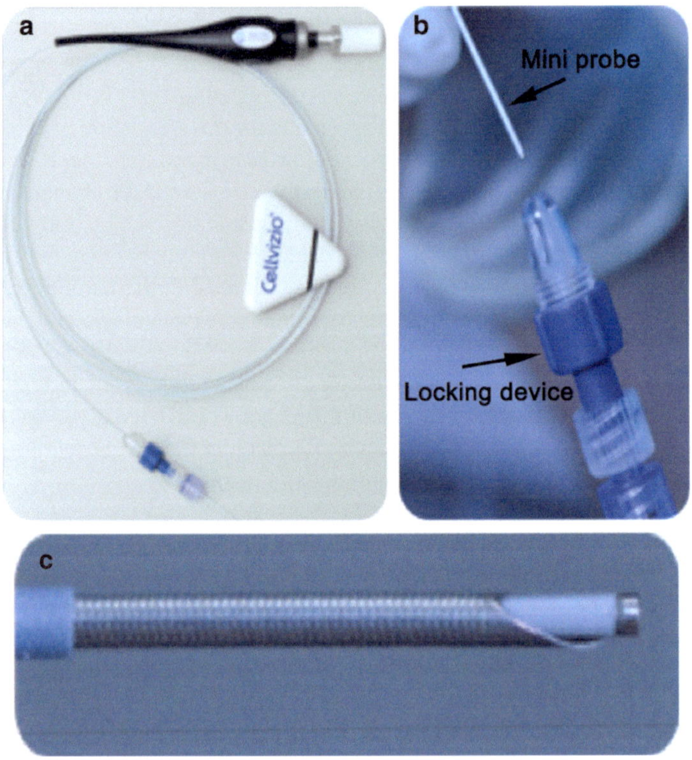

Fig. 13.1 Miniprobe AQ-Flex (**a**), locking device (**b**), miniprobe preloaded in the 19G EUS-Needle (**c**)

by a locking device in the EUS-Needle was guided endosonographically in the target, then the mini-probe was pushed under EUS guidance into the lesion. The intratumoral confocal microscopy examination started after injection of 2.5 mL of fluorescein intra-venously.

nCLE and Pancreatic Cystic Lesion

The first multicenter study was the INSPECT Study [4]; the primary aim of the INSPECT study is to develop descriptive image interpretation criteria and a classification of nCLE findings in pancreatic cysts through a review of prospectively obtained nCLE videos from proven malignant and benign cases and to propose nCLE diagnostic criteria for predicting malignant cysts. Secondary aims include assessing procedure-related adverse events, technical feasibility of nCLE, and developing a first atlas of nCLE images in pancreatic cysts. A total of 66 patients underwent nCLE imaging and images were available for 65, eight of which were subsequently excluded due to insufficient information for consensus reference diagnosis. The presence of epithelial villous structures based on nCLE was associated with pancreatic cystic neoplasm (IPMN) ($P=0.004$) and provided a sensitivity of 59 %, specificity of 100 %, positive predictive value of 100 %, and negative predictive value of 50 % (Fig. 13.2). The overall complication rate was 9 % and included pancreatitis (one mild case, one moderate case), transient abdominal pain ($n=1$), and intracystic bleeding not requiring any further measures ($n=3$). These preliminary data suggested that nCLE has a high specificity in the detection of IPMN, but may be limited by a low sensitivity.

The aim of the second multicenter study published [5] was to define criteria of serous cystadenoma and to try to differentiate mucinous than serous pancreatic lesion using nCLE. The differential diagnosis of solitary pancreatic cystic lesions is frequently difficult. A total of 31 patients with a solitary pancreatic cystic lesion of unknown diagnosis were prospectively included at three centers. EUS-FNA was combined with nCLE. The final diagnosis was based on either a stringent gold

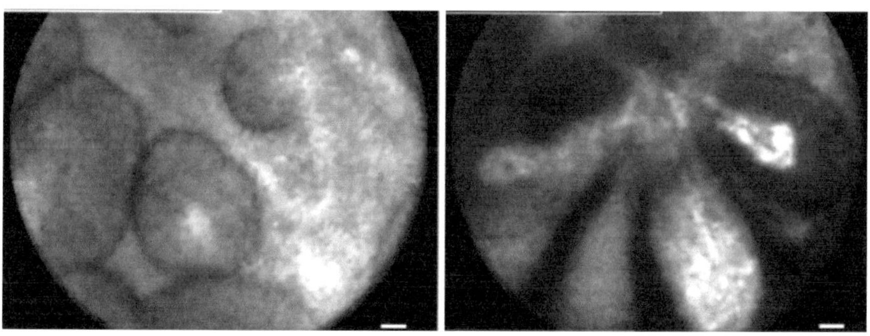

Fig. 13.2 nCLE aspects of IPMN (finger-like projections)

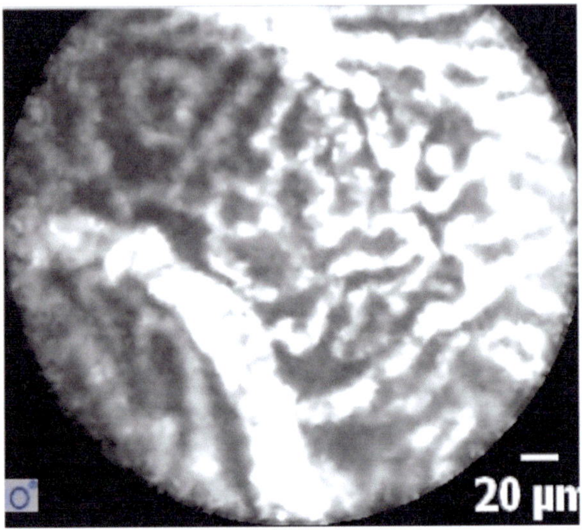

Fig. 13.3 Vascular network typical of a serous cystadenoma

standard (surgical specimen and/or positive cytopathology) or a committee consensus. Six nonblinded investigators reviewed nCLE sequences from patients with the most stringent final diagnosis and identified a single feature that was only present in serous cystadenoma (SCA). The findings were correlated with the pathology of archived specimens. After a training session, four blinded independent observers reviewed a separate independent video set, and the yield and interobserver agreement for the criterion were assessed. A superficial vascular network pattern visualized on nCLE was identified as the criterion. It corresponded on pathological specimen to a dense and subepithelial capillary vascularization only seen in SCA (Fig. 13.3). The accuracy, sensitivity, specificity, positive predictive value, and negative predictive value of this sign for the diagnosis of SCA were 87 %, 69 %, 100 %, 100 %, and 82 %, respectively. Interobserver agreement was substantial ($\kappa=0.77$). This new nCLE criterion seems highly specific for the diagnosis of SCA. The visualization of this criterion could have a direct impact on the management of patients by avoiding unnecessary surgery or follow-up.

The last study [6] was a unicenter trial and combine nCLE with an EUS-guided cystoscopy (DETECT study). The goal of this study was to assess the feasibility, safety, and diagnostic yield of the combination of cystoscopy and nCLE in the clinical diagnosis of pancreatic cystic lesion. Thirty patients were included. The procedure was technically successful with the exception of one probe exchange failure. In two patients (7 %), post-procedure pancreatitis developed. Specific features associated with the clinical diagnosis of mucinous cysts were identified: mucin on cystoscopy and papillary projections and dark rings on nCLE. The sensitivity of cystoscopy was 90 % (9/10), and that of nCLE was 80 % (8/10), and the combination was 100 % (10/10) in 18 high-certainty patients. The combination of dual through-the-needle imaging (cystoscopy and nCLE) of pancreatic cysts appears to have strong concordance with the clinical diagnosis of pancreatic cyst.

nCLE : Pancreatic Solid Masses and Lymph Nodes

The first study published [7] was a feasibility study and the goal was to develop descriptive image interpretation criteria and a classification of nCLE findings in pancreatic masses and lymph nodes through a review of prospectively obtained nCLE videos from proven malignant and benign cases and to propose diagnostic criteria for predicting malignancy. Eleven patients underwent EUS for the staging of a pancreatic mass (three cystic and four solid) or for the diagnosis of celiac and/or mediastinal LN ($n=4$). Benign intraductal papillary mucinous neoplasm (IPMN) was characterized by the aspect of finger-like projections, which correspond to the villous changes of intestinal IPMN type. In pancreatic adenocarcinomas, EUS-CM found vascular leakage with irregular vessels with leakage of fluorescein into the tumor, large dark clumps which correspond to humps of malignant cells. Inflammatory lymph nodes were characterized by the presence of diffuse small cells into a homogeneous stroma with a normal vascularization. At the opposite, nCLE showed in malignant lymph node glandular structures with dark cells, large dark clumps and an important neo-vascularization with huge leakage of fluorescein.

During the UEGW meeting in 2014, a larger series of nCLE in solid pancreatic masses was presented. Thirty-four patients with a pancreatic mass of unknown nature were included prospectively. The localization of the pancreatic masses was: head (17 cases), body (12 cases), and tail (6 cases). Mean size was 30 mm. The puncture of the mass was done in all cases with a 19G puncture needle with the nCLE probe preloaded. After examination of the track of the puncture by nCLE, aspiration was done in the same track to compare images and histological results. No complication occurred during the nCLE procedure or the puncture. A definitive histological diagnosis was obtained in 30/34 patients: adenocarcinoma (21 cases), fibrous stroma adenocarcinoma (1 case), neuroendocrine tumor (4 cases), pseudo-papillary tumor [1], and chronic pancreatitis (3—diagnosis confirmed by a 1-year follow-up). To go further, nCLE sequences were re-visualized by two gastro-enterologists and two pathologists to compare, for each type of lesion, their findings to the pathology specimen. During this review, normal pancreas shows an aspect of coffee beans corresponding to the histological structure of acinis (Fig. 13.4). Adenocarcinomas showed dark cells aggregates with pseudo-glandular aspects and straight hyperdense elements more or less thick (Fig. 13.5). These criteria correlate with the histological structure of those tumors which are characterized by tumoral glands, surrounded by fibrosis in case of fibrous stroma tumor. Neuroendocrine tumors showed a dense network of small vessels on a dark background, which fits with the histological structure based on cord of cells surrounded by vessels and by fibrosis in case of fibrosis area. Chronic pancreatitis showed residual acinis, which corresponds to the pancreatic regression. This preliminary classification of nCLE images obtained in pancreatic masses could help in the differentiation of adenocarcinomas and neuroendocrine tumors and between malignant tumors from normal pancreatic tissue. Regarding pancreatic NET, nCLE aspects are different as a network of vessels around humps of small and round malignant cells (Fig. 13.6).

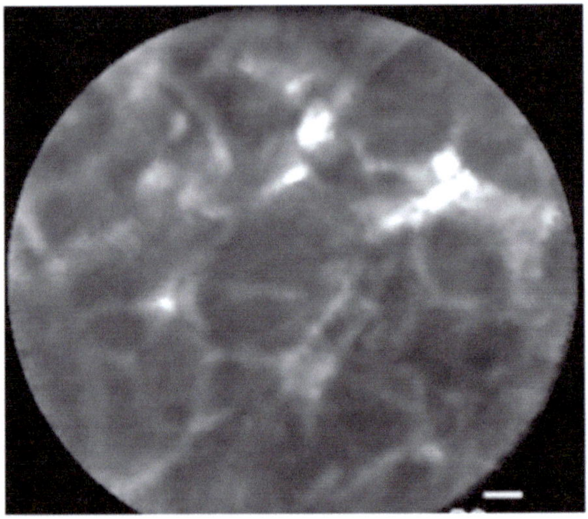

Fig. 13.4 Normal pancreatic tissue (coffee bean aspect: normal acinis)

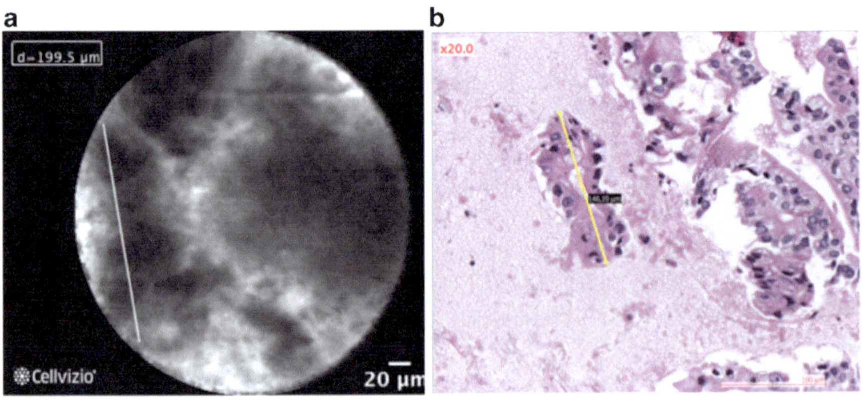

Fig. 13.5 Pancreatic adenocarcinoma : nCLE aspect (**a**) and histology correlation (**b**)

Regarding nCLE and lymph nodes, a presentation during the same meeting was done. Three centres in France (seven investigators) took part in this prospective study. Patients with a suspicious lymph node 1 cm proposed for a EUSFNA were included. In case of multiple lymph nodes, only one of them could be imaged. Seventeen patients with suspicious lymph node were included. The localizations of the lymph nodes were: mediastinal (6 cases), celiac (6 cases), intra-abdominal (3 cases), hepatic hilum (1 case), and hepatic hilum. All had a size superior to 10 mm. A definitive histological diagnosis was obtained in 14/17 patients (seven malignant metastatic LN, seven benign according to a 1-year follow-up).

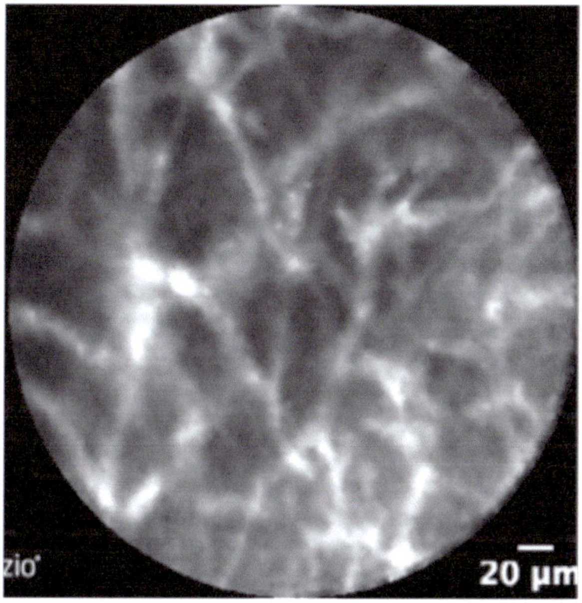

Fig. 13.6 Pancreatic NET: network of vessels around humps of small and round malignant cells

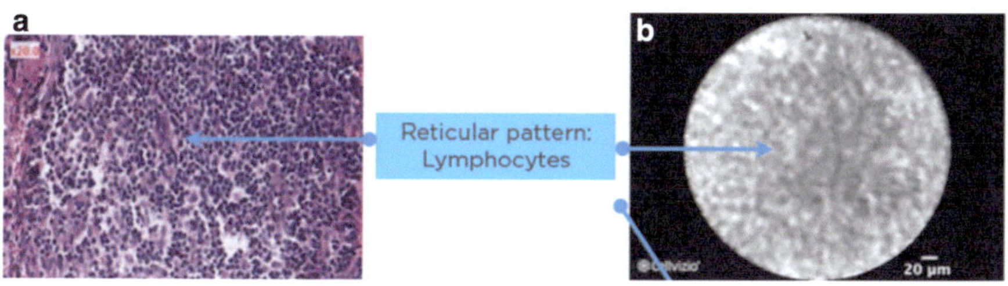

Fig. 13.7 Histology of a normal LN (**a**) and nCLE aspect (**b**)

During this review, all benign or inflammatory lymph nodes showed one sign: a reticular background, which corresponds to the histological structure of lymphocytes (Fig. 13.7). Malignant lymph nodes presented dark clumps or aggregates of dark cells, tumoral glands (Fig. 13.8), and in some cases only a grey background which could histologically correspond to necrosis. Finally, few criteria could be observed in all cases: white bands (blood vessels), macrophages, fat cells, and thin straight bands over a regular dark aggregate, which correspond to the capsula of the lymph node. This preliminary classification of nCLE images obtained in lymph nodes is too preliminary and needs more refinement. More patients should be included in this ongoing study.

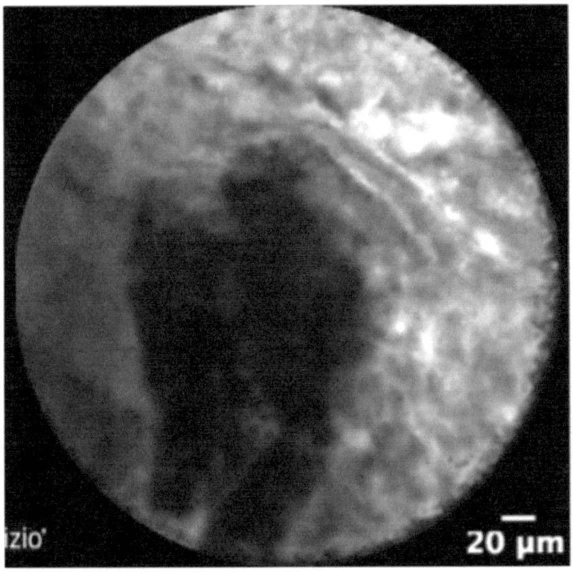

Fig. 13.8 nCLE aspect of a metastatic LN from a prostate carcinoma

References

1. Teubner D, Kiesslich R, Matsumoto T, Rey JW, Hoffman A. Beyond standard image-enhanced endoscopy confocal endomicroscopy. Gastrointest Endosc Clin N Am. 2014;24(3):427–34.
2. Gupta A, Attar BM, Koduru P, Murali AR, Go BT, Agarwal R. Utility of confocal laser endomicroscopy in identifying high-grade dysplasia and adenocarcinoma in Barrett's esophagus: a systematic review and meta-analysis. Eur J Gastroenterol Hepatol. 2014;26(4):369–77.
3. Konda VJ, Aslanian HR, Wallace MB, Siddiqui UD, Hart J, Waxman I. First assessment of needle-based confocal laser endomicroscopy during EUS-FNA procedures of the pancreas (with videos). Gastrointest Endosc. 2011;74(5):1049–60.
4. Konda VJ, Meining A, Jamil LH, Giovannini M, Hwang JH, Wallace MB, Chang KJ, Siddiqui UD, Hart J, Lo SK, Saunders MD, Aslanian HR, Wroblewski K, Waxman I. A pilot study of in vivo identification of pancreatic cystic neoplasms with needle-based confocal laser endomicroscopy under endosonographic guidance. Endoscopy. 2013;45(12):1006–13.
5. Napoléon B, Lemaistre A, Pujol B, Caillol F, Lucidarme D, Bourdariat R, Morellon-Mialhe B, Fumex F, Lefort C, Lepilliez V, Palazzo L, Monges G, Filoche B, Giovannini M. A novel approach to the diagnosis of pancreatic serous cystadenoma: needle-based confocal laser endomicroscopy. Endoscopy. 2015;47(1):26–32.
6. Nakai Y, Iwashita T, Park DH, Samarasena JB, Lee JG, Chang KJ. Diagnosis of pancreatic cysts: EUS-guided, through-the-needle confocal laser-induced endomicroscopy and cystoscopy trial: DETECT study. Gastrointest Endosc. 2015;81(5):1204–14. pii: S0016-5107(14)02381-5.
7. Giovannini M, Caillol F, Poizat F, Bories E, Pesenti C, Monges G, Raoul JL. Feasibility of intratumoral confocal microscopy under endoscopic ultrasound guidance. Endosc Ultrasound. 2012;1(2):80–3.

Index

V.J.A. Konda, I. Waxman (eds.), *Endoscopic Imaging Techniques and Tools*,
DOI 10.1007/978-3-319-30053-5

MIX
Papier aus verantwortungsvollen Quellen
Paper from responsible sources
FSC® C105338

If you have any concerns about our products,
you can contact us on
ProductSafety@springernature.com

In case Publisher is established outside the EU,
the EU authorized representative is:
Springer Nature Customer Service Center GmbH
Europaplatz 3, 69115 Heidelberg, Germany

Printed by Libri Plureos GmbH
in Hamburg, Germany